T0263461

Contemporary Debates and Controversies in Cardiac Electrophysiology, Part II

Guest Editors

RANJAN K. THAKUR, MD, MPH, MBA, FHRS
ANDREA NATALE, MD, FACC, FHRS

CARDIAC ELECTROPHYSIOLOGY CLINICS

www.cardiacEP.theclinics.com

Consulting Editors
RANJAN K. THAKUR, MD, MPH, MBA, FHRS
ANDREA NATALE, MD, FACC, FHRS

September 2012 • Volume 4 • Number 3

SAUNDERS an imprint of ELSEVIER, Inc.

W.B. SAUNDERS COMPANY
A Division of Elsevier Inc.

1600 John F. Kennedy Boulevard • Suite 1800 • Philadelphia, Pennsylvania 19103-2899

http://www.theclinics.com

CARDIAC ELECTROPHYSIOLOGY CLINICS Volume 4, Number 3
September 2012 ISSN 1877-9182, ISBN-13: 978-1-4557-3836-6

Editor: Barbara Cohen-Kligerman
Developmental Editor: Teia Stone

Cardiac Electrophysiology Clinics (ISSN 1877-9182) is published quarterly by Elsevier Inc., 360 Park Avenue South, New York, NY 10010-1710. Months of issue are March, June, September, and December. Subscription prices are $180.00 per year for US individuals, $266.00 per year for US institutions, $95.00 per year for US students and residents, $202.00 per year for Canadian individuals, $297.00 per year for Canadian institutions, $258.00 per year for international individuals, $318.00 per year for international institutions and $136.00 per year for Canadian and foreign students/residents. To receive student/resident rate, orders must be accompanied by name of affilliated institution, date of term, and the signature of program/residency coordinator on institution letterhead. Orders will be billed at individual rate until proof of status is received. Foreign air speed delivery is included in all Clinics subscription prices. All prices are subject to change without notice. **POSTMASTER:** Send address changes to Cardiac Electrophysiology Clinics, Elsevier Health Sciences Division, Subscription Customer Service, 3251 Riverport Lane, Maryland Heights, MO 63043. **Customer Service: 1-800-654-2452 (US and Canada). From outside of the US and Canada, call 314-477-8871. Fax: 314-447-8029. E-mail: JournalsCustomerService-usa@elsevier.com (for print support); JournalsOnlineSupport-usa@elsevier.com (for online support).**

Reprints. For copies of 100 or more of articles in this publication, please contact the Commercial Reprints Department, Elsevier Inc., 360 Park Avenue South, New York, NY 10010-1710. Tel.: 212-633-3812; Fax: 212-462-1935; E-mail: reprints@elsevier.com.

Printed and bound by CPI Group (UK) Ltd, Croydon, CR0 4YY

Transferred to Digital Print 2012

Pre-excited atrial fibrillation with a shortest RR interval of less than 200 ms. Ventricular fibrillation results during pre-excited atrial fibrillation. See "Asymptomatic Wolff-Parkinson–White: Who Should Be Treated?" by Manoj N. Obeyesekere, MBBS, Peter Leong-Sit, MD, Andrew D. Krahn, MD, Lorne J. Gula, MD, MSc, Raymond Yee, MD, Allan C. Skanes, MD, George J. Klein, MD, for further details.

Contributors

CONSULTING EDITORS

RANJAN K. THAKUR, MD, MPH, MBA, FHRS
Professor of Medicine, Director, Arrhythmia Service, Thoracic and Cardiovascular Institute, Sparrow Health System, Michigan State University, Lansing, Michigan

ANDREA NATALE, MD, FACC, FHRS, FESC
Executive Medical Director, Texas Cardiac Arrhythmia Institute, St David's Medical Center, Austin, Texas; Consulting Professor, Division of Cardiology, Stanford University, Palo Alto, California; Adjunct Professor of Medicine, Heart and Vascular Center, Case Western Reserve University, Cleveland, Ohio; Director, Interventional Electrophysiology, Scripps Clinic, San Diego, California; Senior Clinical Director, EP Services, California Pacific Medical Center, San Francisco, California

AUTHORS

AMIN AL-AHMAD, MD, FACC, FHRS, CCDS
Assistant Professor, Stanford Arrhythmia Service, Division of Cardiovascular Medicine, Stanford University, Stanford, California; Director, Cardiac Electrophysiology Laboratory, Associate Director, Cardiac Arrhythmia Service, Stanford University School of Medicine, Stanford, California

ELAD ANTER, MD
Division of Cardiology, Department of Medicine, Beth Israel Deaconess Medical Center, Boston, Massachusetts

RONG BAI, MD, FHRS
Texas Cardiac Arrhythmia Institute, St. David's Medical Center, Austin, Texas; Department of Internal Medicine, Tong-Ji Hospital, Tong-Ji Medical College, Huazhong University of Science and Technology, Wuhan, People's Republic of China

SUNNI A. BARNES, PhD
Institute for Health Care Research and Improvement, Baylor Health Care System, Dallas, Texas

B. BLÜM, MD
Klinik für Kardiologie, Angiologie und Pulmonologie, Klinikum Coburg, Coburg, Germany

FRANK BOGUN, MD
Associate Professor, Division of Cardiovascular Medicine, University of Michigan, Ann Arbor, Michigan

TARA BOURKE, MD
UCLA Cardiac Arrhythmia Center, David Geffen School of Medicine at UCLA, UCLA Health System, Los Angeles, California; Department of Cardiology, Karolinska University Hospital, Stockholm, Sweden

NOEL G. BOYLE, MD, PhD
UCLA Cardiac Arrhythmia Center, David Geffen School of Medicine at UCLA, UCLA Health System, Los Angeles, California

J. BRACHMANN, MD, PhD
Klinik für Kardiologie, Angiologie und Pulmonologie, Klinikum Coburg, Coburg, Germany

J. DAVID BURKHARDT, MD, FHRS
Texas Cardiac Arrhythmia Institute, St. David's Medical Center, Austin, Texas

HUGH CALKINS, MD, FACC, FHRS, FAHA
Section of Cardiac Electrophysiology, Division of Cardiology, Johns Hopkins Medical Institutes, Baltimore, Maryland

DAVID J. CALLANS, MD
Division of Cardiology, Department of Medicine, University of Pennsylvania, Philadelphia, Pennsylvania

DANIEL J. CANTILLON, MD
Assistant Professor, Lerner College of Medicine; Cardiac Electrophysiology and Pacing, Heart and Vascular Institute, Cleveland Clinic, Cleveland, Ohio

ALEXANDRU B. CHICOS, MD
Assistant Professor of Medicine, Division of Cardiology, Department of Internal Medicine, Northwestern University Feinberg School of Medicine, Chicago, Illinois

PAOLO CHINA, MD
Cardiovascular Department, Ospedale dell'Angelo, Mestre-Venice, Italy

AMAN CHUGH, MD
Associate Professor of Medicine, Division of Cardiovascular Medicine, University of Michigan, Ann Arbor, Michigan

ANDREA CORRADO, MD
Cardiovascular Department, Ospedale dell'Angelo, Mestre-Venice, Italy

NICOLAS DERVAL, MD
Hôpital Haut Leveque and Université Bordeaux II, Bordeaux, France

LUIGI DI BIASE, MD, PhD, FHRS
Texas Cardiac Arrhythmia Institute, St. David's Medical Center; Department of Biomedical Engineering, University of Texas, Austin, Texas; Department of Cardiology, University of Foggia, Foggia, Italy

SHEPHAL K. DOSHI, MD
Pacific Heart Institute/St Johns Hospital, Santa Monica, California

JAMES R. EDGERTON, MD, FACS, FACC, FHRS
Director of Research, Education and Training, The Heart Hospital, Baylor Regional Medical Center at Plano, Plano, Texas; Director of Education, Cardiopulmonary Research Science and Technology Institute, Dallas, Texas

BRANDI FALLEY, MS
Institute for Health Care Research and Improvement, Baylor Health Care System, Dallas, Texas

G. JOSEPH GALLINGHOUSE, MD
Texas Cardiac Arrhythmia Institute, St. David's Medical Center, Austin, Texas

HAMID GHANBARI, MD, MPH
Division of Cardiovascular Medicine, University of Michigan, Ann Arbor, Michigan

LORNE J. GULA, MD, MSc
Associate Professor of Medicine, Division of Cardiology, Western University, London, Ontario, Canada

MICHEL HAÏSSAGUERRE, MD
Hôpital Haut Leveque and Université Bordeaux II, Bordeaux, France

MELEZE HOCINI, MD
Hôpital Haut Leveque and Université Bordeaux II, Bordeaux, France

RODNEY P. HORTON, MD
Texas Cardiac Arrhythmia Institute, St. David's Medical Center, Austin, Texas; Department of Biomedical Engineering, University of Texas, Austin, Texas

AMIR S. JADIDI, MD
Hôpital Haut Leveque and Université Bordeaux II, Bordeaux, France

PIERRE JAIS, MD
Hôpital Haut Leveque and Université Bordeaux II, Bordeaux, France

GEORGE J. KLEIN, MD
Professor of Medicine, Division of Cardiology, Western University, London, Ontario, Canada

SEBASTIEN KNECHT, MD
Hôpital Haut Leveque and Université Bordeaux II, Bordeaux, France

BRADLEY P. KNIGHT, MD
Professor of Medicine, Division of Cardiology, Department of Internal Medicine, Northwestern University Feinberg School of Medicine, Chicago, Illinois

YUKI KOMATSU, MD
Hôpital Haut Leveque and Université Bordeaux II, Bordeaux, France

ANDREW D. KRAHN, MD
Professor of Medicine, Division of Cardiology, Western University, London, Ontario, Canada

RAKESH LATCHAMSETTY, MD
Division of Cardiovascular Medicine, University of Michigan, Ann Arbor, Michigan

PETER LEONG-SIT, MD, MSc
Assistant Professor of Medicine, Division of Cardiology, Western University, London, Ontario, Canada

WILLIAM R. LEWIS, MD
Case Western Reserve University School of Medicine, Cleveland, Ohio

XINGPENG LIU, MD
Hôpital Haut Leveque and Université Bordeaux II, Bordeaux, France

MICHELA MADALOSSO, MD
Cardiovascular Department, Ospedale dell'Angelo, Mestre-Venice, Italy

SHINSUKE MIYAZAKI, MD
Hôpital Haut Leveque and Université Bordeaux II, Bordeaux, France

SANGHAMITRA MOHANTY, MD
Texas Cardiac Arrhythmia Institute, St. David's Medical Center, Austin, Texas

JOHN MORIARTY, MD
UCLA Cardiac Arrhythmia Center, David Geffen School of Medicine at UCLA, UCLA Health System, Los Angeles, California

ANDREA NATALE, MD, FACC, FHRS, FESC
Executive Medical Director, Texas Cardiac Arrhythmia Institute, St David's Medical Center, Austin, Texas; Consulting Professor, Division of Cardiology, Stanford University, Palo Alto, California; Adjunct Professor of Medicine, Heart and Vascular Center, Case Western Reserve University, Cleveland, Ohio; Director, Interventional Electrophysiology, Scripps Clinic, San Diego, California; Senior Clinical Director, EP Services, California Pacific Medical Center, San Francisco, California

MATTHEW NEEDLEMAN, MD
Section of Cardiac Electrophysiology, Division of Cardiology, Johns Hopkins Medical Institutes, Baltimore, Maryland

MANOJ N. OBEYESEKERE, MBBS
Clinical Cardiologist, Division of Cardiology, Western University, London, Ontario, Canada

HAKAN ORAL, MD
Division of Cardiovascular Medicine, University of Michigan, Ann Arbor, Michigan

BENZY J. PADANILAM, MD
St. Vincent Medical Group, Indianapolis, Indiana

CARLO PAPPONE, MD
Arrhythmology Department, Maria Cecilia Hospital, Cotignola, Italy

PATRIZIO PASCALE, MD
Hôpital Haut Leveque and Université Bordeaux II, Bordeaux, France

MICHALA E. PEDERSEN, MD
Hôpital Haut Leveque and Université Bordeaux II, Bordeaux, France

LINDSEY M. PHILPOT, MPH
Institute for Health Care Research and Improvement, Baylor Health Care System, Dallas, Texas

ERIC N. PRYSTOWSKY, MD
Director, Electrophysiology Laboratory, St. Vincent Hospital, Indianapolis, Indiana

AGNES PUMP, MD
Texas Cardiac Arrhythmia Institute, St. David's Medical Center, Austin, Texas; Heart Institute, Faculty of Medicine, University of Pecs, Pecs, Hungary

ANTONIO ROSSILLO, MD
Director of EP section and AF Center, Cardiovascular Department, Ospedale dell'Angelo, Mestre-Venice, Italy

LAURENT ROTEN, MD
Hôpital Haut Leveque and Université Bordeaux II, Bordeaux, France

FREDERIC SACHER, MD
Hôpital Haut Leveque and Université Bordeaux II, Bordeaux, France

JAVIER E. SANCHEZ, MD
Texas Cardiac Arrhythmia Institute, St. David's Medical Center; and Seton Heart Institute, Austin, Texas

PASQUALE SANTANGELI, MD
Texas Cardiac Arrhythmia Institute, St. David's Medical Center, Austin, Texas; Department of Cardiology, University of Foggia, Foggia, Italy

VINCENZO SANTINELLI, MD
Arrhythmology Department, Maria Cecilia Hospital, Cotignola, Italy

DANIEL SCHERR, MD
Hôpital Haut Leveque and Université Bordeaux II, Bordeaux, France

S. SCHNUPP, MD
Klinik für Kardiologie, Angiologie und Pulmonologie, Klinikum Coburg, Coburg, Germany

ASHOK J. SHAH, MD
Hôpital Haut Leveque and Université Bordeaux II, Bordeaux, France

KALYANAM SHIVKUMAR, MD, PhD, FHRS
Professor of Medicine & Radiology; and Director, UCLA Cardiac Arrhythmia Center, David Geffen School of Medicine at UCLA, UCLA Health System, Los Angeles, California

ALLAN C. SKANES, MD
Associate Professor of Medicine, Division of Cardiology, Western University, London, Ontario, Canada

KOJIRO TANIMOTO, MD
Instructor, Cardiology Division, Keio University School of Medicine, Shinjuku, Tokyo, Japan

SAKIS THEMISTOCLAKIS, MD
Director of EP section and AF Center, Cardiovascular Department, Ospedale dell'Angelo, Mestre-Venice, Italy

RODERICK TUNG, MD
UCLA Cardiac Arrhythmia Center, Los Angeles, California

PAUL J. WANG, MD, FACC, FHRS
Professor and Director, Cardiac Arrhythmia Service, Division of Cardiovascular Medicine, Stanford University, Stanford, California

STEPHEN B. WILTON, MD
Hôpital Haut Leveque and Université Bordeaux II, Bordeaux, France

RAYMOND YEE, MD
Professor of Medicine, Division of Cardiology, Western University, London, Ontario, Canada

JASON ZAGRODZKY, MD
Texas Cardiac Arrhythmia Institute, St. David's Medical Center, Austin, Texas

Contents

Foreword: "On the Front Lines" Contemporary Debates and Controversies—II xiii

Ranjan K. Thakur and Andrea Natale

Asymptomatic Wolff-Parkinson-White Syndrome: Who Should Be Treated? 273

Manoj N. Obeyesekere, Peter Leong-Sit, Andrew D. Krahn, Lorne J. Gula, Raymond Yee, Allan C. Skanes, and George J. Klein

This article discusses the merits of electrophysiology study (EPS) and/or ablation for asymptomatic preexcitation Wolff-Parkinson-White (WPW) ECG pattern. Sudden deaths in asymptomatic patients are too few to merit broad screening and aggressive intervention. It also discusses the risks of ablation and the low predictive accuracy of EPS. When WPW is an incidental finding, the decision to proceed with investigation and ablation can be made considering patients' situations and preferences. An invasive strategy is targeted at patients concerned about the low risk of life-threatening arrhythmia as a first presentation after a discussion of the risks and benefits.

Asymptomatic Wolff-Parkinson-White Syndrome Should be Ablated 281

Carlo Pappone and Vincenzo Santinelli

Wolff-Parkinson-White syndrome (WPW) is associated with a small but lifetime risk of cardiac arrest and/or sudden cardiac death (SCD). However, the exact risk is not well defined, particularly in asymptomatic persons. Over recent years the authors have collected and reported new follow-up data among a large number of asymptomatic WPW patients, particularly children, intensively followed. These data have significantly contributed to the knowledge and definition of the natural history of WPW from childhood to adulthood. The risk of SCD is higher in asymptomatic children than in adults, and early ablation can be offered only to selected subjects after electrophysiologic testing.

Ablation as First-Line Therapy for Atrial Fibrillation: Yes 287

Pasquale Santangeli, Luigi Di Biase, Amin Al-Ahmad, Rodney Horton, J. David Burkhardt, Javier E. Sanchez, G. Joseph Gallinghouse, Jason Zagrodzky, Rong Bai, Agnes Pump, Sanghamitra Mohanty, William R. Lewis, and Andrea Natale

This article addresses the use of catheter ablation (CA) as first-line therapy for atrial fibrillation (AF). CA increases long-term freedom from AF, reduces hospitalizations, and improves quality of life compared with antiarrhythmic drug (AAD) therapy in patients with symptomatic AF who have already failed one AAD. The role of CA as first-line therapy for AF, however, is still controversial. Evidence from randomized controlled trials shows that CA is definitely superior to AADs as first-line therapy for relatively young patients with paroxysmal AF, with comparable complication rates and results consistently reproducible across different institutions, operators, and types of ablation approaches.

Ablation as First-Line Therapy for Atrial Fibrillation: Not Yet for All 299

Benzy J. Padanilam and Eric N. Prystowsky

Studies have established the superiority of atrial fibrillation ablation in controlling the rhythm compared with medical therapy. The procedure, however, has significant associated risks. Whether ablation therapy would improve the major outcomes of survival and stroke is not yet established. Until this information becomes available, ablation should continue to be used as a second-line option for most patient subgroups when one or more antiarrhythmic medications are ineffective.

Atrial Fibrillation Ablation: Do We Really Need Preprocedural Imaging? **305**

Tara Bourke, John Moriarty, Noel G. Boyle, and Kalyanam Shivkumar

Atrial fibrillation is the most common human arrhythmia, causing significant mortality and morbidity. Because of the potential for complications, it is important that procedures be made as safe and effective as possible by combining safe procedural planning with effective therapy delivery. To change the current approach, large randomized studies are needed to guide the selection of patients who may safely undergo ablation without transesophageal echocardiography to exclude thrombus. For institutions routinely using computed tomography and magnetic resonance imaging to assess pulmonary vein anatomy before procedures, the possibility of excluding intracardiac thrombi using these imaging modalities should be considered.

Postablation Atrial Flutters **317**

Aman Chugh

Mapping and ablation of post–atrial fibrillation (AF) atrial tachycardia (AT) are challenging electrophysiologic procedures. These tachycardias may be caused by multiple mechanisms and may arise from the left or right atrium, or the coronary sinus. The precise mechanism must be defined before ablation because the procedural end point depends on the correct diagnosis. Postablation ATs can be successfully ablated in approximately 90% of patients. Many patients experience recurrence despite rigorous procedural end points. Efforts should focus on decreasing the incidence of AT after AF ablation and identifying patients who require linear ablation during a procedure for persistent AF.

Atrial Fibrillation Ablation in Obese Patients **327**

Matthew Needleman and Hugh Calkins

Despite the increased burden of atrial fibrillation (AF), obese patients have similar, if not slightly improved, mortality, described as the "obesity paradox." Catheter ablation for AF in obese patients is a reasonable option, but patients should be screened for sleep apnea and counseled about the possibility of longer procedure times and repeat procedures to achieve similar success rates. Quality of life will likely improve after successful ablation. Although no statistically significant increases in procedural complications have occurred in obese subjects, patients should be counseled about the increased radiation dose and higher incidence of left atrial thrombus preablation.

Ablation of Persistent Atrial Fibrillation: AF Termination is the End Point **335**

Ashok J. Shah, Shinsuke Miyazaki, Amir S. Jadidi, Xingpeng Liu, Daniel Scherr, Patrizio Pascale, Laurent Roten, Yuki Komatsu, Stephen B. Wilton, Michala E. Pedersen, Sebastien Knecht, Nicolas Derval, Frederic Sacher, Meleze Hocini, Michel Haïssaguerre, and Pierre Jais

This article reviews the literature on various techniques in the ablation of persistent AF, with the aim of highlighting the role of intraprocedural arrhythmia termination, defined as conversion to sinus rhythm or intermediate atrial tachycardia, in the predictability of arrhythmia recurrence. Because arrhythmia termination is not observed universally as a procedural end point, only those studies wherein it has been specifically reported, and its predictive role in arrhythmia recurrence is considered, are described.

Ablation for Atrial Fibrillation: Termination of Atrial Fibrillation is Not the End Point **343**

Pasquale Santangeli, Luigi Di Biase, Amin Al-Ahmad, Rodney Horton, J. David Burkhardt, Javier E. Sanchez, Rong Bai, Agnes Pump, Sanghamitra Mohanty, and Andrea Natale

Permanent pulmonary vein isolation constitutes the main procedural goal of current approaches to atrial fibrillation (AF) catheter ablation, with established effectiveness as a stand-alone procedure in most patients with paroxysmal AF. In patients with AF of longer duration, however, the definition of the optimal procedural end point is still controversial. Based on analysis of data from 16 studies that have assessed the value of AF termination in predicting long-term procedural success, it is concluded that AF termination clearly represents an unreliable procedural end point during ablation of nonparoxysmal AF.

Atrial Fibrillation Ablation Strategy: "Ready Made" or "Tailored"? **353**

Hamid Ghanbari and Hakan Oral

Atrial fibrillation (AF) is the most common arrhythmia leading to hospital admissions. Catheter ablation has evolved as an effective treatment strategy; however, ablation strategies continue to evolve due to the complex and multifactorial nature of atrial fibrillation. A standardized and primarily anatomical approach may not be sufficient to eliminate all mechanisms of atrial fibrillation. A tailored ablation strategy can target specific triggers and drivers of atrial fibrillation; however, it is limited by the accuracy and sensitivity of the methods used in identifying specific mechanisms of atrial fibrillation.

Anticoagulation Issues in Patients with AF **363**

Antonio Rossillo, Andrea Corrado, Paolo China, Michela Madalosso, and Sakis Themistoclakis

The evaluation of the risk of stroke for individual patients with atrial fibrillation (AF) is a crucial factor in the decision to provide anticoagulation therapy. Novel oral anticoagulants, as compared with warfarin, are associated with a lower or similar rate of stroke and systemic embolism and a lower rate of hemorrhagic stroke. These drugs are administered at a fixed dose, have a shorter peak action and half-life, and do not require international normalized ratio monitoring. After a successful AF ablation, oral anticoagulation therapy discontinuation seems to be feasible in patients with a $CHADS_2$ score greater than or equal to 2 and normal left atrial (LA) function. However, larger prospective randomized trials are needed to confirm the safety of this strategy.

AF Ablation: Do You Need a Mapping System for Ablation? **375**

Kojiro Tanimoto, Paul J. Wang, and Amin Al-Ahmad

Radiofrequency ablation has become a mainstay in the therapy for atrial fibrillation (AF). Although there are many different techniques for achieving adequate results, the cornerstone of AF remains pulmonary vein isolation. Three-dimensional (3D) electroanatomical mapping systems play an important role in the reduction of fluoroscopy and the identification of electrical and anatomic landmarks and are used

CARDIAC ELECTROPHYSIOLOGY CLINICS

FORTHCOMING ISSUES

December 2012
Analysis of Complex Arrhythmias—A Case Based Approach
Melvin Scheinman, MD, and
Fred Morady, MD, *Guest Editors*

March 2013
Arrhythmias in Athletes
Domenico Corrado, MD, PhD,
Cristina Basso, MD, PhD, and
Gaetano Thiene, MD, *Guest Editors*

June 2013
Mapping of Atrial Tachycardias Post-Atrial Fibrillation Ablation
Ashok J. Shah, MD, Michel Haissaguerre, MD,
and Shinsuke Miyazaki, MD, PhD, *Guest Editors*

RECENT ISSUES

June 2012
Difficult Decisions in Clinical Electrophysiology—A Case Based Approach
Mark C. Haigney, MD, and
Adam Strickberger, MD, *Guest Editors*

March 2012
Long QT Syndrome
Silvia G. Priori, MD, PhD, *Guest Editor*

December 2011
Contemporary Debates and Controversies in Cardiac Electrophysiology, Part I
Ranjan K. Thakur, MD, and
Andrea Natale, MD, *Guest Editors*

ISSUES OF RELATED INTEREST

Cardiology Clinics May 2012 (Vol. 30, No. 2)
Faces of Right Ventricular Failure
James A. Goldstein, MD, and Jonathan D. Rich, MD, *Guest Editors*
Available at: http://www.cardiology.theclinics.com/

Heart Failure Clinics July 2012 (Vol. 8, No. 3)
Pulmonary Hypertension
Srinivas Murali, MD, and Raymond Benza, MD, *Guest Editors*
Available at: http://www.heartfailure.theclinics.com/

NOW AVAILABLE FOR YOUR iPhone and iPad

Foreword
"On the Front Lines" Contemporary Debates and Controversies—II

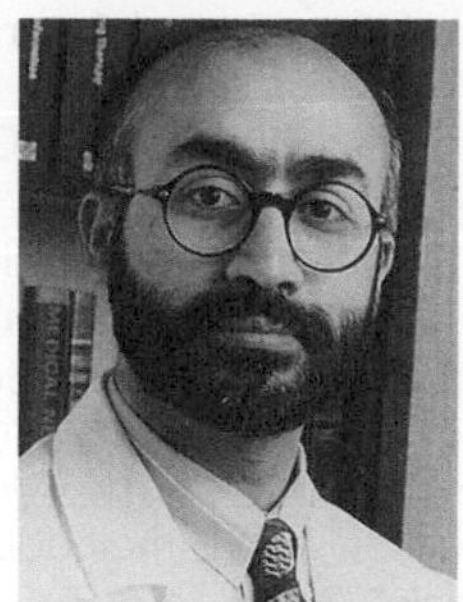

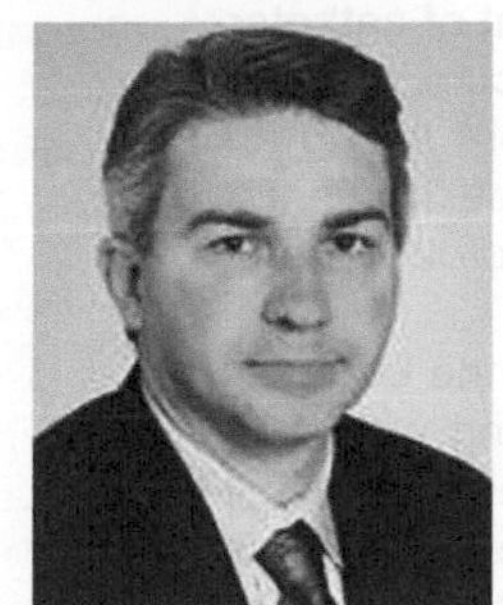

Ranjan K. Thakur, MD, MPH, MBA, FHRS Andrea Natale, MD, FACC, FHRS
Consulting Editors

It is better to debate a question without settling it than to settle a question without debating it.
—Joseph Joubert, French moralist and essayist, 1754-1824

Debates and controversies clarify and spur human understanding and are the essential fuel for scientific progress. So, it is fitting to present both sides of issues and let the reader decide which argument is more convincing based on the current data. Because of the myriad contemporary issues worthy of discussion, this issue of the *Cardiac Electrophysiology Clinics* focuses on issues surrounding ablative therapy. We covered some of the contemporary controversies around device therapy for ventricular arrhythmias in the December 2011 issue of *Cardiac Electrophysiology Clinics*.

Advances in cardiac surgery in the latter part of the 20th century were extended to cardiac arrhythmias once arrhythmias could be reliably induced and studied. Starting in the late 1970s, both supraventricular and ventricular arrhythmias were targeted using surgical techniques. Since diagnosis required placement of intracardiac catheters, catheter-based therapy was a natural extension. Catheter ablation using DC energy (fulguration) was used first, but because of complications, it was quickly supplanted by radiofrequency energy. Although several energy sources are now available, radiofrequency remains synonymous with catheter ablation. Virtually all arrhythmias are now amenable to catheter ablation. While many issues have been studied and settled over the last quarter century, many remain contentious. We have selected a few topics to highlight and debate in the present issue of the *Cardiac Electrophysiology Clinics*. Some examples include:

Wolff-Parkinson-White (WPW) syndrome has intrigued physicians since its initial description. Apart from symptoms, including syncope due to a rapid heart rate, the problem of sudden death due to ventricular fibrillation has been recognized in some patients with WPW syndrome. Fortunately, this is a rare occurrence. Electrocardiographic clues as well as noninvasive tests and electrophysiologic studies can be used to risk stratify these patients at risk for sudden death. Although some patients are symptomatic, others may develop symptoms later in life, or remain totally asymptomatic. The controversy arises as to whether asymptomatic patients with the WPW pattern on ECG should undergo prophylactic ablation. Drs Klein and Pappone present the two arguments.

Catheter ablation for atrial fibrillation (AF) is a proven technique with a reasonable success rate. However, it is generally offered to patients who have failed at least one antiarrhythmic drug. Some believe that AF ablation should be offered as first-line therapy, to at least some patients (eg, highly symptomatic young patients with recurrent paroxysmal AF), whereas others maintain that the current guidelines should be followed in the interest of public

Card Electrophysiol Clin 4 (2012) xiii–xiv
http://dx.doi.org/10.1016/j.ccep.2012.06.010
1877-9182/12/$ – see front matter

health. Dr Natale, who is a very experienced ablater, and Dr Prystowsky, who coauthored the current guidelines, debate the merits of their views.

Atrioventricular junction ablation with pacemaker implantation was a very successful procedure for symptomatic patients with AF who could not be controlled despite antiarrhythmic drugs or rate controlled pharamacologically. The technique was in vogue in the 1990s. The advent of catheter ablation for AF and the possibility of "cure," now or in the future, deterred physicians from taking an irreversible step, especially in younger patients. Dr Knight discusses the role of this procedure in contemporary practice.

These examples illustrate some of the contemporary issues that our field is grappling with. The reader will get a better idea by examining the full table of contents. We endeavored to select topics that are germane to today's practice and contributors who are key opinion leaders. We have learned much from our contributors and we hope that the readership will also benefit from their wisdom in these pages.

Ranjan K. Thakur, MD, MPH, MBA, FHRS
Sparrow Thoracic and Cardiovascular Institute
Michigan State University
1200 East Michigan Avenue, Suite 580
Lansing, MI 48912, USA

Andrea Natale, MD, FACC, FHRS
Texas Cardiac Arrhythmia Institute
Center for Atrial Fibrillation at
St. David's Medical Center
1015 East 32nd Street, Suite 516
Austin, TX 78705, USA

E-mail addresses:
thakur@msu.edu (R.K. Thakur)
andrea.natale@stdavids.com (A. Natale)

Asymptomatic Wolff-Parkinson-White Syndrome
Who Should Be Treated?

Manoj N. Obeyesekere, MBBS, Peter Leong-Sit, MD, MSc*, Andrew D. Krahn, MD, Lorne J. Gula, MD, MSc, Raymond Yee, MD, Allan C. Skanes, MD, George J. Klein, MD

KEYWORDS

• Asymptomatic • Wolff-Parkinson-White • Electrophysiologic study • Ablation • Accessory pathway • Preexcitation

KEY POINTS

- Risk of sudden death as first presentation in truly asymptomatic patients with Wolff-Parkinson-White (WPW) is small.
- Risks associated with routine electrophysiologic study (EPS) and ablation is likely to offset the small benefits on a population level.
- Although it is reasonable to discuss EPS and ablation with the asymptomatic patient with WPW, the evidence suggests that it should not necessarily be advocated.

INTRODUCTION

Recent studies evaluating invasive electrophysiologic study (EPS)-guided risk stratification of asymptomatic patients with Wolff-Parkinson-White (WPW) ECG pattern followed by prophylactic catheter ablation of the accessory pathway, reported several variables, including the inducibility of arrhythmias to predict the development of future symptomatic arrhythmias.[1–4] Ablation of the accessory pathway in these patients decreased the incidence of future symptomatic arrhythmias. Importantly, these studies were not powered to detect a reduction in mortality. Based on these studies, some physicians advocate routine diagnostic EPS to guide management and/or proceed with ablation in all patients with asymptomatic preexcitation. Although ablation in patients with symptomatic WPW syndrome is well established, the management of the asymptomatic individual remains controversial.[5] Guidelines suggest that the low positive predictive value of invasive EPS in conjunction with the cost and procedural morbidity fail to justify routine use in asymptomatic patients.[5]

This article argues that large-scale screening and routine EPS in asymptomatic patients with a WPW ECG pattern is not justified and elaborates on five factors:

1. The risk of sudden death as the first presentation in asymptomatic patients with WPW is exceedingly small, approximating the sudden death rate in the general population.
2. As suggested in the studies, most patients experiencing sudden death are likely to have experienced symptoms of arrhythmia before the sudden death and were not truly asymptomatic.

Disclosures: None.
Division of Cardiology, Western University, 339 Windermere Road, C6-110, London, Ontario N6A 5A5, Canada
* Corresponding author.
E-mail address: pleongs@uwo.ca

Card Electrophysiol Clin 4 (2012) 273–280
http://dx.doi.org/10.1016/j.ccep.2012.05.008
1877-9182/12/$ – see front matter

3. The small but real incidence of procedural complications associated with routine EPS and ablation in asymptomatic individuals will arguably offset the potential benefit of ablation.
4. The predictive accuracy of noninvasive studies or invasive EPS to identify asymptomatic patients at risk of sudden death is low.
5. The cost benefit ratio, although not accurately quantifiable, is undoubtedly exorbitantly high for routinely undertaking EPS and/or ablation in the asymptomatic population.

These factors do not preclude an EPS and possible ablation in well-informed asymptomatic patients who prefer a small procedural risk of serious complications or death against the remote risk of sudden death due to rapidly conducted atrial fibrillation over the accessory pathway that degenerates into ventricular fibrillation (**Fig. 1**). Additionally, in certain circumstances, asymptomatic patients may require EPS for risk stratification and possible catheter ablation (eg, pilots and professional or recreational athletes). Careful deliberation is required when undertaking a diagnostic EPS in asymptomatic patients before proceeding with ablation, based on the location of the accessory pathway and its conduction properties.

EPIDEMIOLOGY

The prevalence of preexcitation on ECG (ie, the WPW pattern) is estimated to be between 0.1 to 0.3%.[6] A critical issue in the discussion of mass screening or routine invasive assessment and treatment is the incidence of sudden death in this broad population. The risk of sudden death in symptomatic patients with WPW syndrome is estimated to be approximately 0.25% per year or 3% to 4% over a lifetime.[7,8] However, sudden death may be the first event in patients with asymptomatic preexcitation.[9] This incidence of sudden death as the first event is not accurately known. The key issue before recommendations regarding EPS or ablation in asymptomatic patients is to confidently establish the sudden death rate associated with asymptomatic preexcitation and balance this risk against the risk, cost, and feasibility of EPS and ablation in this broad population.

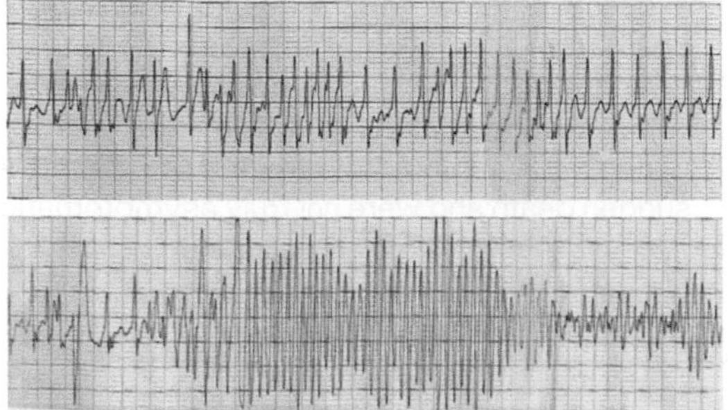

Fig. 1. Preexcited atrial fibrillation with a shortest relative risk interval of less than 200 milliseconds. Ventricular fibrillation results during preexcited atrial fibrillation.

Meta-Analysis of Reports on Sudden Death in Asymptomatic WPW Patients Without Ablation

The authors undertook a meta-analysis of studies reporting on the incidence of sudden death in asymptomatic patients with WPW who did not undergo ablation.[10] This meta-analysis included 20 studies published in the English language and demonstrated an extremely low incidence of sudden death in asymptomatic patients. In total, 10 sudden death episodes (five children, five adults) were reported, involving a total of 11,722 person-years of follow-up and 1869 patients. The combined overall risk of sudden death (in children and adults) was estimated at 1.25 with a 95% CI between 0.57 and 2.19 per 1000 person years of follow-up. Interestingly, seven studies originated from Italy and reported the most sudden deaths (9 out of the 10 sudden deaths). Thus, among the 13 non-Italian studies involving 6991 person years of follow-up, only one sudden death was reported. The risk of sudden death in non-Italian adults and children was estimated at 0.26 (95% CI; 0.06–0.81) and 2.1 (95% CI; 0–8.5) per 1000 person years of follow-up, respectively. The risk of sudden death in Italian adults and children was estimated at 2.5 (95% CI; 0.6–5.9) and 1.9 (95% CI; 0.3–4.9) per 1000 person years of follow-up, respectively. The risk of sudden death was statistically significantly lower in the combined non-Italian (0.4, 95% CI; 0.05–0.9) versus the Italian (2.2, 95% CI; 0.9–4.0) studies ($P<.01$).

The combined overall risk of sudden death was numerically higher in children compared with adults, although the test for interaction was not conventionally significant ($P = .07$). Overall, children had a sudden death event rate of 1.9 (95% CI; 0.6–4.1) compared with 0.9 (95% CI; 0.3–1.8) in adults per 1000 patient years of follow-up. This incidence is comparable with the estimated 0.1% per year risk of death in the general population in Europe, Japan, and the United States.[11] Other studies have reported varied sudden death rates in the general population, still approximating the rates in asymptomatic WPW patients. These studies report incidence rates of 0.13 (ages 35–49),[12] 0.09 (ages 0–35),[13] 0.032 (ages 14–35),[14] and 0.028 (ages 1–35)[15] per 1000 person years of follow up.

If most patients with asymptomatic WPW eventually developed supraventricular tachycardia (SVT) and symptoms, an argument could be made for routine EPS. However, the meta-analysis showed that the overall risk of SVT was 16 events per 1000 person years of follow-up (95% CI; 10–24). This low incidence rate argues against routine EPS. Of course, the lack of a routine EPS in asymptomatic patients does not preclude an EPS to be arranged in the few patients who eventually develop symptoms—a key bedside tip in evaluating and educating asymptomatic patients.

Furthermore, many patients with asymptomatic WPW tend to lose accessory pathway conduction over time.[16] Nine studies involving 7664 person years of follow-up reported on loss of preexcitation in the meta-analysis.[1–4,7,17–20] The incidence of loss of preexcitation was 24.69 per 1000 person years of follow-up (95% CI; 12.18–41.43). Thus, the relatively high incidence of disappearance of preexcitation over time would correspond with a parallel decrease in the risk of potentially life-threatening significant arrhythmia. Of note, the data show that more patients with asymptomatic WPW will lose preexcitation than develop SVT (let alone the rare incidence of sudden death).

Asymptomatic individuals obviously become symptomatic over time with a gradual decrease in the asymptomatic state over the years.[7] It is not surprising that the meta-analysis demonstrated a higher incidence of events in children over their longer life span compared with adults. Children pose a specific challenge in interpreting often nonspecific arrhythmia symptoms, compounded by their inability to articulate these symptoms.[3,4] It is arguable that the higher event rates observed in asymptomatic children reflect the inclusion of children who indeed have had symptoms attributable to arrhythmia not diagnosed as such. In fact, most patients with sudden deaths (6 of 9) had reported symptoms preceding the sudden death event during the course of the study that may have been attributable to SVT.[1,3,4] If so, the true incidence of sudden death in a truly asymptomatic patient is even lower than reported in the meta-analysis. The evolution of clinical status from asymptomatic to symptomatic portends a higher risk for sudden death and these patients obviously should be assessed more vigorously. Children in particular require a high index of suspicion for symptoms and careful monitoring.

COMPLICATIONS AND DEATH ASSOCIATED WITH ACCESSORY PATHWAY ABLATION

The low potential risk of sudden death needs to be weighed against the risk of complications, including death associated with an invasive EPS and ablation. In three large series, death as a consequence of accessory pathway ablation was reported to occur in 0.07%,[21] 0.13%,[22] and 0.19% of cases.[23] Procedure-related complications for accessory pathway ablation in these series were reported to be 1.8%,[21] 4.4%,[22] and 8.2%.[23] Recurrence rates of up to 8% following accessory pathway ablation (and up to 21% in the presence of multiple accessory pathways) may further temper the enthusiasm to ablate asymptomatic patients.[23] The two largest series[21,22] with available data on complication rates and death due to accessory pathway ablation included a total of 7649 patients undergoing ablation of accessory pathways. A total of 7 deaths and 197 complications were reported from these two reports (ie, death rate of 0.9 per 1000 patients undergoing ablation, complication rate of 26 per 1000 patients). Although these series are dated and may overestimate the current incidence of complications, it is also arguable that the incidence of complications is underreported and variable in the community. Less frequent operator exposure to accessory pathway ablation may, in fact, increase the risk of the procedure.

The immediate and long-term risks of EPS and/or catheter ablation in children are also well-recognized.[24] Complication rates range from 3% to 4.2% in children undergoing diagnostic EPS and/or ablation.[24,25] The largest pediatric series reported four procedure-related deaths during 3653 procedures (ie, death rate 1.1 per 1000 procedures).[26]

Another issue relates to procedural radiation exposure, with an estimated risk of fatal malignancy of approximately 0.7 per 1000 procedures.[27] For the pediatric population, the radiation exposure is likely to be more significant because of the larger fraction of the body that is irradiated and the higher radiation sensitivity compared with adults. Malignancy due to radiation exposure approximates 5 in 1000.[28]

Thus, any potential benefit gained by routine EPS and/or ablation must be considered against the small but comparable risks associated with the procedure.

IDENTIFYING HIGH-RISK ASYMPTOMATIC PATIENTS

The very low sudden death rate greatly limits the ability of any diagnostic test to provide clear risk analysis. Not surprisingly, the accuracy of EPS and noninvasive methods in predicting sudden death in this context is poor. For the same reason, a randomized study of prophylactic ablation for asymptomatic WPW would require an enormous sample size that realistically is prohibitive and will not be undertaken. Noninvasive techniques have good sensitivity but low specificity for identifying patients potentially at risk of sudden death. All available invasive parameters (ie, inducibility of atrial fibrillation or SVT, the shortest preexcited QRS coupling interval during atrial fibrillation, and anterograde effective refractory period [ERP] of the accessory pathway) to assess the future sudden death risk or SVT risk also lack specificity but maintain high negative predictive value. It must be remembered that a coin toss will also have excellent negative predictive value if the event rate is very low.[29] Also, the incidence of sudden death, even in the group of patients potentially at risk by virtue of a short anterograde ERP (or a surrogate parameter), is still low. Thus, identifying the low risk patient is less challenging. Identifying the rare person destined to die suddenly from the many with a potential for this by virtue of short ERP is much more challenging. There is no truly high-risk asymptomatic patient with such a low event rate.[30]

Intermittent preexcitation and/or loss of preexcitation during exercise testing suggest a low margin of safety of conduction and a long ERP. Such a patient would not be expected to be able to conduct rapidly over the accessory pathway. Continuous preexcitation during an exercise test identifies potentially at-risk patients with a sensitivity of 80%, a specificity of 29%, and a low predictive accuracy of 12%.[31] The clear loss of preexcitation during monitoring or exercise essentially precludes the need for further assessment. Loss of preexcitation on Holter monitoring also has excellent negative predictive values for predicting future sudden death.[31] Procainamide infusion has been reported as a noninvasive method to identify patients with WPW syndrome who are at risk of sudden death.[32] However, its sensitivity (60%) and specificity (89%) are suboptimal.[33]

In patients resuscitated from sudden death, the shortest preexcited RR interval during atrial fibrillation is very rarely greater than 250 milliseconds and usually less than 200 milliseconds.[9,34,35] Additionally, these patients demonstrate vulnerability to atrial fibrillation and SVT is generally inducible.[1,2] Although the shortest preexcited RR interval in atrial fibrillation has a high negative predictive value for predicting sudden death, its positive predictive value remains low with approximately one-third of asymptomatic WPW patients having values less than 250 milliseconds (**Fig. 2**).[36] An anterograde ERP of less than 250 milliseconds has been

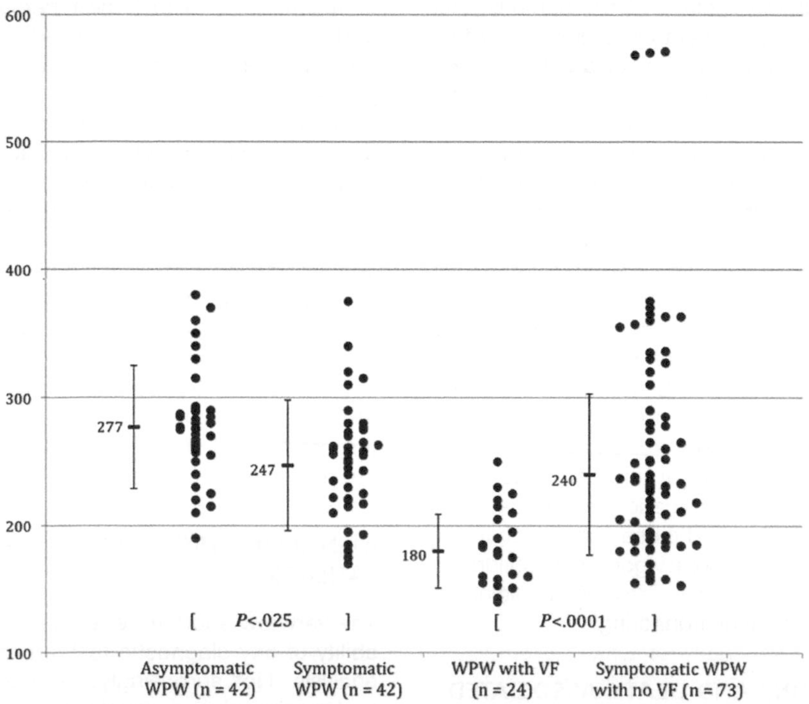

Fig. 2. Scatter plot demonstrating shortest preexcited RR intervals (milliseconds) in atrial fibrillation in four groups: asymptomatic WPW patients, symptomatic WPW patients, symptomatic WPW patients with ventricular fibrillation, and symptomatic WPW patients without ventricular fibrillation. Mean values shown and standard deviation bars. (*Adapted from* Milstein S, Sharma AD, Klein GJ. Electrophysiologic profile of asymptomatic Wolff-Parkinson-White pattern. Am J Cardiol 1986;57:1097–100; and Klein GJ, Bashore TM, Sellers TD, et al. Ventricular fibrillation in the Wolff-Parkinson-White syndrome. N Engl J Med 1979;301:1080–5.)

reported to be an independent predictor of sudden death (along with multiple accessory pathways).[4] However, asymptomatic patients generally have a longer anterograde ERP compared with symptomatic patients.[4,37] An anterograde ERP of less than 250 milliseconds is observed in up to 30% and has been reported to have a low predictive accuracy, as one would expect.[35,37,38]

A recent study sought to identify high-risk asymptomatic patients with invasive EPS for risk stratification.[1] The combination of anterograde ERP of the accessory pathway less than 250 milliseconds and inducible arrhythmias was reported to have a sensitivity of 94%, a positive predictive value of 47%, and a negative predictive value of 94% for predicting future arrhythmic events over a mean follow-up of 38 months. Three sudden deaths of 212 patients were reported in this study (two aborted) and 84% remained completely asymptomatic. Fifty nine percent of inducible patients became symptomatic over the follow-up for SVT or atrial fibrillation. All three patients with sudden death had high-risk features identified at EPS (defined as inducibility of atrial fibrillation and SVT, an anterograde effective refractory period of the accessory pathway of less than 250 milliseconds, and the shortest preexcited RR interval of less than 250 ms). All three patients also had multiple accessory pathways.[1] However, at the time of their sudden death, none were truly asymptomatic. Each had developed symptomatic arrhythmias before their sudden death. Another study also highlights the low specificity and positive predictive value of EPS for predicting sudden death—specificity of 48.3% and a low predictive accuracy (18.9%) when using the shortest preexcited RR interval of less than 250 milliseconds.[31]

The diagnostic utility of inducibility of SVT for predicting future SVT is also disputed. In another study, inducibility of SVT in asymptomatic patients did not predict future SVT events and no sudden deaths were observed over a 4.3-year follow-up period.[19] Thus, the inducibility of SVT has been reported to have positive predictive values that vary widely between 0% to 70% and negative predictive values generally greater than 95% at predicting subsequent SVT.[1,19]

The inducibility of atrial fibrillation at EPS has also been used to risk stratify patients.[1] The authors' meta-analysis of asymptomatic WPW patients revealed a low incidence of spontaneous atrial fibrillation in this population. Nine studies of asymptomatic WPW patients, involving 3654 person years of follow-up reported on subsequent atrial fibrillation (mean age range 7–36) in the meta-analysis.[1–4,19,20,38–40] The risk of atrial fibrillation was estimated at 9.25 per 1000 person years of follow-up (95% CI; 3.37–18.00).[16]

A diagnostic EPS is most reassuring (because of high negative predictive values) when invasive variables reveal the absence of inducibility of SVT, a shortest preexcited RR interval of more than 250 milliseconds, and a long anterograde ERP. In select circumstances when diagnostic EPS is undertaken in the asymptomatic patient, the presence of catheters within the heart may lead to a psychological momentum that leads to catheter ablation in the absence of a strong indication. The location of the accessory pathway needs to be considered in this situation (left vs right, proximity to the atrioventricular node) because of site-specific potential for complications.

PROPHYLACTIC ABLATION IN ASYMPTOMATIC PATIENTS

Only two studies have evaluated the effect of prophylactic ablation in asymptomatic WPW patients in randomized control trials.[2,3]

In the first study involving 224 asymptomatic adult patients (older than 13 years of age) who underwent invasive EPS, 87 had inducible arrhythmias. Of these inducible patients, patients less than 35 years of age were deemed high-risk and underwent randomization to catheter ablation (n = 37) versus observation only (high risk controls, n = 35).[2] Among the high-risk controls, the 5-year rate of any arrhythmic event was 77% compared with 7% in the ablation group. One resuscitated sudden death occurred in a patient in the high-risk control group (EPS had demonstrated multiple left-sided and right-sided accessory pathways, inducibility of SVT that had deteriorated to atrial fibrillation, and a shortest preexcited RR interval of less than 200 milliseconds). Major complications occurred in 4 of 224 patients (2%).

Another study evaluated prophylactic ablation in asymptomatic children (5–12 years of age).[3] Sixty out of the 165 children who underwent EPS had inducible SVT or atrial fibrillation and were considered as high risk. From these high-risk children, 47 were randomized to either observation (n = 27) or accessory pathway ablation (n = 20). In the ablation group, one SVT event occurred during a median follow-up of 34 months. In the high-risk control group, one sudden death and two ventricular fibrillation events occurred (both aborted). The study also reported that these three patients might have had nonspecific symptoms due to SVT prior to the sudden death. Therefore, at the time of their sudden death, none may have been truly asymptomatic. All three children had multiple accessory pathways, inducible SVT, and atrial fibrillation.

Complications included anesthesia related (3%), EPS related (3%), and those related to catheter ablation (15%). A subsequent study of asymptomatic WPW children also reported on the high prevalence of probable arrhythmic symptoms before the occurrence of life-threatening arrhythmia.[4] This study demonstrated the occurrence of symptoms during and related to atrial fibrillation in three patients before deterioration into ventricular fibrillation, allowing presentation to hospital; none died.

In summary, these studies suggest that inducibility of arrhythmia during EPS,[1–3] an anterograde ERP of less than 250 milliseconds, and multiple accessory pathways[4] predict future symptomatic arrhythmia. Prophylactic ablation in these potentially at-risk patients reduces the incidence of subsequent arrhythmic events.[1–3] The authors also suggest that life-threatening arrhythmias are reduced by prophylactic ablation[3] even though none of these studies were powered to detect a reduction in mortality or life-threatening arrhythmia. In these studies, unheralded sudden death was not likely the initial presentation because symptoms were likely due to SVT in most patients before sudden death and most life-threatening arrhythmias were aborted.

Expert consensus guidelines do not advocate routine diagnostic EPS (or ablation) in asymptomatic patients because a large body of evidence points to a benign outcome in asymptomatic patients. A well-informed asymptomatic individual should be offered the choice of proceeding with EPS and potential ablation and accepting procedural risk or waiting for development of symptoms and accepting a very small risk of sudden death as the first symptom.

INDICATIONS FOR EPS IN ASYMPTOMATIC INDIVIDUALS

In specific circumstances, a diagnostic EPS and prophylactic accessory pathway ablation may be reasonable in the asymptomatic individual for occupational or other specific requirements (eg, professional and/or recreational reasons; ie, pilots and professional athletes) (**Fig. 3**). The preference of the patient and their appreciation of life-long versus procedural risk are paramount. The evidence does not warrant a blanket recommendation.

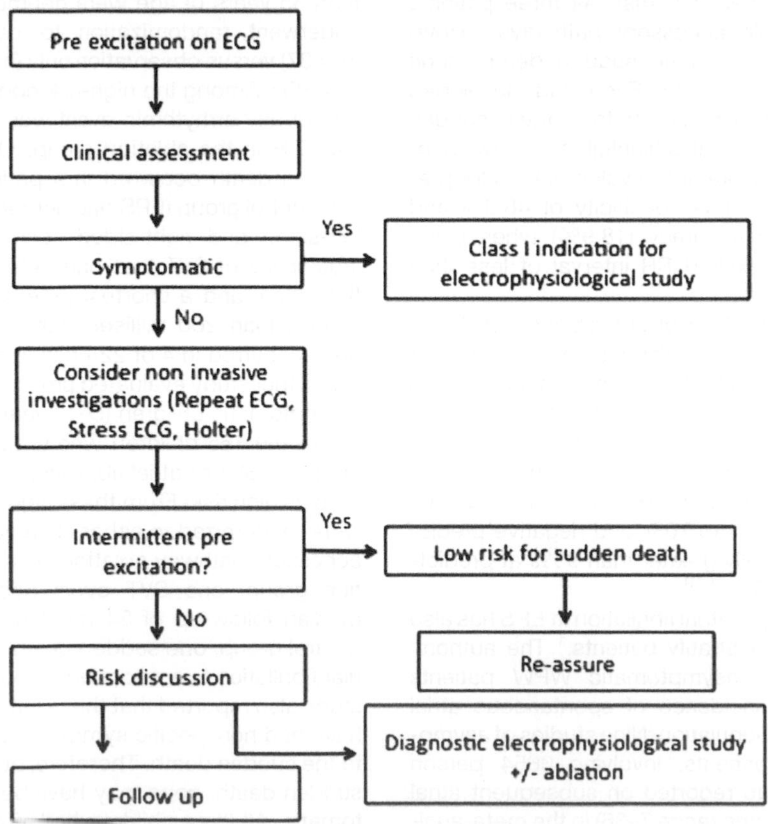

Fig. 3. A summary algorithmic approach to the patient with preexcitation.

A carefully informed patient (or parent) must choose between the very small risk of sudden death versus the success and complication rates associated with EPS and ablation.

COST EFFECTIVENESS OF ACCESSORY PATHWAY ABLATION

Considering the very low event rate, it is difficult to imagine that routine ablation based on invasive EPS assessment would be cost effective. A Markov simulation cost analysis supports ablation in symptomatic patients with Wolff-Parkinson-White syndrome, but also supported the practice of observing asymptomatic patients.[41] In asymptomatic patients, routine ablation resulted in the cost for a quality-adjusted life year gained from $174,000 in 20-year-olds to $540,000 in 60-year-olds. This compared with symptomatic patients for whom the cost per quality-adjusted life year gained ranged from $6600 in 20-year-olds to $19,000 in 60-year-olds.

SUMMARY

The risk of sudden death as the first presentation in truly asymptomatic patients with WPW is exceedingly small. The risks associated with routine EPS and ablation in these patients is likely to offset the small benefit of ablation on a population basis. The very low event rate severely challenges any diagnostic test to provide accurate risk stratification and the predictive accuracy of even short ERP at invasive EPS to identify asymptomatic patients at risk of sudden death is low. These factors argue against any strong recommendation to a patient for routine diagnostic EPS with a view to ablation. The well-informed patient must ultimately decide whether they are more comfortable with a very small long-term risk of unheralded sudden death or a short-term procedural risk that is probably at least comparable with the former.

REFERENCES

1. Pappone C, Santinelli V, Rosanio S, et al. Usefulness of invasive electrophysiologic testing to stratify the risk of arrhythmic events in asymptomatic patients with Wolff-Parkinson-White pattern: results from a large prospective long-term follow-up study. J Am Coll Cardiol 2003;41:239–44.
2. Pappone C, Santinelli V, Manguso F, et al. A randomized study of prophylactic catheter ablation in asymptomatic patients with the Wolff-Parkinson-White syndrome. N Engl J Med 2003;349:1803–11.
3. Pappone C, Manguso F, Santinelli R, et al. Radiofrequency ablation in children with asymptomatic Wolff-Parkinson-White syndrome. N Engl J Med 2004;351:1197–205.
4. Santinelli V, Radinovic A, Manguso F, et al. The natural history of asymptomatic ventricular preexcitation a long-term prospective follow-up study of 184 asymptomatic children. J Am Coll Cardiol 2009;53:275–80.
5. Blomstrom-Lundqvist C, Scheinman MM, Aliot EM, et al. ACC/AHA/ESC guidelines for the management of patients with supraventricular arrhythmias—executive summary: a report of the American College of Cardiology/American Heart Association Task Force on Practice Guidelines and the European Society of Cardiology Committee for Practice Guidelines (Writing Committee to Develop Guidelines for the Management of Patients With Supraventricular Arrhythmias). Circulation 2003;108:1871–909.
6. Hiss RG, Lamb LE. Electrocardiographic findings in 122,043 individuals. Circulation 1962;25:947–61.
7. Munger TM, Packer DL, Hammill SC, et al. A population study of the natural history of Wolff-Parkinson-White syndrome in Olmsted County, Minnesota, 1953–1989. Circulation 1993;87:866–73.
8. Flensted-Jensen E. Wolff-Parkinson-White syndrome. A long-term follow-up of 47 cases. Acta Med Scand 1969;186:65–74.
9. Klein GJ, Bashore TM, Sellers TD, et al. Ventricular fibrillation in the Wolff-Parkinson-White syndrome. N Engl J Med 1979;301:1080–5.
10. Obeyesekere MN, Leong-Sit P, Massel D, et al. Risk of arrhythmia and sudden death in patients with asymptomatic preexcitation: a meta-analysis. Circulation 2012;125:2308–15.
11. Smith TW, Cain ME. Sudden cardiac death: epidemiologic and financial worldwide perspective. J Interv Card Electrophysiol 2006;17:199–203.
12. Morentin B, Audicana C. Population-based study of out-of-hospital sudden cardiovascular death: incidence and causes of death in middle-aged adults. Rev Esp Cardiol 2011;64:28–34.
13. Lim Z, Gibbs K, Potts JE, et al. A review of sudden unexpected death in the young in British Columbia. Can J Cardiol 2010;26:22–6.
14. Morris VB, Keelan T, Leen E, et al. Sudden cardiac death in the young: a 1-year post-mortem analysis in the Republic of Ireland. Ir J Med Sci 2009;178:257–61.
15. Winkel BG, Holst AG, Theilade J, et al. Nationwide study of sudden cardiac death in persons aged 1-35 years. Eur Heart J 2011;32:983–90.
16. Obeyesekere MN, Leong-Sit P, Massel D, et al. Incidence of atrial fibrillation and prevalence of intermittent pre-excitation in asymptomatic Wolff-Parkinson-White patients: A meta-analysis. Int J Cardiol 2012. [Epub ahead of print].

17. Fitzsimmons PJ, McWhirter PD, Peterson DW, et al. The natural history of Wolff-Parkinson-White syndrome in 228 military aviators: a long-term follow-up of 22 years. Am Heart J 2001;142:530–6.
18. Klein GJ, Yee R, Sharma AD. Longitudinal electrophysiologic assessment of asymptomatic patients with the Wolff-Parkinson-White electrocardiographic pattern. N Engl J Med 1989;320:1229–33.
19. Leitch JW, Klein GJ, Yee R, et al. Prognostic value of electrophysiology testing in asymptomatic patients with Wolff-Parkinson-White pattern. Circulation 1990; 82:1718–23.
20. Sarubbi B, Scognamiglio G, Limongelli G, et al. Asymptomatic ventricular pre-excitation in children and adolescents: a 15 year follow up study. Heart 2003;89:215–7.
21. Scheinman MM. NASPE Survey on Catheter Ablation. Pacing Clin Electrophysiol 1995;18:1474–8.
22. Hindricks G. The Multicentre European Radiofrequency Survey (MERFS): complications of radiofrequency catheter ablation of arrhythmias. The Multicentre European Radiofrequency Survey (MERFS) investigators of the Working Group on Arrhythmias of the European Society of Cardiology. Eur Heart J 1993;14:1644–53.
23. Calkins H, Yong P, Miller JM, et al. Catheter ablation of accessory pathways, atrioventricular nodal reentrant tachycardia, and the atrioventricular junction: final results of a prospective, multicenter clinical trial. The Atakr Multicenter Investigators Group. Circulation 1999;99:262–70.
24. Kugler JD, Danford DA, Houston KA, et al. Pediatric radiofrequency catheter ablation registry success, fluoroscopy time, and complication rate for supraventricular tachycardia: comparison of early and recent eras. J Cardiovasc Electrophysiol 2002;13:336–41.
25. Kugler JD, Danford DA, Deal BJ, et al. Radiofrequency catheter ablation for tachyarrhythmias in children and adolescents. The Pediatric Electrophysiology Society. N Engl J Med 1994;330:1481–7.
26. Kugler JD, Danford DA, Houston K, et al. Radiofrequency catheter ablation for paroxysmal supraventricular tachycardia in children and adolescents without structural heart disease. Pediatric EP Society, Radiofrequency Catheter Ablation Registry. Am J Cardiol 1997;80:1438–43.
27. Calkins H, Niklason L, Sousa J, et al. Radiation exposure during radiofrequency catheter ablation of accessory atrioventricular connections. Circulation 1991;84:2376–82.
28. Bacher K, Bogaert E, Lapere R, et al. Patient-specific dose and radiation risk estimation in pediatric cardiac catheterization. Circulation 2005;111: 83–9.
29. Goldberger JJ. The coin toss: implications for risk stratification for sudden cardiac death. Am Heart J 2010;160:3–7.
30. Delise P, Sciarra L. Asymptomatic Wolff-Parkinson-White: what to do. Extensive ablation or not? J Cardiovasc Med (Hagerstown) 2007;8:668–74.
31. Sharma AD, Yee R, Guiraudon G, et al. Sensitivity and specificity of invasive and noninvasive testing for risk of sudden death in Wolff-Parkinson-White syndrome. J Am Coll Cardiol 1987;10:373–81.
32. Wellens HJ, Braat S, Brugada P, et al. Use of procainamide in patients with the Wolff-Parkinson-White syndrome to disclose a short refractory period of the accessory pathway. Am J Cardiol 1982;50:1087–9.
33. Boahene KA, Klein GJ, Sharma AD, et al. Value of a revised procainamide test in the Wolff-Parkinson-White syndrome. Am J Cardiol 1990;65:195–200.
34. Timmermans C, Smeets JL, Rodriguez LM, et al. Aborted sudden death in the Wolff-Parkinson-White syndrome. Am J Cardiol 1995;76:492–4.
35. Satoh M, Aizawa Y, Funazaki T, et al. Electrophysiologic evaluation of asymptomatic patients with the Wolff-Parkinson-White pattern. Pacing Clin Electrophysiol 1989;12:413–20.
36. Klein GJ, Prystowsky EN, Yee R, et al. Asymptomatic Wolff-Parkinson-White. Should we intervene? Circulation 1989;80:1902–5.
37. Milstein S, Sharma AD, Klein GJ. Electrophysiologic profile of asymptomatic Wolff-Parkinson-White pattern. Am J Cardiol 1986;57:1097–100.
38. Brembilla-Perrot B, Chometon F, Groben L, et al. Interest of non-invasive and semi-invasive testings in asymptomatic children with pre-excitation syndrome. Europace 2007;9:837–43.
39. Fazio G, Mossuto C, Basile I, et al. Asymptomatic ventricular pre-excitation in children. J Cardiovasc Med (Hagerstown) 2009;10:59–63.
40. Beckman KJ, Gallastegui JL, Bauman JL, et al. The predictive value of electrophysiologic studies in untreated patients with Wolff-Parkinson-White syndrome. J Am Coll Cardiol 1990;15:640–7.
41. Hogenhuis W, Stevens SK, Wang P, et al. Cost-effectiveness of radiofrequency ablation compared with other strategies in Wolff-Parkinson-White syndrome. Circulation 1993;88:II437–46.

Asymptomatic Wolff-Parkinson-White Syndrome Should be Ablated

Carlo Pappone, MD*, Vincenzo Santinelli, MD

KEYWORDS

• Wolff-Parkinson-White syndrome • Sudden cardiac death • Pediatric patients • Catheter ablation

KEY POINTS

- Asymptomatic pediatric patients with Wolff-Parkinson-White syndrome (WPW) are at higher risk of sudden cardiac death than are adult asymptomatic patients.
- Most asymptomatic WPW patients have essentially no risk and a good outcome; only the subgroup of children is at high risk, requiring early catheter ablation.
- Intrinsic electrophysiologic properties of accessory pathways, rather than symptoms, predict the risk.
- Liberal indications for catheter ablation as currently suggested by guidelines is justified only for patients with symptomatic ventricular preexcitation, and is aimed at improving the patient's quality of life by eliminating symptoms associated with arrhythmia recurrences and/or chronic antiarrhythmic drug therapy.

INTRODUCTION

It is about 100 years since Wolff, Parkinson, and White reported the syndrome bearing their name,[1] and the earliest reports of sudden cardiac death (SCD) in patients with Wolff-Parkinson-White syndrome (WPW) were published in the late 1930s.[2,3] Subsequently, although the occurrence of cardiac arrest and/or SCD in asymptomatic patients with a WPW pattern on the electrocardiogram (ECG) has been well documented by several prospective, randomized cohort studies and alarming reports,[4–34] the true incidence of SCD in asymptomatic WPW patients is undefined. In the last years the authors have substantially contributed to the understanding and knowledge of the natural history of the syndrome, and the available data is proving useful in the management of asymptomatic subjects with ventricular preexcitation.[4,5,21,22,35,36] This article discusses how to manage the asymptomatic WPW patient in the era of the widespread use of catheter ablation.

THE NATURAL HISTORY OF WPW

Prior Anecdotal Follow-Up Studies on Asymptomatic WPW

Knowledge of the natural history of WPW is crucial in defining outcomes and predictors of outcome, which require a clear definition of end points, a large number of patients prospectively enrolled, and adequate follow-up monitoring, particularly for initially asymptomatic WPW patients. Unfortunately, prior available natural history studies have reported a small number of patients, many of whom were retrospectively analyzed without adequate monitoring and with follow-up periods that were too short, considering the lifetime risk of the syndrome and the supposed low event rates of WPW.[4–23] Based on these limited data, it is not surprising that decreased estimations of the true SCD event rates have been reported.[4–23] Of course it is not easy to incidentally detect, enroll, and intensively follow a large number of asymptomatic subjects.

Arrhythmology Department, Maria Cecilia Hospital, Via Corriera 1, 48010 Cotignola, Italy
* Corresponding author. Department of Electrophysiology, Maria Cecilia Hospital, Via Corriera 1, 48010 Cotignola, Italy.
E-mail address: cpappone@gvmnet.it

Card Electrophysiol Clin 4 (2012) 281–285
http://dx.doi.org/10.1016/j.ccep.2012.06.006

Recent Follow-Up Studies on Asymptomatic WPW

The authors' experience of the asymptomatic WPW population represents an important recognized contribution to the knowledge of the natural history of the syndrome.[4,5,21,22,37,38] The major message is that asymptomatic WPW syndrome in the pediatric population is not as benign as previously supposed, and that asymptomatic children are at higher risk of SCD than are asymptomatic adults.[4,5] The authors have previously demonstrated the ability of electrophysiologic testing (EPT) to stratify asymptomatic patients,[21] and that prophylactic catheter ablation in asymptomatic WPW patients (children and adults) reduces the likelihood of arrhythmia.[22] Another study in children between 5 and 12 years of age also suggested that early catheter ablation significantly reduces symptoms.[37] The authors' experience began in 1980 with a pilot study enrolling the first 20 asymptomatic WPW patients who underwent sequential transesophageal electrophysiologic testing to assess a potential relationship between sustained arrhythmia inducibility and outcome.[39] Since 1990 to date, asymptomatic WPW patients have been increasingly referred from all over Italy for risk evaluation, and follow-up data have now been accumulated on about 500 asymptomatic patients with a median age of 26 years. These data, by virtue of their magnitude, have contributed toward better delineating the natural history of the disease from childhood to adulthood. Because SCD is a relatively rare event, the authors have used as primary end point of outcome a conservative and inclusive surrogate of death: documented extremely rapid preexcited atrial fibrillation resulting in syncope, presyncope, cardiac arrest, and/or SCD (collectively termed as malignant arrhythmia). This end point allows one to perform a multivariate analysis for independent predictors of outcome. A recent meta-analysis by Obeyesekere and colleagues[40] reports the incidence of SCD among 20 selected studies on the asymptomatic pediatric[5–10] or adult[4,11–23] population with ventricular preexcitation, which also included the authors' experience.[4,5,21,22] One of the main findings of this meta-analysis was that asymptomatic children have a higher event rate of SCD compared with asymptomatic adults, which indicates that the risk of cardiac arrest and/or SCD in the asymptomatic patient population indeed begins in the early stages of life, as first reported by Santinelli and colleagues.[5] These findings are important because they suggest that a higher index of suspicion for arrhythmia is warranted in the pediatric population, with careful follow-up and intensive monitoring for arrhythmia to prevent SCD. The data also suggest that most previous natural history studies on both symptomatic and asymptomatic WPW population are inconclusive and that older current guidelines should be revisited.[41]

SCD IN THE ASYMPTOMATIC WPW POPULATION

Although the recent meta-analysis by Obeyesekere and colleagues[40] has found only 10 cases of SCD in 20 selected studies involving either children (5 cases of SCD in 6 studies) or adults (5 cases of SCD in 14 studies), several alarming anecdotal reports have documented the occurrence of devastating, fatal arrhythmias and/or SCD in many asymptomatic subjects, particularly in the pediatric population.[24–35] In 1979, Klein and colleagues[25] raised concerns for asymptomatic patients with WPW by documenting ventricular fibrillation in 3 pediatric subjects (ages 8–16 years) who presented with cardiac arrest. In 1993, Russell and colleagues[26] described 256 pediatric patients with WPW, 6 of whom had presented with a life-threatening arrhythmia as the first manifestation of their preexcitation syndrome. Among this group of 256 patients, 60 (23.4%) were asymptomatic. In 1995, Deal and colleagues,[27] representing the Pediatric Electrophysiology Society, reported 42 SCDs in children with WPW and of these, in 20 (mean age, 11 years) SCD was the presenting symptom. In one of the largest reports of children who had WPW and experienced cardiac arrest, Bromberg and colleagues[28] in 1996 described 60 patients who underwent surgical elimination of WPW in the era before widespread use of radiofrequency ablation. Ten children had experienced a clinical cardiac arrest and of these, only 1 had a history of syncope or atrial fibrillation. In this group of patients, a shortest RR interval of less than 220 milliseconds during atrial fibrillation (AF) was more sensitive than clinical history for identifying those at risk of SCD. Dubin and colleagues[29] assessed 100 pediatric patients with WPW and documented that asymptomatic subjects had statistically the same recognized EPT risk profile as the symptomatic ones, theorizing that the risk of SCD in asymptomatic patients may be higher than previously suspected. All these data and reports reflect the current clinical practice of pediatric electrophysiologists, with the majority (84%) using EPT for risk stratification in the asymptomatic population. Campbell and colleagues[30] surveyed the members of the Pediatric and Congenital Electrophysiology Society study groups. Of the 43 respondents (of whom 37 had been performing ablation for >5 years),

36 used EPT to risk-stratify children with asymptomatic WPW syndrome. Most (33 of 43, 77%) would also perform ablation on children with a shortest preexcited RR during AF of less than 240 milliseconds, and 19 of 43 (44%) would have ablated those with an anterograde effective refractory period (ERP) of accessory pathways (AP) of less than 240 milliseconds. Only 11 of 43 (26%) would ablate those with inducible sustained ventricular tachycardia alone. Special considerations of ablation was given by these electrophysiologists to subjects considering high-risk careers, competitive athletes, and those with coexisting congenital heart disease, asthma, and attention-deficit disorder likely to require medical management with drugs.

SCD IN ASYMPTOMATIC VERSUS SYMPTOMATIC WPW SUBJECTS

It is unclear how high is the risk of SCD in the whole WPW population, and whether symptomatic patients are at higher risk of SCD than the asymptomatic ones. It is well known that most cases of ventricular fibrillation with aborted sudden death and/or SCD have been reported in symptomatic patients. However, many other cases of SCD or cardiac arrest caused by malignant arrhythmias have been reported as occurring in often young, otherwise healthy asymptomatic subjects, particularly children, and many others continue to die unexpectedly despite the availability of catheter ablation as definitive cure. The strategy and management of the asymptomatic patients is now significantly affected by the availability of EPT and catheter ablation. However, both EPT and catheter ablation are invasive procedures with potential complications for the asymptomatic patient; as a result, careful and objective risk-benefit analysis is necessary. The population-based study of the natural history of WPW by Munger and colleagues[18] reported 53 asymptomatic subjects with a mean age of 33 years and no case of SCD. However, they described two cases of SCD in the symptomatic group, one of whom had had specified "symptoms" only during infancy, remaining completely asymptomatic from infancy up to 23 years when he experienced SCD during athletic competition. This intriguing case further suggests that SCD may unexpectedly occur in a patient who has been asymptomatic throughout life from infancy to adulthood. Of note, of the asymptomatic group, Munger and colleagues[18] also report that 21% of the initially asymptomatic group became symptomatic and 2 required surgery because of incapacitating symptoms. These findings taken together strongly confirm that the lifetime risk of SCD may be due to intrinsic electrophysiologic properties of accessory pathways rather than to the mere presence of symptoms. In the last 15 years the morbidity and poor quality of life associated with recurrent cardiac arrhythmias and the need for chronic antiarrhythmic drug therapy have justified the widespread use of catheter-ablation therapy for all symptomatic WPW patients regardless of risk assessment, as suggested by guidelines.[41] As a result, nowadays the most important steps in the management of a patient with WPW are the recognition of the condition and subsequent referral of the patient to an electrophysiologist for curative catheter ablation. At present, early catheter ablation in asymptomatic WPW subjects may be justified only in selected asymptomatic WPW patients found to be at risk of malignant arrhythmias and/or SCD, but predictors of the risk are necessary.

PREDICTORS OF THE RISK

Previous longitudinal studies on the natural history of WPW do not report independent predictors of the risk of SCD, and catheter ablation in the asymptomatic WPW population to prevent malignant arrhythmias and/or SCD has not been justified by guidelines.[41] Noninvasive risk stratification with Holter monitoring, exercise stress testing, and pharmacologic testing should be performed before invasive studies are considered, but sensitivity and specificity of noninvasive testing has been shown to be poor.[42] Transesophageal EPT is a semi-invasive technique, but is not entirely risk free because it is painful and requires use of heavy sedation. Risk stratification by independent predictors requires a well-defined primary end point of outcome (malignant arrhythmias and/or SCD) with an adequate number of events for a multivariate analysis, which in a patient population supposed to be at low risk needs a large number of enrolled patients and intensive and adequate lengths of follow-up to detect such events. To date only 2 prospective natural history studies on asymptomatic WPW have fully fulfilled these criteria, enrolling about 500 asymptomatic WPW patients, and the results have been recently published.[4,5] Multivariate analysis demonstrated that short anterograde ERP of the AP (<240 ms) and multiple accessory pathways are able to predict the occurrence of malignant arrhythmias and ventricular fibrillation in asymptomatic children with accessory pathways. The authors have demonstrated for the first time that the risk of malignant arrhythmias and/or SCD is higher in the pediatric population, beginning early in life, with minimal or no risk in the adult asymptomatic population.[4,5] In addition, a pooled analysis of the overall asymptomatic and symptomatic WPW population has shown high negative and positive predictive values for risk factors using as end point ventricular fibrillation (Pappone and Santinelli, personal communication, 2012). As stated by Balaji[43] in his editorial comment to the authors' article,[5] one big impediment to settling the controversy about the management of asymptomatic WPW in children is our ignorance about the natural history of asymptomatic WPW from childhood to adulthood, resulting from the fact that it is very difficult to detect, enroll, and intensively follow a large number of asymptomatic children or young adults. Experience indicates that the natural history of WPW is more complex and that the risk of cardiac arrest or SCD is higher in the pediatric population, depending mostly on intrinsic properties of accessory pathways rather than on symptoms alone. As a result, catheter ablation should be contextually performed after EPT only in a minority of younger patients, particularly children, incidentally found with a WPW pattern on the ECG, to prevent malignant arrhythmias and/or sudden death.

SUMMARY

The natural history of asymptomatic WPW is more complex than previously reported. The asymptomatic pediatric population is at higher risk of SCD than the adult asymptomatic population. The vast majority of the asymptomatic WPW population has essentially no risk and a good outcome, whereas only the subgroup of children is at high risk, requiring early catheter ablation. Intrinsic electrophysiologic properties of accessory pathways, rather than symptoms, predict the risk. Liberal indications for catheter ablation as currently suggested by guidelines is justified only for patients with symptomatic ventricular preexcitation, and is aimed at improving the patient's quality of life by eliminating symptoms associated with arrhythmia recurrences and/or chronic antiarrhythmic drug therapy.

REFERENCES

1. Wolff L, Parkinson J, White PD. Bundle-branch block with short P-R interval in healthy young people prone to paroxysmal tachycardia. Am Heart J 1930;5:685–704.
2. Wood FC, Wolferth CC, Geckeler GD. Histologic demonstration of accessory muscular connections between auricle and ventricle in a case of short P-R interval and prolonged QRS complex. Am Heart J 1943;25:454–62.
3. Kimball JL, Burch G. The prognosis of the Wolff-Parkinson-White syndrome. Ann Intern Med 1947;27:239–42.
4. Santinelli V, Radinovic A, Manguso F, et al. Asymptomatic ventricular preexcitation. A long-term prospective follow-up study of 293 adult patients. Circ Arrhythm Electrophysiol 2009;2:102–7.
5. Santinelli V, Radinovic A, Manguso F, et al. The natural history of asymptomatic ventricular pre-excitation a long-term prospective follow-up study of 184 asymptomatic children. J Am Coll Cardiol 2009;53:275–80.
6. Fazio G, Mossuto C, Basile I, et al. Asymptomatic ventricular preexcitation in children. J Cardiovasc Med (Hagerstown) 2009;10:59–63.
7. Inoue K, Igarashi H, Fukushige J, et al. Long-term prospective study on the natural history of Wolff-Parkinson-White syndrome detected during a heart screening program at school. Acta Paediatr 2000;89:542–5.
8. Sarubbi B, Scognamiglio G, Limongelli G, et al. Asymptomatic ventricular preexcitation in children and adolescents: a 15 year follow-up study. Heart 2003;89:215–7.
9. Vignati G, Balla E, Maurii L, et al. Clinical and electrophysiologic evaluation of the Wolff-Parkinson-White syndrome in children: impact on approaches to management. Cardiol Young 2000;10:367–75.
10. Brembilla-Perrot B, Chometon F, Groben L, et al. Interest of non-invasive and semi-invasive testing in asymptomatic children with pre-excitation syndrome. Europace 2007;9:837–43.
11. Milstein S, Sharma AD, Klein GJ. Electrophysiologic profile of asymptomatic Wolff-Parkinson-White pattern. Am J Cardiol 1986;57:1097–100.
12. Klein GL, Yee R, Sharma AD. Longitudinal electrophysiologic assessment of asymptomatic patients with the Wolff Parkinson White electrocardiographic pattern. N Engl J Med 1989;320:1229–33.
13. Satoh M, Aizawa Y, Funazaki T, et al. Electrophysiologic evaluation of asymptomatic patients with the Wolff-Parkinson-White pattern. Pacing Clin Electrophysiol 1989;12:413–20.
14. Beckman BJ, Gallastegui JL, Bauman JL, et al. The predictive value of electrophysiologic studies in untreated patients with Wolff-Parkinson-White syndrome. J Am Coll Cardiol 1990;15:640–7.
15. Leitch JW, Klein GJ, Yee R, et al. Prognostic value of electrophysiology testing in asymptomatic patients with Wolff-Parkinson-White pattern. Circulation 1990;82:1718–23.
16. Fukatani M, Tanigawa M, Mori M, et al. Prediction of a fatal atrial fibrillation in patients with asymptomatic Wolff-Parkinson-White pattern. Jpn Circ J 1990;54:1331–9.
17. Brembilla-Perrot B, Ghawi R. Electrophysiological characteristics of asymptomatic Wolff-Parkinson-White syndrome. Eur Heart J 1993;14:511–5.

18. Munger TM, Packer DL, Hammill SC, et al. A population study of the natural history of Wolff-Parkinson-White syndrome in Olmsted country, Minnesota, 1953-1989. Circulation 1993;87:866–73.
19. Fitzsimmons PJ, McWhirter PD, Peterson DW, et al. The natural history of Wolff-Parkinson-White syndrome in 228 military aviators: a long-term follow-up of 22 years. Am Heart J 2001;142:530–6.
20. Gouvedenos JA, Katsouras CS, Graekas G, et al. Ventricular pre-excitation in the general population: a study on the mode of presentation and clinical course. Heart 2000;83:29–34.
21. Pappone C, Santinelli V, Rosario S, et al. Usefulness of invasive electrophysiologic testing to stratify the risk of arrhythmic events in asymptomatic patients with Wolff-Parkinson-White pattern. J Am Coll Cardiol 2003;41:239–44.
22. Pappone C, Santinelli V, Manguso F, et al. A randomized study of prophylactic catheter ablation in asymptomatic patients with the Wolff-Parkinson-White syndrome. N Engl J Med 2003;349:1803–11.
23. Smith RF. The Wolff-Parkinson-White syndrome as an aviation risk. Circulation 1964;29:672–9.
24. Dreifus LS, Haiat R, Watanabe Y, et al. Ventricular fibrillation: a possible mechanism of sudden death in patients with Wolff-Parkinson-White syndrome. Circulation 1971;43:520–7.
25. Klein GL, Bashore TM, Sellers TD, et al. Ventricular fibrillation in the Wolff Parkinson White syndrome. N Engl J Med 1979;15:1080–5.
26. Russell MV, Dorostkar PC, Macdonald D. Incidence of catastrophic events associated with the Wolff-Parkinson-White syndrome in young patients: diagnostic and therapeutic dilemma. Circulation 1993; 88:2608.
27. Deal BJ, Dick M, Beerman L, et al. Cardiac arrest in young patients with Wolff-Parkinson-White syndrome [abstract]. Pacing Clin Electrophysiol 1995; 18(Pt II):815.
28. Bromberg BI, Lindsay BD, Cain ME, et al. Impact of clinical history and electrophysiologic characterization of accessory pathways on management strategies to reduce sudden death among children with Wolff-Parkinson-White syndrome. J Am Coll Cardiol 1996;27:690–5.
29. Dubin AM, Collins KK, Chiesa N, et al. The use of electrophysiologic testing to assess risk in children with Wolff-Parkinson-White syndrome. Cardiol Young 2002;12:248–52.
30. Campbell RM, Strieper MJ, Frias PA, et al. Survey of current practice of pediatric electrophysiologists for asymptomatic Wolff-Parkinson-White syndrome. Pediatrics 2003;111:e245–7.
31. Prystowsky EN, Fananapazir L, Packer DL, et al. Wolff-Parkinson-White syndrome and sudden cardiac death. Cardiology 1987;74(Suppl 2):67–71.
32. Cosio FG, Benson DW Jr, Anderson RW, et al. Onset of atrial fibrillation during antidromic tachycardia: association with sudden cardiac arrest and ventricular fibrillation in a patient with Wolff-Parkinson-White syndrome. Am J Cardiol 1982;50:353–9.
33. Timmermanns C, Smeets JL, Rodriguez LM, et al. Aborted sudden death in the Wolff-Parkinson-White syndrome. Am J Cardiol 1995;76:492–4.
34. Montoya P, Brugada P, Smeets J, et al. Ventricular fibrillation in the Wolff-Parkinson-White syndrome. Eur Heart J 1991;12:144–50.
35. Attoyan C, Haissaguerre M, Dartigues JF, et al. Ventricular fibrillation in the Wolff-Parkinson-White syndrome. Predictive factors. Arch Mal Coeur Vaiss 1994;87:889–97.
36. Wiedermann CJ, Becker AE, Hopperwieser T, et al. Sudden death in young competitive athlete with Wolff-Parkinson-White syndrome. Eur Heart J 1987; 8:651–5.
37. Pappone C, Manguso F, Santinelli V, et al. Radiofrequency ablation in children with asymptomatic Wolff-Parkinson-White syndrome. N Engl J Med 2004;351:1197–205.
38. Pappone C, Vicedomini G, Manguso F, et al. Risk of malignant arrhythmias in initially symptomatic patients with the Wolff-Parkinson-White syndrome: results of a prospective long-term electrophysiological follow-up study. Circulation 2012;125:661–8.
39. Santinelli V, Turco P, de Paola M, et al. Long-term assessment of asymptomatic patients with ventricular preexcitation: a pilot study [abstract]. Circulation 1990;82(Suppl III):318.
40. Obeyesekere MN, Leong-Sit P, Massel D, et al. Risk of arrhythmia and sudden death in patients with asymptomatic preexcitation. A meta-analysis. Circulation 2012;125:2308–15.
41. Blomstrom-Lundqvist C, Scheinman MM, Aliot EM, et al. American College of Cardiology; American Heart Association Task Force on Practice Guidelines; European Society of Cardiology Committee for Practice Guidelines. Writing Committee to Develop Guidelines for the Management of Patients with Supraventricular Arrhythmias. Circulation 2003; 108:1871–909.
42. Sharma AD, Yee R, Guiraudon G, et al. Sensitivity and specificity of invasive and noninvasive testing for risk of sudden death in Wolff-Parkinson-White syndrome. J Am Coll Cardiol 1987;10:373–81.
43. Balaji S. Asymptomatic Wolff-Parkinson-White syndrome in children. J Am Coll Cardiol 2009;53:281–3.

Ablation as First-Line Therapy for Atrial Fibrillation: Yes

Pasquale Santangeli, MD[a,b], Luigi Di Biase, MD, PhD, FHRS[a,b], Amin Al-Ahmad, MD, FHRS[c], Rodney Horton, MD[a], J. David Burkhardt, MD[a], Javier E. Sanchez, MD[a], G. Joseph Gallinghouse, MD[a], Jason Zagrodzky, MD[a], Rong Bai, MD, FHRS[a,d], Agnes Pump, MD[a,e], Sanghamitra Mohanty, MD[a], William R. Lewis, MD[f], Andrea Natale, MD, FHRS, FESC[a,c,f,g,h,*]

KEYWORDS

• Atrial fibrillation • Catheter ablation • First-line therapy

KEY POINTS

- Two randomized controlled trials and 2 consecutive case series, including a total of 451 patients, have consistently shown that catheter ablation (CA) is superior to antiarrhythmic drug (AAD) therapy as first-line rhythm-control therapy for paroxysmal atrial fibrillation (AF).
- In these patients, the risk of complications with CA is entirely comparable with that of AAD therapy.
- The results are consistently reproducible across different institutions, operators, and types of ablation approaches.
- CA should be preferred to antiarrhythmic drug therapy as first-line therapy for paroxysmal AF.

INTRODUCTION

Atrial fibrillation (AF) is the most common arrhythmia encountered in clinical practice, affecting 1% of the general population and up to 10% of patients older than 80 years.[1] AF has a significant impact on morbidity, mainly related to symptoms, heart failure, and thromboembolic events, and is the most frequent arrhythmic cause of hospital admission in the United States.[2,3] In addition, AF is associated with excess mortality independently of thromboembolic complications.[4,5] Based on these premises, achieving a definite cure for this arrhythmia is highly desirable, and as such would have profound social and economic implications.

In recent years, multiple clinical trials have clearly demonstrated the superiority of catheter ablation (CA) over antiarrhythmic drug (AAD) therapy in terms of long-term freedom from AF, improvement in quality of life, and reduction of hospitalizations.[6,7] The great majority of such trials have evaluated CA in patients who have already failed at least one AAD.[8] The extent to which CA might be valuable as first-line therapy in patients with AF is still considered a controversial issue.

In a previous article published 6 years ago, Verma and Natale[9] defended the thesis in favor of CA as first-line therapy for AF based on the results of an early trial by the same investigators

[a] Texas Cardiac Arrhythmia Institute, St David's Medical Center, 3000 North I-35, Suite 720, Austin, TX 78705, USA; [b] University of Foggia, Foggia, Italy; [c] Division of Cardiology, Stanford University, 300 Pasteur Drive, MC 5319 A260, Stanford, CA, USA; [d] Department of Internal Medicine, Tong-Ji Hospital, Tong-Ji Medical College, Huazhong University of Science and Technology, Wuhan, China; [e] Heart Institute, Faculty of Medicine, University of Pecs, Pecs, Hungary; [f] Heart and Vascular Center, Case Western Reserve University School of Medicine, 2500 MetroHealth Drive, Cleveland, OH 44109, USA; [g] Interventional Electrophysiology, Scripps Clinic, San Diego, CA, USA; [h] EP Services, California Pacific Medical Center, San Francisco, CA, USA
* Corresponding author.
E-mail address: dr.natale@gmail.com

Card Electrophysiol Clin 4 (2012) 287–297
http://dx.doi.org/10.1016/j.ccep.2012.05.011
1877-9182/12/$ – see front matter

(ie, Radiofrequency Ablation vs Antiarrhythmic drugs as First-line Treatment of symptomatic atrial fibrillation [RAAFT])[10] as well as on additional considerations, including the survival benefit of effective sinus rhythm maintenance,[11–13] the ineffectiveness of AADs for the rhythm-control of AF,[14–16] and the significant risks associated with AAD therapy.[17–19] In an antagonist article, Padanilam and Prystowsky[20] argued that, unlike other arrhythmic conditions such as the Wolff-Parkinson-White syndrome, there was insufficient evidence supporting CA as first-line therapy for AF because of the lack of definite knowledge regarding the efficacy and short-term and long-term risks of CA in this setting, as well as the cost-effectiveness of such a strategy and the reproducibility of the results across different institutions and operators.

Of note, over the last 6 years such lack of evidence has been largely fulfilled, and herein the authors provide quantitative data supporting CA as first-line therapy for AF, shifting the paradigm of treatment evaluation from expert opinions to an actual numbers-based appraisal of the evidence.

CA AS FIRST-LINE THERAPY FOR AF: FULFILLING THE GAPS IN THE EVIDENCE

To date, 2 multicenter randomized trials and 2 consecutive case series have evaluated the benefit of CA as first-line therapy for AF. The baseline clinical characteristics and outcomes of these studies are summarized in **Tables 1** and **2**.[10,21–23]

RANDOMIZED TRIALS ON CA AS FIRST-LINE THERAPY FOR AF: RAAFT-1, MANTRA-PAF, RAAFT-2

In the early RAAFT trial,[10] 70 patients (mean age 54 years) with monthly symptomatic episodes of AF for at least 3 months (96% paroxysmal AF) were randomly assigned to CA or AAD therapy. Four different Institutions (1 in the United States, 1 in Germany, and 2 in Italy) participated in this trial, all adopting a standardized CA protocol consisting of pulmonary vein antrum isolation guided by intracardiac echocardiography, with confirmation of electrical isolation through a circular mapping catheter.[10] Of note, in this early trial only solid-tipped 8-mm ablation catheters were used because irrigated-tip catheters were not yet approved for AF ablation. The outcomes assessed in this trial were recurrence of AF, hospitalization, and quality of life at 1-year follow-up. At the end of follow-up, 63% of patients assigned to AAD therapy experienced at least 1 recurrence of symptomatic AF, as compared with 13% of those assigned to the pulmonary vein antrum isolation (PVAI) treatment arm (**Fig. 1**), accounting for 80% relative risk reduction with CA ($P<.001$). Translating such figures into treatment effects, the corresponding number of patients who need to be treated (NNT) with CA to prevent one episode

Table 1
Characteristics of studies evaluating CA as first-line therapy for AF

	Study[Ref]			
	RAAFT[10]	MANTRA-PAF[22]	Tanner et al[23]	Namdar et al[21]
Year	2005	2011	2011	2011
No. of patients	70	294	72	18
Randomized	Yes	Yes	No	No
Design	CA vs AADs in pts with AF	CA vs AADs in pts with paroxysmal AF	First-line CA vs CA of drug-refractory AF	First-line CA of paroxysmal AF
CA approach	PVAI guided by ICE, 8-mm NIC	CPVA or PVI, OIC or 8-mm NIC	PVI with OIC	PVI, cryoballoon
Primary end point	AF recurrences	AF burden	AF recurrences	AF recurrences
No. of institutions	4	10	1	3
Follow-up (mo)	12	24	12	14

Abbreviations: AADs, antiarrhythmic drugs; AF, atrial fibrillation; CA, catheter ablation; ICE, intracardiac echocardiography; NIC, nonirrigated ablation catheter; OIC, open-irrigated ablation catheter; pts, patients; PVAI, pulmonary vein antrum isolation.

Table 2
Characteristics of patients included in studies evaluating CA as first-line therapy for AF and reported study outcomes

	Study[Ref]						
	RAAFT[10]		MANTRA-PAF[22]		Tanner et al[23]		Namdar et al[21]
	CA	AADs	CA	AADs	FL/CA	SL/CA	Cryoballoon
Age, y	53 ± 8	54 ± 8	56 ± 9	54 ± 10	58 ± 11	59 ± 9	44 ± 9
Paroxysmal AF, %	97	95	100	100	74	67	100
LA size, cm	4.1 ± 0.8	4.2 ± 0.7	4.0 ± 0.6	4.0 ± 0.5	4.3 ± 0.6	4.4 ± 0.7	3.9 ± 0.4
LVEF, % or % of pts >60%	53 ± 5	54 ± 6	79	82	62 ± 7[a]	59 ± 10[a]	58 ± 3
Structural HD and HTN, %	25	28	38	47	43	45	0
AF recurrence at FU, %	13[a]	63[a]	15[a]	29[a]	22[a]	36[a]	11
Complications (%)							
Death	0	0	2.1	2.7	0	0	0
Stroke/TIA	0	0	1.4	0.7	0	0.7	0
Cardiac tamponade	0	0	2.1	0	1.1	1.5	0
Bleeding	6.3	2.9	1.4	0	2.4	1.9	6
Bradycardia	0[a]	8.6[a]	0	0.7	0	0	0
PV stenosis	6.2	0	0.7	0	0	0.2	0
Other	0	0	11.6	14.9	4.5	2.1	6

Abbreviations: AADs, antiarrhythmic drugs; AF, atrial fibrillation; CA, catheter ablation; FL, first-line; FU, follow-up; HD, heart disease; HTN, hypertension; LVEF, left ventricular ejection fraction; pts, patients; PV, pulmonary vein; SL, second-line (drug-refractory AF); TIA, transient ischemic attack.
[a] $P<.05$.

of recurrent AF at 1 year was only 2. Furthermore, PVAI was associated with a significantly lower rate of hospitalization (9% vs 54%, $P<.001$), and better quality of life. With regard to complications, the pooled rate of CA-related complications was 12.5% (2 patients with mild/moderate pulmonary vein stenosis, and 2 patients with bleeding complications), which was similar to that observed in

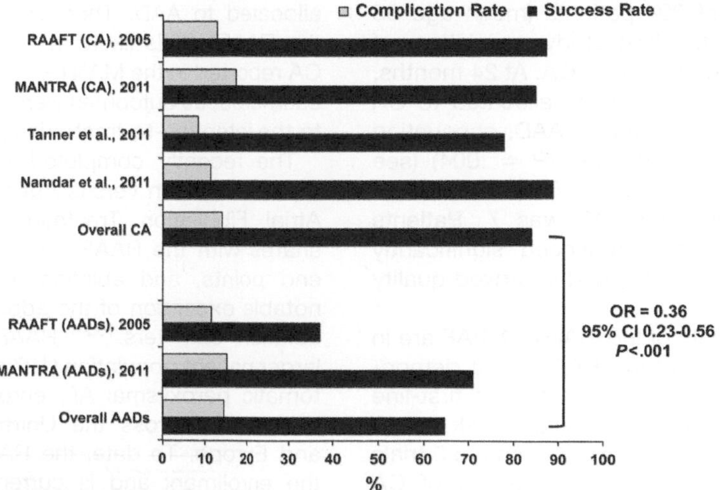

Fig. 1. Plot showing individual and pooled success and complication rates of catheter ablation (CA) and antiarrhythmic drug therapy (AADs) in studies evaluating CA as first-line therapy for atrial fibrillation.

the AAD group (11.5%; 1 patient experiencing a bleeding complication, and 3 with drug-induced bradycardia) (see **Fig. 1**). The RAAFT was the first randomized trial to show the feasibility, safety, and effectiveness of CA as first-line therapy in patients with symptomatic paroxysmal AF. The high rate of crossover to CA in patients initially assigned to AAD (51%)[10] further strengthened the efficacy of CA as first-line therapy.

Following the encouraging results of the RAAFT, 2 larger multicenter randomized trials on CA as first-line therapy for AF have been designed and conducted.[24,25] The Medical ANtiarrhythmic Treatment or Radiofrequency Ablation in Paroxysmal Atrial Fibrillation (MANTRA-PAF) trial compared CA with AAD therapy as first-line therapy for symptomatic paroxysmal AF.[25] A total of 10 Institutions in Europe (Scandinavia and Germany) participated in the trial. At variance with the RAAFT, the ablation techniques adopted in the MANTRA-PAF were heterogeneous, and included pulmonary vein isolation guided by circular mapping catheter or circumferential pulmonary vein ablation guided by a 3-dimensional electroanatomic mapping system (CARTO; Biosense-Webster, Diamond Bar, CA), at the discretion of the enrolling Institution. The MANTRA-PAF was expected to randomize 300 patients followed up for 24 months. The primary study end point was cumulative AF burden (symptomatic and asymptomatic) during 7-day Holter recordings after 3, 6, 12, 18, and 24 months of follow-up. Freedom from any AF after 24 months, quality of life, and burden of symptomatic AF were included among the secondary end points. The results of the MANTRA-PAF were presented at the 2011 American Heart Association annual meeting,[22] although the study has not yet been published.

Overall, a total of 294 patients (mean age 55 years) constituted the final study population, of whom 146 were randomized to CA. At 24 months, AF recurred in 15% of patients allocated to CA and in 29% of those receiving AAD, accounting for 48% relative risk reduction (P = .004) (see **Fig. 1**). The corresponding NNT with CA to prevent one episode of recurrent AF was 7. Patients assigned to CA also experienced significantly lower AF burden (P = .007) and improved quality of life.[22]

Although the results of the MANTRA-PAF are in line with the findings of the RAAFT and demonstrate the superiority of CA over AAD as first-line therapy for AF, a comparison of relative risk reductions and of the NNT with CA between the 2 trials shows nearly 2-fold lower effectiveness of CA in the MANTRA-PAF compared with the RAAFT (see **Fig. 1**). This finding might be explained by the adoption of obsolete ablation techniques in the MANTRA-PAF, with discretional use of circumferential ablation without confirmation of pulmonary vein isolation with a circular mapping catheter. Indeed, lack of verification of pulmonary vein electrical isolation by means of a circular mapping catheter is known to negatively affect the long-term outcomes of CA procedures, as consistently demonstrated in several randomized trials comparing circumferential pulmonary vein ablation with pulmonary vein isolation,[26,27] and as can be also derived from an indirect analysis of treatment effects in randomized trials comparing CA with AAD therapy (**Fig. 2**).[7,10,28–30] With regard to complications, CA was shown to have a similar rate of complications compared with AAD therapy (ie, 17% vs 15%) (see **Table 2**). Of note, a total of 7 deaths were reported in the trial, 3 occurring in the CA arm and 4 in the AAD group, and no details were provided with regard to the causes of death. Among the most relevant complications occurring in the CA group, 2 stroke/transient ischemic attacks, 3 cardiac tamponades, and 1 perforation during the transseptal puncture were reported. Again, although the complication rates were similar to those occurring in the AAD group, it is entirely plausible that the complications reported in the CA arm would have been minimized if state-of-the-art ablation strategies were consistently adopted in the trial, including performing procedures without therapeutic warfarin discontinuation,[31,32] using intracardiac echocardiography to assist the transseptal puncture, catheter manipulation, and radiofrequency power titration.[33] Also in the MANTRA-PAF, the rate of crossover to CA in patients initially assigned to AAD therapy was considerable, and accounted for 36% of patients allocated to AAD. Therefore, as is the case for the RAAFT, it is likely that the actual benefit of CA reported in the MANTRA-PAF has been underestimated, as outcomes were evaluated according to the intention-to-treat principle.

The recently completed First Line Radiofrequency Ablation versus Antiarrhythmic Drugs for Atrial Fibrillation Treatment 2 (RAAFT-2) trial shares with the RAAFT similar inclusion criteria, end points, and ablation techniques, with the notable exception of the adoption of irrigated-tip ablation catheters.[10,24] RAAFT-2 focuses on a larger patient population (127 patients) with symptomatic paroxysmal AF, enrolled in 15 different Institutions across the United States, Canada, and Europe. To date, the RAAFT-2 has finished the enrollment and is currently completing the follow-up. The results of the RAAFT-2 will be presented during 2012.

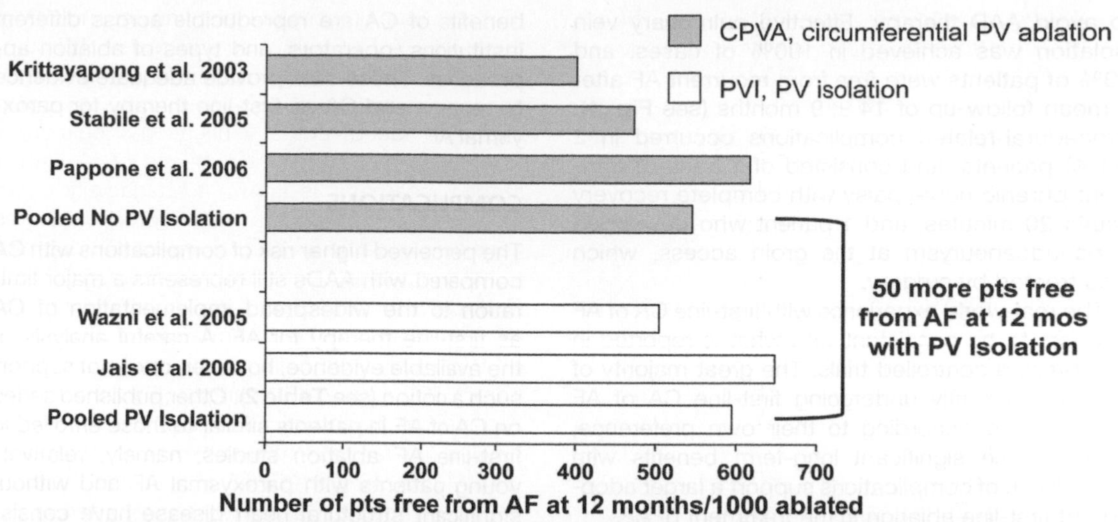

Trial[Ref.#]	Year	N. of pts	% of PAF	LVEF, %	LA diam.	FU	Abl. Tech.	Isolation
Krittayaphong et al.[30]	2003	30	67	63	39	12	CPVA	No
Wazni et al.[10]	2005	70	96	54	42	12	PVI	Yes
Stabile et al.[28]	2005	137	67	59	46	12	CPVA	No
Pappone et al.[29]	2006	198	100	61	39	12	CPVA	No
Jais et al.[7]	2008	112	100	64	40	12	PVI	Yes

Fig. 2. Evidence that confirmation of pulmonary vein isolation (PVI) with a circular mapping catheter improves the outcome. The plot depicts an indirect comparison of treatment effects in trials evaluating catheter ablation versus antiarrhythmic drug therapy in patients who have already failed at least 1 antiarrhythmic drug (second-line ablation). More than 50 patients are free from atrial fibrillation recurrence at 1 year if PVI is confirmed through a circular mapping catheter. Abl. Tech., ablation technique; FU, follow-up; LA diam., left atrial diameter; LVEF, left ventricular ejection fraction; N, number; PAF, paroxysmal atrial fibrillation.

CASE SERIES ON CA AS FIRST-LINE THERAPY FOR AF: FROM RANDOMIZED TRIALS TO THE REAL WORLD

Beyond randomized trials, the value of first-line therapy with CA has been evaluated in 2 consecutive European case series.[21,23] Tanner and colleagues[23] reported their experience on first-line ablation of AF in a consecutive series of patients referred to their institution for CA of symptomatic paroxysmal or persistent AF. Between 2001 and 2009, a total of 72 out of 434 (17%) patients were selected for first-line CA of AF, predominantly attributable to patient preference. Pulmonary vein isolation guided by recordings from a circular mapping catheter was the ablation approach adopted in this study. The baseline characteristics and outcomes of included patients were compared with those of the remaining 362 patients undergoing CA of drug-refractory AF. Patients selected for first-line CA were similar to those undergoing CA of drug-refractory AF with regard to age (57.6 ± 11.4 vs 58.6 ± 9.4, P = .51), baseline comorbidities (hypertension, diabetes, and stroke/transient ischemic attack), presence of structural heart disease, and type of AF (74% with paroxysmal AF in the first-line CA group versus 67% in the CA of drug-refractory AF group, P = .26). On the other hand, patients selected for CA as first-line therapy had higher left ventricular ejection fraction (62% ± 7% vs 59% ± 10%, P = .02). After a follow-up of 12 months the success reached 78% in the first-line CA group (see **Fig. 1**), compared with 64% in patients undergoing CA of drug-refractory AF (P = .03). The overall complication rate in the first-line CA group was 8% (P = .58 for comparison with CA of drug-refractory AF) (see **Table 2**).

In another consecutive case series including 3 institutions, Namdar and colleagues[21] evaluated the benefit of first-line ablation of paroxysmal AF with the cryoballoon technology. A total of 18 patients (mean age 44 years) were selected to undergo the procedure, based on their preference to avoid AAD therapy. Effective pulmonary vein isolation was achieved in 100% of cases, and 89% of patients were free from recurrent AF after a mean follow-up of 14 $\pm$ 9 months (see **Fig. 1**). Procedural-related complications occurred in 2 (11%) patients, and consisted of 1 case of transient phrenic nerve palsy with complete recovery within 20 minutes, and 1 patient who developed a pseudoaneurysm at the groin access, which was treated by surgery.

The real-world experience with first-line CA of AF appears to be consistent with what is reported in randomized controlled trials. The great majority of patients currently undergoing first-line CA of AF are selected according to their own preference, although the significant long-term benefits with a small risk of complications support a larger adoption of first-line ablation in the treatment of AF.

QUANTITATIVE DATA SYNTHESIS: CA AS FIRST-LINE THERAPY FOR AF

Pooling together the available evidence, a total of 451 patients (95% with paroxysmal AF, mean age range 44–58 years) have been included in studies evaluating CA as first-line therapy for AF. Overall, 18 different institutions and multiple operators across the United States, Canada, and Europe have participated in these studies, with a wide range of CA approaches, including pulmonary vein isolation confirmed by a circular mapping catheter, circumferential pulmonary vein ablation, and cryoballoon ablation.

After a mean follow-up of 16 months (range 12–24 months), the pooled success rate of CA was 84%, compared with 65% in the AAD group (odds ratio 0.36, 95% confidence interval 0.23–0.56; $P<.001$). These figures account for 23% relative risk reduction of recurrent AF with CA, and for an NNT with CA to prevent one episode of recurrent AF of 5 (see **Fig. 1**). Furthermore, the pooled complication rate in the CA group was similar to that reported in the AAD group (ie, 13.8% vs 14.2%), and could even become lower than AAD therapy if state-of-the-art ablation techniques were consistently adopted across the included studies. For instance, in the authors' most recent report of CA without therapeutic warfarin discontinuation and with intracardiac echocardiography monitoring, the total periprocedural complication rate was of 4.9%,[32] that is, 3-fold lower than that reported in the AAD group of the studies referenced here.

First-line CA is definitely more effective than AADs in achieving long-term freedom from recurrent arrhythmia in patients with paroxysmal AF, with comparable complication rates. The benefits of CA are reproducible across different institutions, operators, and types of ablation approaches. These data provide adequate evidence to recommend CA as first-line therapy for paroxysmal AF.

COMPLICATIONS

The perceived higher risk of complications with CA compared with AADs still represents a major limitation to the widespread implementation of CA as first-line therapy for AF. A careful analysis of the available evidence, however, does not support such a notion (see **Table 2**). Other published series on CA of AF in patients similar to those enrolled in first-line AF ablation studies, namely, relatively young patients with paroxysmal AF and without significant structural heart disease have consistently reported a low rate of complications.[34,35] Leong-Sit and colleagues[35] assessed the efficacy and risk of CA of AF in 232 young patients (<45 years), presenting predominantly with paroxysmal AF. Of note, only 2 complications were observed in this group of patients, comprising 1 case of arteriovenous fistula and of 1 case of groin hematoma. Similar findings have been reported by Lee and colleagues[34] in a consecutive series of 500 CA procedures performed on patients with low prevalence of structural heart disease. Overall, major complications occurred only in 4 (0.8%) procedures, and consisted of 2 cases of esophageal hematoma caused by the transesophageal echo probe, 1 case of pharyngeal trauma, and 1 case of retroperitoneal hematoma. Putting such results into perspective, the risk of complications with CA of AF is very low, especially in relatively young patients without significant structural heart disease, which further supports the benefit of CA early in the treatment of AF.

COST-EFFECTIVENESS OF CA AS FIRST-LINE THERAPY FOR AF

Khaykin and colleagues[36] evaluated the cost-effectiveness of CA as first-line therapy for AF based on the results from the RAAFT. The cost-comparison analysis was conducted from the perspective of a publicly funded health care payer, using Canadian health care cost estimates. The investigators found that despite the initial higher costs associated with CA, the higher rate of AF recurrences in the AAD therapy arm leading to a higher hospitalization rate counterbalanced the initial costs of CA, with CA being cost neutral after 2 years of follow-up (**Fig. 3**). It bears emphasis that the analysis by Khaykin and colleagues[36] might actually underestimate the cost-effectiveness of

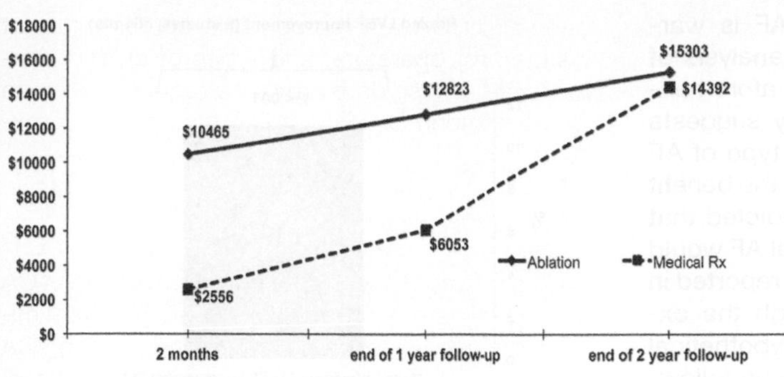

Fig. 3. Cost comparison of first-line catheter ablation versus antiarrhythmic drug therapy based on the outcomes of the RAAFT.[10] Catheter ablation appears to be cost neutral after 2 years of follow-up. (*Data from* Khaykin Y, Wang X, Natale A, et al. Cost comparison of ablation versus antiarrhythmic drugs as first-line therapy for atrial fibrillation: an economic evaluation of the RAAFT pilot study. J Cardiovasc Electrophysiol 2009;20(1):7–12.)

CA as first-line therapy for AF in current cohorts of patients. For instance, all the procedures performed in the RAAFT patients adopted a periprocedural discontinuation of warfarin therapy, with periprocedural bridging with low molecular weight heparin and a preprocedural transesophageal echocardiogram, which account for additional up-front costs of $10,651. On the other hand, AF patients currently undergoing CA typically maintain therapeutic warfarin therapy during the periprocedural period,[31] thus avoiding the additional costs of bridging with low molecular weight heparin and of transesophageal echocardiography if they have consistently been in therapeutic range during the 4 weeks before the procedure.[31]

AREAS OF UNCERTAINTY

CA as a First-Line Therapy for Elderly Patients with AF

Patients enrolled in studies evaluating the role of CA as first-line therapy for paroxysmal AF were relatively young (mean age range 44–58 years).[10,21–23] AF is an age-dependent disease, with a prevalence reaching 10% in people older than 80 years.[37,38] Because of the significant underrepresentation of the elderly population with AF in trials evaluating CA as first-line therapy, it would be inappropriate to generalize the reported efficacy and safety results to elderly patients with AF (**Fig. 4**). On the other hand, evidence already exists suggesting no significant interaction between advancing age and the safety and efficacy of CA procedures.[39–41] Further data on the safety and efficacy of CA procedures in the elderly are certainly warranted, and a properly designed trial of first-line CA versus AADs in this age subgroup is necessary before recommending first-line CA in these patients.

CA as a First-Line Therapy for Nonparoxysmal AF

As already mentioned, 95% of patients enrolled in studies evaluating the role of CA as first-line therapy for AF had paroxysmal AF. The extent to which the results of such studies might be applicable to nonparoxysmal AF patients is unclear and warrants further properly designed trials. However, some evidence already exists supporting the benefit of CA compared with AAD therapy in patients with chronic AF. Oral and colleagues[42] randomly assigned 146 patients with chronic AF to amiodarone and electrical cardioversion or in combination with circumferential pulmonary vein ablation. At 1 year, 74% of patients in the ablation group and 58% of those in the amiodarone group were free of recurrent AF ($P = .05$ for comparison). Of note, 77% of patients initially assigned to amiodarone actually crossed over to CA for recurrent AF during follow-up, which further support the incremental effectiveness of CA compared with AADs in patients with chronic AF.

Based on these findings and on the results of first-line CA in patients with paroxysmal AF, a properly designed trial to evaluate the role of CA as

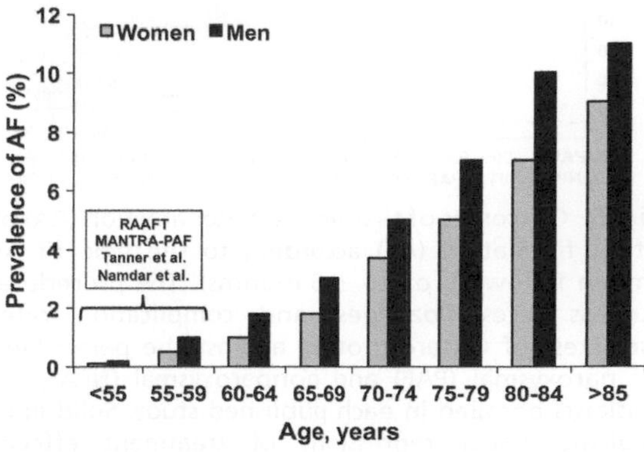

Fig. 4. Despite the higher prevalence of atrial fibrillation in elderly patients, trials evaluating first-line catheter ablation have enrolled only relatively young patients. (*Data from* Go AS, Hylek EM, Phillips KA, et al. Prevalence of diagnosed atrial fibrillation in adults: national implications for rhythm management and stroke prevention: the AnTicoagulation and Risk Factors in Atrial Fibrillation (ATRIA) Study. JAMA 2001;285(18):2370–5.)

first-line therapy for nonparoxysmal AF is warranted. In this regard, an exploratory analysis of the treatment effects reported in the aforementioned studies on first-line CA therapy suggests no significant interaction between the type of AF (ie, paroxysmal vs nonparoxysmal) and the benefit of CA (**Fig. 5**). Therefore, it can be predicted that a trial on first-line CA for nonparoxysmal AF would produce results similar to those already reported in the setting of paroxysmal AF, although the expected success rate of CA in such a hypothetical trial would drop to around 50% at a mean follow-up of 16 ± 6 months (see **Fig. 5**).

CA as a First-Line Therapy for Patients with AF and Left Ventricular Dysfunction

Treatment of AF in patients with left ventricular dysfunction represents a major challenge. Class I sodium-channel–blocking AADs should be avoided in this setting, because of their negative inotropic effects and potential for proarrhythmia and increased mortality.[43,44] Among class III antiarrhythmic agents, dofetilide has the potential to reduce hospitalizations in patients with AF and heart failure,[45] although proarrhythmia caused by drug-induced QT prolongation is a major concern. Amiodarone still remains the best choice among AADs, largely because of its safety in terms of cardiac side effects.[46,47] However, noncardiac

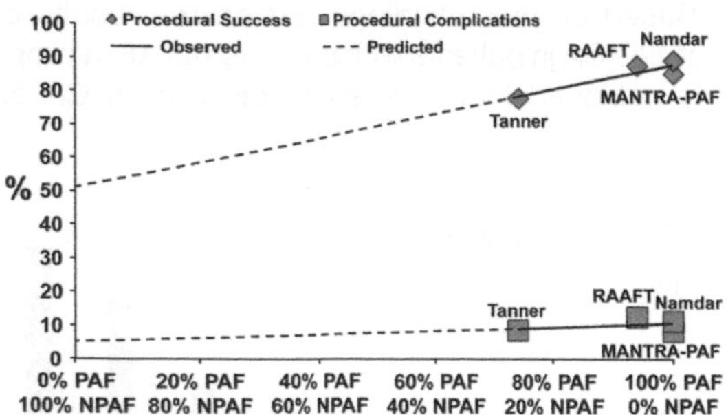

Fig. 5. Outcomes of first-line catheter ablation (CA) of atrial fibrillation (AF) according to the type of AF (mean follow-up of 16 ± 6 months). The procedural success rates (*lozenges*) and complication rates (*squares*) of CA are plotted against the percentage of paroxysmal (PAF) and nonparoxysmal (NPAF) AF patients enrolled in each published study. Solid lines indicate linear regressions of treatment effects. Extrapolation of regression lines (*dotted lines*) to a population of only NPAF patients (0% PAF, 100% NPAF) shows the predicted outcomes of first-line ablation in NPAF. In particular, the predicted success rate at 16 ± 6 months is approximately 50%, with an overall periprocedural complication rate of less than 10%. This analysis supports the benefit of first-line ablation also in NPAF patients.

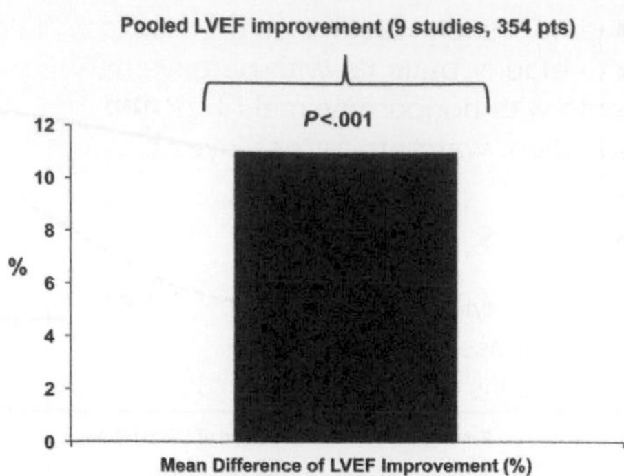

Fig. 6. Pooled random-effect meta-analysis of mean differences of left ventricular ejection fraction (LVEF), comparing baseline LVEF with LVEF after catheter ablation of AF in 9 published studies (follow-up range 6–16 months).[49–57] Analysis shows a significant 11% improvement of LVEF at follow-up ($P<.001$).

toxicity remains an issue with amiodarone, limiting its usefulness in the long term.[48]

To date, a total of 9 studies (2 randomized trials and 7 observational studies) have evaluated the benefit of CA in patients with AF and left ventricular dysfunction,[49–57] including a total of 354 patients with left ventricular dysfunction (range of ejection fraction 35%–43%) and both paroxysmal and persistent AF. Follow-up ranged from 6 months[49,51,53–55] to 16 months.[56] All studies reported a significant improvement of ejection fraction at follow-up, accounting for an overall average improvement of 11% ($P<.001$) compared with baseline values, when performing a pooled random effect meta-analysis of mean differences (**Fig. 6**).

There is highly consistent evidence supporting the benefit of AF ablation in patients with left ventricular dysfunction, which is associated with a significant improvement of left ventricular ejection fraction. No AAD has ever demonstrated such a benefit in clinical studies. First-line CA in patients with left ventricular dysfunction has a strong background rationale, and a prospective randomized comparison with AAD therapy is warranted.

SUMMARY

In relatively young patients with paroxysmal AF, first-line therapy with CA is definitely more effective than AADs for the long-term maintenance of sinus rhythm, with comparable rates of adverse effects. The incremental benefit of CA over AADs is consistently reproducible among different institutions, multiple operators, and different ablation approaches, with a better cost-effectiveness profile.

Whether such results might be generalized also to elderly patients with paroxysmal AF, or to patients with nonparoxysmal AF or left ventricular dysfunction, warrants further investigations.

REFERENCES

1. Go AS, Hylek EM, Phillips KA, et al. Prevalence of diagnosed atrial fibrillation in adults: national implications for rhythm management and stroke prevention: the AnTicoagulation and Risk Factors in Atrial Fibrillation (ATRIA) Study. JAMA 2001; 285(18):2370–5.
2. Friberg J, Buch P, Scharling H, et al. Rising rates of hospital admissions for atrial fibrillation. Epidemiology 2003;14(6):666–72.
3. Bialy D, Lehmann H, Schumacher DN, et al. Hospitalization for arrhythmias in the United States: importance of atrial fibrillation. J Am Coll Cardiol 1992; 19(3):41A. 41.
4. Benjamin EJ, Wolf PA, D'Agostino RB, et al. Impact of atrial fibrillation on the risk of death: the Framingham Heart Study. Circulation 1998;98(10):946–52.
5. Wolf PA, Abbott RD, Kannel WB. Atrial fibrillation as an independent risk factor for stroke: the Framingham Study. Stroke 1991;22(8):983–8.
6. Wilber DJ, Pappone C, Neuzil P, et al. Comparison of antiarrhythmic drug therapy and radiofrequency catheter ablation in patients with paroxysmal atrial fibrillation: a randomized controlled trial. JAMA 2010;303(4):333–40.
7. Jais P, Cauchemez B, Macle L, et al. Catheter ablation versus antiarrhythmic drugs for atrial fibrillation: the A4 study. Circulation 2008;118(24):2498–505.
8. Calkins H, Reynolds MR, Spector P, et al. Treatment of atrial fibrillation with antiarrhythmic drugs or radiofrequency ablation: two systematic literature reviews and meta-analyses. Circ Arrhythm Electrophysiol 2009;2(4):349–61.
9. Verma A, Natale A. Should atrial fibrillation ablation be considered first-line therapy for some patients? Why atrial fibrillation ablation should be considered first-line therapy for some patients. Circulation 2005;112(8):1214–22 [discussion: 1231].
10. Wazni OM, Marrouche NF, Martin DO, et al. Radiofrequency ablation vs antiarrhythmic drugs as first-line treatment of symptomatic atrial fibrillation: a randomized trial. JAMA 2005;293(21):2634–40.
11. Corley SD, Epstein AE, DiMarco JP, et al. Relationships between sinus rhythm, treatment, and survival in the Atrial Fibrillation Follow-Up Investigation of Rhythm Management (AFFIRM) Study. Circulation 2004;109(12):1509–13.
12. Pedersen OD, Brendorp B, Elming H, et al. Does conversion and prevention of atrial fibrillation enhance survival in patients with left ventricular dysfunction? Evidence from the Danish Investigations of Arrhythmia and Mortality ON Dofetilide/(DIAMOND) study. Card Electrophysiol Rev 2003;7(3): 220–4.
13. Deedwania PC, Singh BN, Ellenbogen K, et al. Spontaneous conversion and maintenance of sinus rhythm by amiodarone in patients with heart failure and atrial fibrillation: observations from the veterans affairs congestive heart failure survival trial of antiarrhythmic therapy (CHF-STAT). The Department of Veterans Affairs CHF-STAT Investigators. Circulation 1998;98(23):2574–9.
14. Wyse DG, Waldo AL, DiMarco JP, et al. A comparison of rate control and rhythm control in patients with atrial fibrillation. N Engl J Med 2002;347(23): 1825–33.
15. Hagens VE, Ranchor AV, Van Sonderen E, et al. Effect of rate or rhythm control on quality of life in persistent atrial fibrillation. Results from the Rate Control Versus Electrical Cardioversion (RACE) Study. J Am Coll Cardiol 2004;43(2):241–7.
16. Carlsson J, Miketic S, Windeler J, et al. Randomized trial of rate-control versus rhythm-control in persistent atrial fibrillation: the Strategies of Treatment of Atrial Fibrillation (STAF) study. J Am Coll Cardiol 2003;41(10):1690–6.
17. Roy D, Talajic M, Dorian P, et al. Amiodarone to prevent recurrence of atrial fibrillation. Canadian Trial of Atrial Fibrillation Investigators. N Engl J Med 2000;342(13):913–20.
18. Preliminary report: effect of encainide and flecainide on mortality in a randomized trial of arrhythmia suppression after myocardial infarction. The Cardiac Arrhythmia Suppression Trial (CAST) Investigators. N Engl J Med 1989;321(6):406–12.
19. Waldo AL, Camm AJ, deRuyter H, et al. Effect of d-sotalol on mortality in patients with left ventricular dysfunction after recent and remote myocardial infarction. The SWORD Investigators. Survival With Oral d-Sotalol. Lancet 1996;348(9019):7–12.
20. Padanilam BJ, Prystowsky EN. Should atrial fibrillation ablation be considered first-line therapy for some patients? Should ablation be first-line therapy and for whom? The antagonist position. Circulation 2005;112(8):1223–9 [discussion: 1230].
21. Namdar M, Chierchia GB, Westra S, et al. Isolating the pulmonary veins as first-line therapy in patients with lone paroxysmal atrial fibrillation using the Cryoballoon. Europace 2012;14(2):197–203.
22. Nielsen J, Johannessen A, Raatikainen P, et al. A randomized multicenter comparison of radiofrequency ablation and antiarrhythmic drug therapy as first-line treatment in 294 patients with paroxysmal atrial fibrillation. Presented at the AHA 2011 Scientific Session (LBCT.03). Available at: http://my.americanheart.org/idc/groups/ahamah-public/@wcm/@sop/@scon/documents/downloadable/ucm_433720.pdf. Accessed January 2012.

23. Tanner H, Makowski K, Roten L, et al. Catheter ablation of atrial fibrillation as first-line therapy—a single-centre experience. Europace 2011;13(5):646–53.
24. First Line Radiofrequency Ablation Versus Antiarrhythmic Drugs for Atrial Fibrillation Treatment (The RAAFT-2 Study). NCT00392054. Available at: http://clinicaltrials.gov/ct2/show/NCT00392054.
25. Jons C, Hansen PS, Johannessen A, et al. The Medical ANtiarrhythmic Treatment or Radiofrequency Ablation in Paroxysmal Atrial Fibrillation (MANTRA-PAF) trial: clinical rationale, study design, and implementation. Europace 2009;11(7):917–23.
26. Khaykin Y, Skanes A, Champagne J, et al. A randomized controlled trial of the efficacy and safety of electroanatomic circumferential pulmonary vein ablation supplemented by ablation of complex fractionated atrial electrograms versus potential-guided pulmonary vein antrum isolation guided by intracardiac ultrasound. Circ Arrhythm Electrophysiol 2009;2(5):481–7.
27. Tamborero D, Mont L, Berruezo A, et al. Circumferential pulmonary vein ablation: does use of a circular mapping catheter improve results? A prospective randomized study. Heart Rhythm 2010;7(5):612–8.
28. Stabile G, Bertaglia E, Senatore G, et al. Catheter ablation treatment in patients with drug-refractory atrial fibrillation: a prospective, multi-centre, randomized, controlled study (Catheter Ablation For The Cure Of Atrial Fibrillation Study). Eur Heart J 2006;27(2):216–21.
29. Pappone C, Augello G, Sala S, et al. A randomized trial of circumferential pulmonary vein ablation versus antiarrhythmic drug therapy in paroxysmal atrial fibrillation: the APAF Study. J Am Coll Cardiol 2006;48(11):2340–7.
30. Krittayaphong R, Raungrattanaamporn O, Bhuripanyo K, et al. A randomized clinical trial of the efficacy of radiofrequency catheter ablation and amiodarone in the treatment of symptomatic atrial fibrillation. J Med Assoc Thai 2003;86(Suppl 1):S8–16.
31. Santangeli P, Di Biase L, Sanchez JE, et al. Atrial fibrillation ablation without interruption of anticoagulation. Cardiol Res Pract 2011;2011:837841.
32. Di Biase L, Burkhardt JD, Mohanty P, et al. Periprocedural stroke and management of major bleeding complications in patients undergoing catheter ablation of atrial fibrillation: the impact of periprocedural therapeutic international normalized ratio. Circulation 2010;121(23):2550–6.
33. Santangeli P, Di Biase L, Pelargonio G, et al. Catheter ablation of atrial fibrillation: randomized controlled trials and registries, a look back and the view forward. J Interv Card Electrophysiol 2011;31(1):69–80.
34. Lee G, Sparks PB, Morton JB, et al. Low risk of major complications associated with pulmonary vein antral isolation for atrial fibrillation: results of 500 consecutive ablation procedures in patients with low prevalence of structural heart disease from a single center. J Cardiovasc Electrophysiol 2011;22(2):163–8.
35. Leong-Sit P, Zado E, Callans DJ, et al. Efficacy and risk of atrial fibrillation ablation before 45 years of age. Circ Arrhythm Electrophysiol 2010;3(5):452–7.
36. Khaykin Y, Wang X, Natale A, et al. Cost comparison of ablation versus antiarrhythmic drugs as first-line therapy for atrial fibrillation: an economic evaluation of the RAAFT pilot study. J Cardiovasc Electrophysiol 2009;20(1):7–12.
37. Heeringa J, van der Kuip DA, Hofman A, et al. Prevalence, incidence and lifetime risk of atrial fibrillation: the Rotterdam study. Eur Heart J 2006;27(8):949–53.
38. Kopecky SL, Gersh BJ, McGoon MD, et al. The natural history of lone atrial fibrillation. A population-based study over three decades. N Engl J Med 1987;317(11):669–74.
39. Zado E, Callans DJ, Riley M, et al. Long-term clinical efficacy and risk of catheter ablation for atrial fibrillation in the elderly. J Cardiovasc Electrophysiol 2008;19(6):621–6.
40. Corrado A, Patel D, Riedlbauchova L, et al. Efficacy, safety, and outcome of atrial fibrillation ablation in septuagenarians. J Cardiovasc Electrophysiol 2008;19(8):807–11.
41. Santangeli P, Biase LD, Mohanty P, et al. Catheter ablation of atrial fibrillation in octogenarians: safety and outcomes. J Cardiovasc Electrophysiol 2012. [Epub ahead of print].
42. Oral H, Pappone C, Chugh A, et al. Circumferential pulmonary-vein ablation for chronic atrial fibrillation. N Engl J Med 2006;354(9):934–41.
43. Flaker GC, Blackshear JL, McBride R, et al. Antiarrhythmic drug therapy and cardiac mortality in atrial fibrillation. The Stroke Prevention in Atrial Fibrillation Investigators. J Am Coll Cardiol 1992;20(3):527–32.
44. Stevenson WG, Stevenson LW, Middlekauff HR, et al. Improving survival for patients with atrial fibrillation and advanced heart failure. J Am Coll Cardiol 1996;28(6):1458–63.
45. Torp-Pedersen C, Moller M, Bloch-Thomsen PE, et al. Dofetilide in patients with congestive heart failure and left ventricular dysfunction. Danish Investigations of Arrhythmia and Mortality on Dofetilide Study Group. N Engl J Med 1999;341(12):857–65.
46. Singh SN, Fletcher RD, Fisher SG, et al. Amiodarone in patients with congestive heart failure and asymptomatic ventricular arrhythmia. Survival Trial of Antiarrhythmic Therapy in Congestive Heart Failure. N Engl J Med 1995;333(2):77–82.
47. Nul DR, Doval HC, Grancelli HO, et al. Heart rate is a marker of amiodarone mortality reduction in severe heart failure. The GESICA-GEMA Investigators. Grupo de Estudio de la Sobrevida en la Insuficiencia Cardiaca

en Argentina-Grupo de Estudios Multicentricos en Argentina. J Am Coll Cardiol 1997;29(6):1199–205.
48. Effect of prophylactic amiodarone on mortality after acute myocardial infarction and in congestive heart failure: meta-analysis of individual data from 6500 patients in randomised trials. Amiodarone Trials Meta-Analysis Investigators. Lancet 1997;350(9089): 1417–24.
49. Chen MS, Marrouche NF, Khaykin Y, et al. Pulmonary vein isolation for the treatment of atrial fibrillation in patients with impaired systolic function. J Am Coll Cardiol 2004;43(6):1004–9.
50. Hsu LF, Jais P, Sanders P, et al. Catheter ablation for atrial fibrillation in congestive heart failure. N Engl J Med 2004;351(23):2373–83.
51. Gentlesk PJ, Sauer WH, Gerstenfeld EP, et al. Reversal of left ventricular dysfunction following ablation of atrial fibrillation. J Cardiovasc Electrophysiol 2007;18(1):9–14.
52. Efremidis M, Sideris A, Xydonas S, et al. Ablation of atrial fibrillation in patients with heart failure: reversal of atrial and ventricular remodelling. Hellenic J Cardiol 2008;49(1):19–25.
53. Lutomsky BA, Rostock T, Koops A, et al. Catheter ablation of paroxysmal atrial fibrillation improves cardiac function: a prospective study on the impact of atrial fibrillation ablation on left ventricular function assessed by magnetic resonance imaging. Europace 2008;10(5):593–9.
54. Khan MN, Jais P, Cummings J, et al. Pulmonary-vein isolation for atrial fibrillation in patients with heart failure. N Engl J Med 2008;359(17):1778–85.
55. De Potter T, Berruezo A, Mont L, et al. Left ventricular systolic dysfunction by itself does not influence outcome of atrial fibrillation ablation. Europace 2010; 12(1):24–9.
56. Choi AD, Hematpour K, Kukin M, et al. Ablation vs medical therapy in the setting of symptomatic atrial fibrillation and left ventricular dysfunction. Congest Heart Fail 2010;16(1):10–4.
57. MacDonald MR, Connelly DT, Hawkins NM, et al. Radiofrequency ablation for persistent atrial fibrillation in patients with advanced heart failure and severe left ventricular systolic dysfunction: a randomised controlled trial. Heart 2011;97(9): 740–7.

Ablation as First-Line Therapy for Atrial Fibrillation

Not Yet for All

Benzy J. Padanilam, MD*, Eric N. Prystowsky, MD

KEYWORDS

• Atrial fibrillation • Ablation • First-line therapy • Antiarrhythmic medications

KEY POINTS

- Studies have established that atrial fibrillation (AF) ablation is superior to medical therapy in controlling the rhythm; however, its use is not justified in all patients before antiarrhythmic medications are tried because of the associated procedural risks.
- The risks of AF ablation may be worth taking if future studies establish improved survival and stroke risk in patients undergoing AF ablation.
- Until improved survival and stroke risk are established, AF ablation should continue to be used as a second-line option for most patient subgroups when one or more antiarrhythmic medications are ineffective.

Three major goals of atrial fibrillation (AF) management are

- Symptom control
- Prevention of cardiomyopathy
- Prevention of stroke[1,2]

AF may be managed using 2 general strategies: rate control or rhythm control. No definitive evidence showing reduction in mortality, stroke, or tachycardia-mediated cardiomyopathy when rhythm control is compared with rate control strategy has been presented.[3] The major reason to pursue sinus rhythm in patients with AF, thus, is to improve their symptoms and quality of life. Ablation therapy is being increasingly used for the treatment of symptomatic AF[4] and it is a generally accepted option for AF refractory to antiarrhythmic medications.[1] The question being debated, however, is whether the current state of AF ablation has reached the stature to be used as a first-line therapy ahead of antiarrhythmic medications.

DETERMINANTS OF FIRST-LINE THERAPY

The criteria for a new invasive therapy to achieve first-line status should be stringent and prove superiority above existing medical therapy. There are 3 metrics that should be evaluated before any new treatment can be considered a first-line option[5]:

1. Superior outcomes of the proposed treatment
2. Acceptable short-term and long-term risks
3. Cost-effectiveness

The evidence supporting the efficacy and safety of AF ablation derives mostly from single-center reports, registries, meta-analyses, and a few small prospective randomized multicenter trials. The following discussion reviews the data on catheter ablation of AF as it pertains to the 3 metrics determining first-line therapy. As the authors show for most subgroups of patients, the evidence does not support catheter ablation as a first-line therapy for AF.

St Vincent Medical Group, 8333 Naab Road, #400, Indianapolis, IN 46260, USA
* Corresponding author.
E-mail address: bjpadani@stvincent.org

Card Electrophysiol Clin 4 (2012) 299–304
http://dx.doi.org/10.1016/j.ccep.2012.06.003
1877-9182/12/$ – see front matter © 2012 Published by Elsevier Inc.

OUTCOMES: CATHETER ABLATION VERSUS MEDICAL THERAPY

Multiple randomized trials have demonstrated a modest but highly significant efficacy for antiarrhythmic medications in AF rhythm control without affecting survival or risk of stroke.[6] The limited long-term efficacy and high incidence of side effects of antiarrhythmic medications has prompted physicians to consider nonpharmacologic therapies for AF.

Ever since the initial description of pulmonary vein ablation by Haissaguerre and colleagues[7] in 1998, several single-center, nonrandomized ablation experiences with varied outcomes have been published. Prospective randomized controlled trials comparing medical therapy with ablation therapy have been few and the number of patients enrolled has been very small (**Table 1**).[8–11] These trials collectively have shown the superior efficacy of ablation in eliminating AF in patients with structurally normal hearts who have failed at least one antiarrhythmic medication. One of these trials,[8] which included a total of 70 patients, did look at ablation as a first-line therapy and showed less AF recurrence, less hospitalizations, and better quality of life in the ablation group.

Unfortunately, these trials were underpowered to determine the important outcomes of survival and stroke. Because AF is associated with a decreased survival and increased risk of stroke,[12] it is indeed possible that a nonpharmacologic therapy eliminating AF could result in improved long-term outcomes.[13] Although nonrandomized studies suggest a survival benefit in patients undergoing catheter ablation,[14] a meta-analysis of randomized controlled trials showed similar survival and stroke risks in the ablation and drug groups.[15] Several larger studies,[16–21] including the Catheter Ablation Versus Anti-arrhythmic Drug Therapy for Atrial Fibrillation (CABANA) trial,[16] are underway to answer these questions (**Table 2**). The ongoing Safety of AF Ablation Registry Initiative (SAFARI) could also provide a real-world picture of the state of the procedure. Would it not be prudent to wait for the results of these ongoing trials before considering a first-line overall status for a procedure associated with at least a 0.15% risk of death and a 0.94% risk of transient ischemic attack/stroke[4]?

In summary, although catheter ablation may very well be a more effective therapy to control AF, the invasive nature of the treatment, along with the procedural risks, makes it a less attractive option to the simpler antiarrhythmic medication therapy in most patient subgroups.

LONG-TERM EFFICACY

An area of concern is the lack of long-term efficacy of pulmonary vein ablation techniques. Several reports have claimed more than 80% cure rates with circumferential pulmonary vein ablation techniques during short mean follow-up periods ranging from 6 to 14 months. The long-term prospective follow-up, however, indicates low arrhythmia-free survival rates after a single catheter ablation procedure of 40%, 37%, and 29% at 1, 2, and 5 years, respectively.[22] Better long-term outcomes are reported when more than one procedure is undertaken.[22,23]

Another troubling problem is the significant variance of success among laboratories using similar ablation techniques.[24,25] The procedures are technically challenging and highly operator dependent, which may explain the differences in the outcomes. In addition to the pulmonary vein ablation techniques, some investigators propose ablation of the superior vena cava, coronary sinus, cavotricuspid isthmus, complex fractionated electrograms, and linear lesions in the left atrium. Whether these adjunctive ablations improve outcomes and which patients should be targeted for them needs more investigation. Making efficacy of AF ablation even harder to define is the well-known occurrence of asymptomatic AF.[26] Studies reporting only symptomatic AF episodes after ablation could overestimate success, especially during short-term follow-up. In a study of 60 patients who became asymptomatic following pulmonary vein ablation,

Table 1
Randomized controlled trials of antiarrhythmic drug versus ablation therapy for paroxysmal AF

Study Author (Reference)	Year	Design	Number of Patients	Primary End Points (%)
Wazni et al,[8]	2005	Drugs vs ablation as first line	70	AF recurrence (87 vs 37), quality of life, hospitalizations
Jais et al,[9]	2008	Drugs vs ablation as second line	112	AF recurrence (89 vs 23)
Wilber et al,[10]	2010	Drugs vs ablation as second line	167	AF recurrence (66 vs 16)
Packer et al,[11]	2010	Drugs vs ablation as second line	245	AF recurrence (69.9 vs 7.3)

Table 2
Ongoing randomized trials of AF ablation versus medical therapy

Study, Year (Reference)	Patient Characteristics	Number of Patients	Primary End Points
CABANA,[16] 2009	AF with risk factors	3000	Total mortality
AATAC-HF,[17] 2008	Persistent/permanent AF, dual-chamber ICD/CRTD, EF $\leq$40%	120	Time to AF recurrence >15s
CASTLE-AF,[18] 2008	AF, EF $\leq$35%, CHF-class $\geq$II, dual-chamber ICD	420	Total mortality, hospitalizations for CHF
SARA,[19] 2009	Persistent AF, EF $\geq$30%, left atrium <5.0 cm	208	AF $\geq$24-h duration
MANTRA-PAF,[20] 2005	Paroxysmal AF, EF $\geq$40%, severe left atrial enlargement	300	AF recurrence
RAAFT-2,[21] 2006	Paroxysmal AF, EF $\geq$40%, left atrium $\leq$5.5 cm	400	AF recurrence, safety of ablation and AADs

Abbreviations: AAD, Antiarrhythmic Drugs; AATAC-HF, Ablation vs Amiodarone for Treatment of AFib in Patients with CHF and an ICD; CASTLE-AF, Catheter Ablation Versus Standard Conventional Treatment in Patients With Left Ventricular Dysfunction and Atrial Fibrillation; CHF, Congestive Heart Failure; CRTD, Cardiac Resynchronization Therapy Defibrillator; EF, ejection fraction; ICD, Implantable Cardioverter Defibrillator; MANTRA-PAF, Radiofrequency Ablation Versus Antiarrhythmic Drug Treatment in Paroxysmal Atrial Fibrillation; RAAFT-2, First Line Radiofrequency Ablation Versus Antiarrhythmic Drugs for Atrial Fibrillation Treatment; SARA, Study of Ablation Versus antiaRrhythmic Drugs in Persistent Atrial Fibrillation.

12% reported symptoms and documented AF when given an event recorder almost 2 years following the ablation.[27] It is possible that radiofrequency ablation may change symptomatic AF to asymptomatic AF in some patients.[28,29] This possibility is important not only to quantify the true success of the procedure but also for decisions regarding anticoagulation in patients at a high risk for stroke. In the Atrial Fibrillation Follow-up Investigation of Rhythm Management (AFFIRM) trial, the risk of thromboembolism persisted in patients who were clinically maintaining sinus rhythm with antiarrhythmic medications, perhaps because of the clinically undetected episodes of AF in these patients.[3] Patients cured of symptomatic AF after a radiofrequency ablation procedure could be in an analogous situation.

COMPLICATIONS OF ABLATION

Few therapies, pharmacologic or otherwise, can be administered without safety concerns. The use of antiarrhythmic medications other than amiodarone is rarely associated with organ toxicity or life-threatening proarrhythmia in patients with structurally normal hearts with normal electrocardiograms. Unfortunately, complications of ablation can occur in any patient, including those with normal hearts; previously unknown complications may emerge with changes in techniques, wider ablation experience, or longer follow-up. A worldwide survey of AF ablations from 2003 to 2006 indicates a wider use of the procedure and a lack of improvement in procedure-related complications with experience.[4] Major complications were reported in 4.5% of patients (**Table 3**). The lack of improved safety, even in centers that had gained more experience, could be related to the procedure being offered to an older and sicker population.

Death

The previously mentioned worldwide survey of 85 institutions performing 20,825 AF ablations reported 25 procedure-related deaths (0.15%). Cardiac tamponade and atrio-esophageal fistula were the two most common complications that resulted in death.

Cardiac Perforation and Tamponade

The transseptal puncture procedure and the extensive ablations performed in the left atrium in a fully anticoagulated state may set patients up for cardiac perforation and tamponade. Patients have also been reported to present with delayed (days or weeks after ablation) tamponade. It is hoped that the use of intracardiac echocardiography for transseptal punctures and new catheter technologies with contact force sensors and endoscopic tissue visualization will reduce the incidence of cardiac perforation.

Table 3
Major complications associated with 20,825 AF ablation procedures

Type of Complication	Number of Patients	Rate (%)
Death	25	0.15
Tamponade	213	1.31
Pneumothorax	15	0.09
Hemothorax	4	0.02
Sepsis, abscess, endocarditis	2	0.01
Permanent diaphragmatic paralysis	28	0.17
Femoral pseudoaneurysm	152	0.93
A-V fistulae	88	0.54
Valve damage/requiring surgery	11/7	0.07
Atrio-esophageal fistulae	6	0.04
Stroke	37	0.23
Transient ischemic attack	115	0.71
PV stenosis requiring intervention	48	0.29
Total	741	4.54

Abbreviations: A-V, arterio-venous; PV, pulmonary vein.
Data from Cappato R, Calkins H, Chen SA, et al. Updated worldwide survey on the methods, efficacy, and safety of catheter ablation for human atrial fibrillation. Circ Arrhythm Electrophysiol 2010;3(1):32–8.

Pulmonary Vein Stenosis

Pulmonary vein stenosis of variable degree was commonly seen after focal ablation inside the pulmonary veins. The incidence of this complication has been dramatically reduced by changes in technique, including the reduction in power delivery and limiting ablations to the pulmonary vein ostia.[30] The true incidence is likely underreported unless postprocedure imaging techniques are used because pulmonary vein stenosis can be asymptomatic.[31] The long-term effects of even mild to moderate pulmonary vein stenosis are unclear.

Thromboembolism

Embolic stroke is a well-recognized complication of pulmonary vein ablation. The incidence has varied from 0% to 5%.[7,32] The use of open irrigated tip ablation catheters and uninterrupted warfarin anticoagulation during ablation may reduce the incidence of stroke without a significant increase in hemorrhagic complications.[33,34] It should be noted that clinically silent cerebral embolism may occur in a large percent of patients undergoing AF ablation. Gaita and colleagues[35] reported that magnetic resonance imaging detected cerebral lesions in 14.0% of patients, with only 0.4% having a clinically manifest event following AF ablation. The silent cerebral lesions may vary among the ablation technologies used, with multielectrode ablation catheters showing an increased incidence compared with irrigated radio frequency (RF) and cryoballoon ablation.[36]

Atrio-Esophageal Fistula

Radiofrequency applications to the posterior left atrium can lead to esophageal injury caused by their close anatomic relationship. Left atrium to esophagus fistula has occurred after intraoperative radiofrequency ablation of AF[37] and after catheter ablation.[38,39] This rare (0.04%) complication[4] carries a high fatality rate. Patients usually present with sudden neurologic symptoms or endocarditis after an initial unremarkable postoperative course. Survival, which requires prompt surgical intervention, may be associated with significant morbidity caused by complications, such as stroke. Risk factors for this potentially fatal complication have not been established.[37] Different strategies have been adopted to reduce its occurrence. Avoiding the use of high powers of RF energy on the posterior left atrium, localization of the esophagus during the procedure using various methods (barium swallow, intracardiac echo (ICE), 3-dimensional map), and monitoring of temperatures with an esophageal probe[40] are some of the proposed methods. However, the true incidence and strategies to prevent this complication during catheter ablation require further study.

Left Atrial Flutter

Reentrant rhythms may originate following circumferential pulmonary vein ablations and linear left atrial ablations in 2.5% to 20.0% of patients.[25,41] Macroreentry involving the left atrial roof or mitral isthmus and localized reentry can be mapped and ablated successfully in most patients,[42] although repeat procedures may be necessary.

SUMMARY

In order for an invasive treatment to be considered a first-line therapy over an established medical option, the burden of proof should be high. The procedural outcomes must show superiority, acceptable risks, and cost-effectiveness. In the case of AF ablation, studies have established its superiority in controlling the rhythm compared with medical therapy. However, that in itself would not justify its use in all patients before trying antiarrhythmic medications because of the associated procedural risks.

These risks may be worth taking if future studies establish improved survival and stroke risk in patients undergoing AF ablation. Until then, it should continue to be used as a second-line option for most patient subgroups when one or more antiarrhythmic medications are ineffective.

Are there circumstances when catheter ablation might be considered as an initial therapy? The authors think so. Patients with highly symptomatic paroxysmal AF with minimal to no structural heart disease, who are intolerant or unwilling to try antiarrhythmic medications, may be considered for primary ablation. Patients with AF and sinus node dysfunction who require a permanent pacemaker before trying antiarrhythmic medications may be considered for primary ablation. Significant improvement in sinus node function was reported, eliminating the need for pacing after ablation of AF in such patients.[43] The long-term morbidity associated with a pacemaker in addition to the risks related to antiarrhythmic drug therapy might tilt the balance in favor of ablation as a first-line treatment in these selected patients. Another situation may be patients with cardiomyopathies in whom the only appropriate antiarrhythmic agent is amiodarone. Although clinical judgment is important in deciding the best course of therapy in these individual circumstances, catheter ablation should not be the first-line therapy for most patients with AF.

REFERENCES

1. Calkins H, Brugada J, Packer DL, et al. HRS/EHRA/ECAS expert consensus statement on catheter and surgical ablation of atrial fibrillation: recommendations for personnel, policy, procedures and follow-up. A report of the Heart Rhythm Society (HRS) Task Force on Catheter and Surgical Ablation of Atrial Fibrillation developed in partnership with the European Heart Rhythm Association (EHRA) and the European Cardiac Arrhythmia Society (ECAS); in collaboration with the American College of Cardiology (ACC), American Heart Association (AHA), and the Society of Thoracic Surgeons (STS). Europace 2007;9(6):335–79.
2. Padanilam BJ, Prystowsky EN. Atrial fibrillation: goals of therapy and management strategies to achieve the goals. Cardiol Clin 2009;27(1):189–200.
3. Wyse DG, Waldo AL, DiMarco JP, et al, Atrial Fibrillation Follow-up Investigation of Rhythm Management (AFFIRM) Investigators. A comparison of rate control and rhythm control in patients with atrial fibrillation. N Engl J Med 2002;347(23):1825–33.
4. Cappato R, Calkins H, Chen SA, et al. Updated worldwide survey on the methods, efficacy, and safety of catheter ablation for human atrial fibrillation. Circ Arrhythm Electrophysiol 2010;3(1):32–8.
5. Padanilam BJ, Prystowsky EN. Should atrial fibrillation ablation be considered first-line therapy for some patients? Should ablation be first-line therapy and for whom? The antagonist position. Circulation 2005;112(8):1223–9.
6. Nichol G, McAlister F, Pham B, et al. Meta-analysis of randomised controlled trials of the effectiveness of antiarrhythmic agents at promoting sinus rhythm in patients with atrial fibrillation. Heart 2002;87(6):535–43.
7. Haissaguerre M, Jais P, Shah DC, et al. Spontaneous initiation of atrial fibrillation by ectopic beats originating in the pulmonary veins. N Engl J Med 1998;339(10):659–66.
8. Wazni OM, Marrouche NF, Martin DO, et al. Radiofrequency ablation vs antiarrhythmic drugs as first-line treatment of symptomatic atrial fibrillation: a randomized trial. JAMA 2005;293:2634–40.
9. Jais P, Cauchemez B, Macle L, et al. Catheter ablation versus antiarrhythmic drugs for atrial fibrillation: the A4 study. Circulation 2008;118:2498–505.
10. Wilber DJ, Pappone C, Neuzil P, et al. Comparison of antiarrhythmic drug therapy and radiofrequency catheter ablation in patients with paroxysmal atrial fibrillation: a randomized controlled trial. JAMA 2010;303:333–40.
11. Packer DL, Irwin JM, Champagne J, et al. Cryoballoon ablation of pulmonary veins for paroxysmal atrial fibrillation: first results of the North American Arctic Front Stop-AF clinical trial. American College of Cardiology Annual Scientific Session. Atlanta, March 15, 2010.
12. Benjamin EJ, Wolf PA, D'Agostino RB, et al. Impact of atrial fibrillation on the risk of death: the Framingham Heart Study. Circulation 1998;98(10):946–52.
13. Corley SD, Epstein AE, DiMarco JP, et al, AFFIRM Investigators. Relationships between sinus rhythm, treatment, and survival in the Atrial Fibrillation Follow-Up Investigation of Rhythm Management (AFFIRM) study. Circulation 2004;109(12):1509–13.
14. Pappone C, Rosanio S, Augello G, et al. Mortality, morbidity, and quality of life after circumferential pulmonary vein ablation for atrial fibrillation: outcomes from a controlled nonrandomized long-term study. J Am Coll Cardiol 2003;42(2):185–97.
15. Dagres N, Varounis C, Flevari P, et al. Mortality after catheter ablation for atrial fibrillation compared with antiarrhythmic drug therapy. A meta-analysis of randomized trials. Am Heart J 2009;158(1):15–20.
16. U.S. National Institutes of Health. Catheter Ablation Versus Anti-arrhythmic Drug Therapy for Atrial Fibrillation trial (CABANA). 2009. Available at: http://www.clinicaltrials.gov/. Accessed January 2012.
17. U.S. National Institutes of Health. Ablation vs Amiodarone for Treatment of AFib in Patients with CHF and an ICD (AATAC-HF). 2008. Available at: http://www.clinicaltrials.gov/.

18. U.S. National Institutes of Health. Catheter Ablation Versus Standard Conventional Treatment in Patients With Left Ventricular Dysfunction and Atrial Fibrillation (CASTLE-AF). 2008. Available at: http://www.clinicaltrials.gov/.
19. Study of Ablation Versus antiaRrhythmic Drugs in Persistent Atrial Fibrillation (SARA). 2009. Available at: http://clinicaltrials.gov/.
20. U.S. National Institutes of Health. Radiofrequency Ablation (RFA) versus Antiarrhythmic Drug Treatment in Paroxysmal Atrial Fibrillation (MANTRA-PAF). 2005. Available at: http://clinicaltrials.gov/.
21. U.S. National Institutes of Health. First Line Radiofrequency Ablation Versus Antiarrhythmic Drugs for Atrial Fibrillation Treatment (The RAAFT Study). 2006. Available at: http://www.clinicaltrials.gov/.
22. Weerasooriya R, Khairy P, Litalien J, et al. Catheter ablation for atrial fibrillation: are results maintained at 5 years of follow-up? J Am Coll Cardiol 2011; 57(2):160–6.
23. Hussein AA, Saliba WI, Martin DO, et al. Natural history and long-term outcomes of ablated atrial fibrillation. Circ Arrhythm Electrophysiol 2011;4(3): 271–8.
24. Deisenhofer I, Schneider MA, Bohlen-Knauf M, et al. Circumferential mapping and electric isolation of pulmonary veins in patients with atrial fibrillation. Am J Cardiol 2003;91(2):159–63.
25. Kanagaratnam L, Tomassoni G, Schweikert R, et al. Empirical pulmonary vein isolation in patients with chronic atrial fibrillation using a three-dimensional nonfluoroscopic mapping system: long-term follow-up. Pacing Clin Electrophysiol 2001;24(12):1774–9.
26. Israel CW, Gronefeld G, Ehrlich JR, et al. Long-term risk of recurrent atrial fibrillation as documented by an implantable monitoring device: implications for optimal patient care. J Am Coll Cardiol 2004;43(1): 47–52.
27. Oral H, Veerareddy S, Good E, et al. Prevalence of asymptomatic recurrences of atrial fibrillation after successful radiofrequency catheter ablation. J Cardiovasc Electrophysiol 2004;15:920–4.
28. Wokhlu A, Monahan KH, Hodge DO, et al. Long-term quality of life after ablation of atrial fibrillation: the impact of recurrence, symptom relief, and placebo effect. J Am Coll Cardiol 2010;55:2308–16.
29. Prystowsky EN, Padanilam BJ. All's well that ends well, or is it? J Am Coll Cardiol 2010;55:2317–8.
30. Haissaguerre M, Shah DC, Jais P, et al. Electrophysiological breakthroughs from the left atrium to the pulmonary veins. Circulation 2000;102(20):2463–5.
31. Saad EB, Rossillo A, Saad CP, et al. Pulmonary vein stenosis after radiofrequency ablation of atrial fibrillation: functional characterization, evolution, and influence of the ablation strategy. Circulation 2003, 108(25):3102–7.
32. Mangrum JM, Mounsey JP, Kok LC, et al. Intracardiac echocardiography-guided, anatomically based radiofrequency ablation of focal atrial fibrillation originating from pulmonary veins. J Am Coll Cardiol 2002;39(12):1964–72.
33. Wazni OM, Beheiry S, Fahmy T, et al. Atrial fibrillation ablation in patients with therapeutic international normalized ratio: comparison of strategies of anticoagulation management in the periprocedural period. Circulation 2007;116(22):2531–4.
34. Di Biase L, Burkhardt JD, Mohanty P, et al. Periprocedural stroke and management of major bleeding complications in patients undergoing catheter ablation of atrial fibrillation: the impact of periprocedural therapeutic international normalized ratio. Circulation 2010;121(23):2550–6.
35. Gaita F, Caponi D, Pianelli M, et al. Radiofrequency catheter ablation of atrial fibrillation: a cause of silent thromboembolism? Magnetic resonance imaging assessment of cerebral thromboembolism in patients undergoing ablation of atrial fibrillation. Circulation 2010;122(17):1667–73.
36. Gaita F, Leclercq JF, Schumacher B, et al. Incidence of silent cerebral thromboembolic lesions after atrial fibrillation ablation may change according to technology used: comparison of irrigated radiofrequency, multipolar nonirrigated catheter and cryoballoon. J Cardiovasc Electrophysiol 2011; 22(9):961–8.
37. Doll N, Borger MA, Fabricius A, et al. Esophageal perforation during left atrial radiofrequency ablation: is the risk too high? J Thorac Cardiovasc Surg 2003; 125(4):836–42.
38. Pappone C, Oral H, Santinelli V, et al. Atrio-esophageal fistula as a complication of percutaneous transcatheter ablation of atrial fibrillation. Circulation 2004;109(22):2724–6.
39. Scanavacca M, Avila A, Parga J, et al. Left atrial-esophageal fistula following radiofrequency catheter ablation of atrial fibrillation. J Cardiovasc Electrophysiol 2004;15:960–2.
40. Cummings JE, Schweikert RA, Saliba WI, et al. Assessment of temperature, proximity, and course of the esophagus during radiofrequency ablation within the left atrium. Circulation 2005;112(4):459–64.
41. Oral H, Scharf C, Chugh A, et al. Catheter ablation for paroxysmal atrial fibrillation: segmental pulmonary vein ostial ablation versus left atrial ablation. Circulation 2003;108(19):2355–60.
42. Jaïs P, Matsuo S, Knecht S, et al. A deductive mapping strategy for atrial tachycardia following atrial fibrillation ablation: importance of localized reentry. J Cardiovasc Electrophysiol 2009;20(5):480–91.
43. Hocini M, Sanders P, Deisenhofer I, et al. Reverse remodeling of sinus node function after catheter ablation of atrial fibrillation in patients with prolonged sinus pauses. Circulation 2003;108(10):1172–5.

Atrial Fibrillation Ablation
Do We Really Need Preprocedural Imaging?

Tara Bourke, MD[a,b], John Moriarty, MD[a], Noel G. Boyle, MD, PhD[a], Kalyanam Shivkumar, MD, PhD[a,*]

KEYWORDS

• Atrial fibrillation • Ablation • Preprocedural imaging

KEY POINTS

- The need for exclusion of LA thrombus with preprocedural imaging is not necessarily determined only by the type of AF but needs to be determined on an individual-patient basis taking into account factors such as cardiovascular risks, CHADS2 score, history of prior CVA, and the presence of LA dilatation and structural heart disease.
- The yield of LA thrombus identification with TEE among patients with paroxysmal AF who are in sinus rhythm at the time of ablation is low, particularly in patients without structural heart disease or risk factors for stroke.
- Data suggests that a screening TEE before PVI should be performed in patients with a CHADS2 score greater than or equal to 1, and in patients with a CHADS2 score of 0 when AF is persistent and therapeutic anticoagulation has not been maintained for 4 weeks before the procedure.
- Although not the gold standard, intracardiac thrombi can be effectively identified using modalities other than TEE including cardiac CT and MRI.
- To change the current approach, large randomized studies are needed to guide the selection of patients who may safely undergo ablation without TEE to exclude thrombus.

INTRODUCTION

Atrial fibrillation (AF) is the most common human arrhythmia, causing significant mortality and morbidity.[1] It has been estimated that 2.2 million people in the United States and 4.5 million in the European Union have paroxysmal or persistent AF.[2] AF carries a considerable degree of morbidity, including cardioembolic stroke, and is a risk factor for death independently of associated cardiovascular diseases.[3,4] Hospital admissions for AF have increased by 66% in the last 2 decades[5–8] because of factors including population aging, increasing prevalence of chronic heart disease, and increased diagnosis secondary to the use of ambulatory monitoring devices. The financial burden of AF on public health services is significant,[9,10] making the need to find effective treatment options imperative.

In the past decade, catheter ablation has emerged as a promising approach for treating AF.[11–14] Catheter ablation is a potentially curative treatment of AF, with significantly higher efficacy than antiarrhythmic drugs[15] and none of the long-term adverse effects. The potential for procedure-related complications has led to the implementation of practices (many of which have not been validated) before and during procedures intended to reduce them. As ablation techniques have evolved, so too has the use of imaging modalities used to plan and perform these

Supported by the NHLBI (R01HL084261) to KS.
Conflicts of interest: None.
[a] UCLA Cardiac Arrhythmia Center, David Geffen School of Medicine at UCLA, UCLA Health System, 100 UCLA Medical Plaza, Suite 660, Los Angeles, CA 90095, USA; [b] Department of Cardiology, Karolinska University Hospital, 141 86 Stockholm, Sweden
* Corresponding author.
E-mail address: kshivkumar@mednet.ucla.edu

Card Electrophysiol Clin 4 (2012) 305–315
http://dx.doi.org/10.1016/j.ccep.2012.05.002

procedures. Irrespective of the ablation approach used, or the type of AF being treated, for all cases a thorough understanding of the anatomy of the left atrium (LA) and adjacent structures is valuable for performing successful catheter ablation and avoiding complications. Just as techniques for catheter ablation should be tailored to specific patients and their type of AF, so too does the type of imaging need to be tailored to each patient. This article discusses the indications and usefulness of several preprocedural imaging techniques currently used in AF ablation.

COMPLICATIONS OF CATHETER-BASED ABLATION

To consider the relative merits of any imaging modality, the focus should first be on the potential procedural complications that may be encountered during or after the procedure and on how these may be affected by imaging studies. Major complications during AF ablation include pulmonary vein (PV) stenosis, thromboembolism, atrioesophageal fistula, and phrenic nerve paralysis.[13]

1. PV stenosis. Initial ablation approaches targeted ectopy within the PVs and was associated with an unacceptably high rate of PV stenosis, delivery of radiofrequency (RF) within the PVs is no longer advised and instead current approaches target areas outside the veins to isolate the ostia from the remainder of the LA conducting tissue. The rate of redo procedures in AF procedures is high, especially in patients with persistent AF. Preprocedural imaging to define PV anatomy can identify the presence of asymptomatic PV stenosis resulting from prior instrumentation and act as a point of reference in the event of development of symptoms with subsequent procedures (**Fig. 1**).
2. Embolic stroke. Embolic stroke is among the most serious and preventable complications of catheter-based ablation procedures in patients with AF. The incidence varies from 0% to 7%.[13,16–19] Embolic stroke may be caused by the dislodgement of a preformed thrombus, identifiable with several forms of preprocedural imaging; be caused by the intraprocedural formation of thrombus; or introduction of air. Precautions taken during procedures to avoid this complication include (1) administering a loading dose of heparin before or immediately on septal puncture (because thrombi can form on the transseptal sheath almost immediately after crossing the septum), (2) infusing heparinized saline continuously through the transseptal sheaths, (3) withdrawing the sheath to the right atrium once a catheter is positioned in the LA, and (4) the use of single-catheter techniques that may also reduce this risk of systemic embolization of thrombus formed on a sheath. A higher intensity of anticoagulation during the procedure reduces the risk of thrombus formation during ablation.[20] LA thrombus occurs in 11.2% and 2.8% of patients with an activated clotting time of 250 to 300 and greater than 300 seconds, respectively. Continuation of periprocedural warfarin anticoagulation has recently been proposed as a means of minimizing periprocedural interruption of anticoagulation, although this approach has not yet been shown to reduce the risk of cerebrovascular accident (CVA).[21] However, early CVAs may

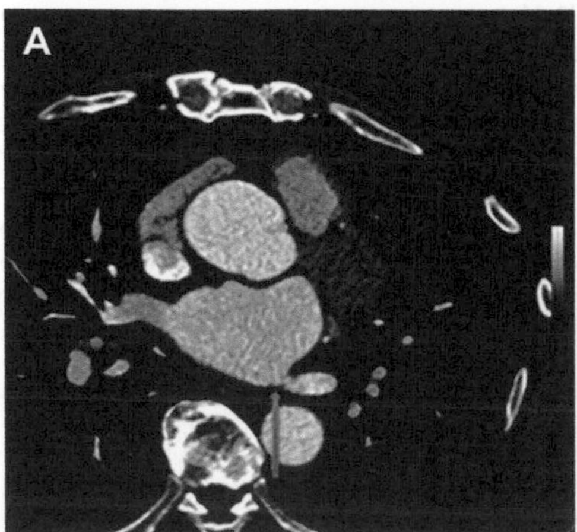

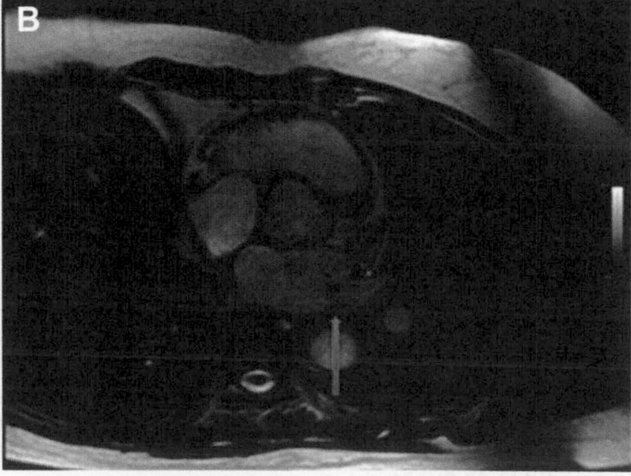

Fig. 1. (*A*) Axial reconstruction of contrast-enhanced electrocardiogram-gated cardiac computed tomography shows a moderately tight stenosis of the left superior PV (*arrow*) as it enters the LA. (*B*) Axial noncontrast steady state free precession in the same patient. Magnetic resonance imaging (MRI) of the heart shows a tight stenosis of the left superior PV (*arrow*) at the orifice into the LA.

occur even in the face of therapeutic anticoagulation, indicating that there is an inherent procedure-related risk of CVA that cannot be completely eliminated by appropriate anticoagulation and careful catheter and sheath management (this includes the risk of air emboli).[17]

3. Atrioesophageal fistula. Although rare, atrioesophageal fistula has been reported with both the circumferential approach[22] and the PV ablation techniques,[23] and is frequently fatal. The proximity of the esophagus to mediastinal structures can be noted on computed tomography (CT) or magnetic resonance imaging (MRI) scans (**Fig. 2**) performed to assess PV anatomy or identify intracardiac thrombi before procedures; however, most steps taken to prevent this outcome are taken during procedures. This complication is more likely to occur when extensive ablative lesions are applied to the posterior LA wall, increasing the risk of atrial perforation. Ablation at a reduced output of 25 W in the posterior wall has been advised to avoid this potentially fatal complication. Other precautions taken during the procedure include the use of esophageal barium as well as temperature monitoring in the esophagus during lesion formation in the posterior LA wall. The typical manifestations include sudden neurologic symptoms or endocarditis.
4. Phrenic nerve injury. The reported prevalence of phrenic nerve injury as a complication of AF ablation is 0.11% to 0.48%.[13,24] Precautions to prevent this complication are taken during procedures. Because of the anatomic proximity of the phrenic nerves, high-output pacing should be performed before ablation at the posteroseptal superior vena cava, anteroinferior right superior pulmonary vein ostium, or left atrial appendage roof, and, in case of diaphragmatic stimulation, energy application should be avoided. Phrenic nerve injury should be suspected if decreased diaphragmatic excursions, cough, or hiccoughs occur during RF delivery.

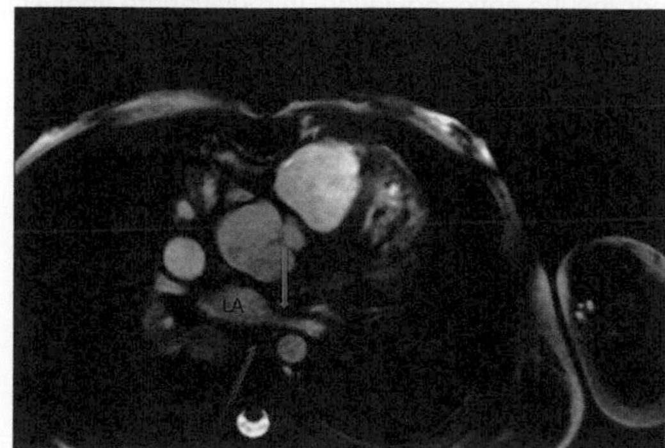

Fig. 2. Cardiac MRI shows the left inferior PV (*blue arrow*) entering the LA in close contact with the esophagus (*red arrow*). Because of the proximity of the esophagus to the LA, care is required to prevent thermal injury or perforation during ablation.

PREPROCEDURAL TRANSESOPHAGEAL ECHOCARDIOGRAPHY

1. Detection of intracardiac thrombi. Transesophageal echocardiography (TEE) provides high-quality images of cardiac structure[25] and function.[26] It is the most sensitive and specific technique to detect sources and potential mechanisms for cardiogenic embolism,[27] surpassing transthoracic echocardiography.[28] TEE features associated with thromboembolism in patients with nonvalvular AF include LA/left atrial appendage (LAA) thrombus, LA/LAA spontaneous echo contrast (SEC), reduced LAA flow velocity, and aortic atheromatous abnormalities (**Figs. 3** and **4**).[29] Current guidelines suggest that the management of patients with AF at the time of the procedure should be the same as that for a cardioversion.[30] Patients should have TEE performed within 48 hours of the procedure regardless of whether or not they have been anticoagulated with warfarin. Detection of LA/LAA thrombus in the setting of stroke or systemic embolism is convincing evidence of a cardiogenic mechanism.[31] Detection of LA/LAA thrombus stands as a contraindication to elective AF ablation procedures. The absence of a detectable thrombus does not preclude stroke after cardioversion in the absence of anticoagulation therapy. For low-risk lone paroxysmal AF with prior anticoagulation, there is uncertainty about the usefulness of performing routine thrombus detection. In this case, TTE can be used to stratify risk in patients before performing TEE with a very high negative predictive value (NPV).[32]
2. Determination of LA size, cardiac function, and cardiac anatomy. LA dimensions, which can independently predict the procedural termination of AF with catheter ablation,[33] can be accurately assessed during a TEE to screen for thrombi. In addition, TEE is the most accurate modality to detect the presence of a patent foramen ovale,[34] and can reliably detect septal abnormalities including bowing or aneurysm formation, which may be helpful during the procedure. However, it has been shown that septal anatomy is more accurately visualized on CT.[35] PV isolation is the cornerstone of all ablation strategies for both paroxysmal and persistent AF, and therefore an accurate

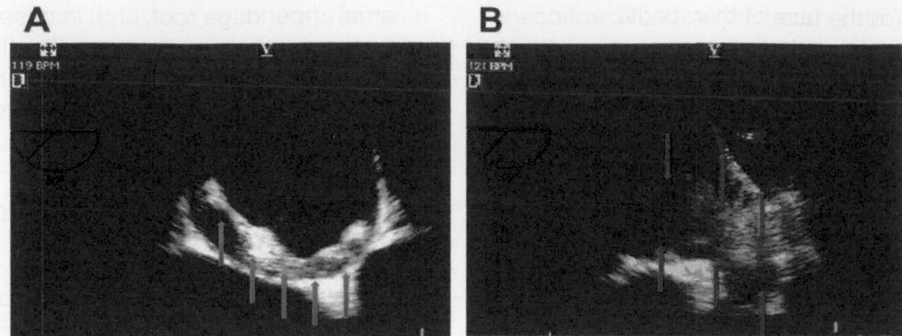

Fig. 3. (*A*) TEE showing layered thrombus (*blue arrows*) lining the LA of a patient newly diagnosed with persistent AF. (*B*) Thrombus filled LAA (*red arrows*) of the same patient.

knowledge of an individual's PV anatomy is useful before the procedure. Although TEE can provide an assessment of PV diameter, the most accurate measure is provided by CT scanning or MRI.[36]

CURRENT GUIDELINES

The Heart Rhythm Society Consensus Statement on catheter ablation of AF recommends preablation TEE to exclude LA thrombus in patients with persistent AF; no specific recommendation is made for patients with paroxysmal AF.[30] However, the use of TEE to assess atrial thrombus before AF ablation is variable. Recent data suggest that preablation TEE is routinely used in up to 72% of centers performing catheter ablation of AF.[13] However, TEE requires moderate sedation and, at times, esophageal intubation (and is usually used for the purpose of thrombus identification), and may not allow complete visualization and assessment of all of the PVs or their precise relationship to other thoracic structures. Before catheter ablation for AF, patients frequently undergo evaluation with TEE to rule out intracardiac thrombus and either CT or MRI to evaluate PV anatomy, resulting in increased procedural costs and potential for increased complications. In addition, although CT/MRI images can be used to assist mapping and ablation as well as the development of complications, TEE is generally not used during procedures. This article reviews the evidence for different imaging modalities in this patient population.

INCIDENCE AND PREDICTORS OF PERIPROCEDURAL CVA IN PATIENTS UNDERGOING CATHETER ABLATION OF AF

Although a successful AF ablation procedure may reduce the occurrence of future stroke, periprocedural stroke, and transient ischemic attack, CVAs remain among the most serious complications of catheter ablation of AF. The incidence and predictors of left atrial thrombus in patients undergoing AF ablation have been reported in several studies. McCready and colleagues[37] assessed a cohort of 635 patients who underwent TEE before AF ablation. All patients were on warfarin for a minimum of 4 weeks and 52% had persistent AF. The incidence of thrombus was 12/635 (1.9%) despite therapeutic anticoagulation. In multivariate analysis,

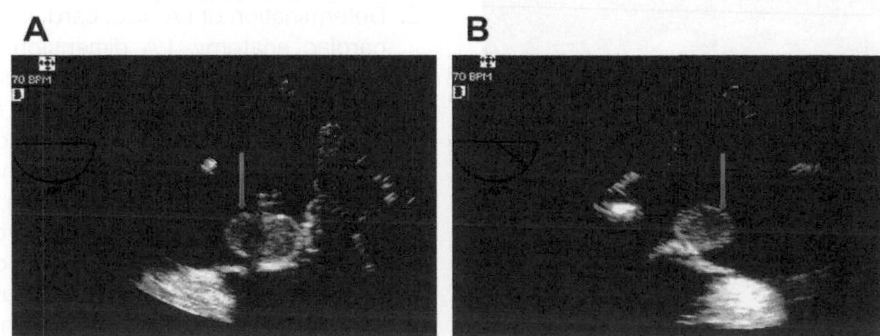

Fig. 4. (*A, B*) TEE shows 2 views of a mobile LA thrombus (*blue arrows*) in a 70-year-old woman with a history of paroxysmal AF and a $CHADS_2$ (congestive heart failure, hypertension, age 75 years or older, diabetes mellitus, priorstrokeortransient ischemic attack) score of 2. Thrombus resolved completely within 6 weeks of therapeutic anticoagulation.

hypertension (odds ratio [OR] = 14.2), age greater than 75 years (OR = 8.1), and cardiomyopathy (OR = 10.5) were independently associated with thrombus, whereas LA size greater than 50 mm and type of AF were not associated with LA thrombus. They concluded that, in patients presenting for AF ablation, LA thrombus was only seen in those with clinical risk factors, and that, although TEE is indicated in patients with risk factors, it may be unnecessary in patients without clinical risk factors. Scherr and colleagues[38] reported findings on 732 patients undergoing pulmonary vein isolation (PVI). Prevalence of thrombus was 1.6%, 48% had persistent AF, and all had been anticoagulated for 4 weeks or longer. In multivariate analysis a $CHADS_2$ (congestive heart failure, hypertension, age 75 years or older, diabetes mellitus, priorstrokeortransient ischemic attack) score greater than or equal to 2 and larger LA diameter were independent predictors of LA thrombus in this patient population, whereas type of AF or rhythm at the time of TEE was not. The risk of LA thrombus is low in patients with a $CHADS_2$ score of 0 and in patients with an LA diameter less than 4.5 cm.

The role of $CHADS_2$ score in patients with AF before PVI was also reported by Puwanant and colleagues,[19] who assessed the presence of thrombus, sludge, and SEC. Prevalence of thrombus in 1058 patients was 0.6%, 18% had persistent AF, and 73% were anticoagulated. In a multivariate model, history of congestive heart failure and left ventricular ejection fraction less than 35% were significantly associated with sludge/thrombus. The prevalence of thrombus/sludge/SEC increased with ascending $CHADS_2$ scores. No patient with a $CHADS_2$ score of 0 had LA/LAA sludge/thrombus. Based on these, data the investigators suggested that a screening TEE before PVI should be performed in patients with a $CHADS_2$ score greater than or equal to 1, and in patients with a $CHADS_2$ score of 0 when AF is persistent and therapeutic anticoagulation has not been maintained for 4 weeks before the procedure. $CHADS_2$ score was not found to be independently predictive in a study on 446 patients in which advancing age, persistent AF, and structure were the independent predictors of LA thrombus.[39]

A study by Calvo and colleagues[40] reported a low incidence of thrombi detected with TEE (6 of 408 patients, 1.47%) in their cohort of 408 patients undergoing PVI. Oral anticoagulation was used in 67% (patients with a $CHADS_2$ score $\geq$2) and AF was persistent in 41%. They noted that patients in whom thrombus was identified were more likely to have larger LA diameter, persistent AF, structural heart disease, and be female. The likelihood of thrombus increased with the number of these factors present (<0.001). Five of the patients with thrombi were receiving oral anticoagulation before ablation; the $CHADS_2$ score was less than 2 in 5 and 2 in 1 patient, and patients with LA thrombus had persistent AF and large LA diameters. The investigators concluded that TEE before AF ablation might not be needed in patients with paroxysmal AF and no LA dilatation or structural heart disease.

The incidence and predictors of periprocedural CVA in the AF ablation population have also been reported. In 529 patients,[41] periprocedural ischemic CVA was seen in 1.4% (10 patients), 50% were in persistent AF, and 94% on warfarin for 4 weeks or longer. The risk of CVA increased with the patients' $CHADS_2$ scores: a $CHADS_2$ score greater than or equal to 2 conferred a 9-fold higher risk of CVA than patients with a $CHADS_2$ score less than or equal to 1 (P<.001). In addition, the risk of stroke was very low in patients with a $CHADS_2$ score of 0. Their findings further suggest that patient-specific factors seem to play a significant role in determining the procedural CVA risk. The importance of the $CHADS_2$ score in relation to CVA was also reported by Bunch and colleagues.[42] They reported no periprocedural or postprocedural strokes in 123 patients with $CHADS_2$ scores of 0 to 1 despite the use of only aspirin rather than warfarin.

ASSESSING INTRACARDIAC THROMBUS USING CT

Although 64-slice CT scanning has been used to identify LA thrombus, TEE remains the gold standard. Patients referred for RF PV antral isolation often undergo contrast-enhanced multidetector CT (MDCT) to assess PV and left atrial anatomy as well as TEE to detect intra-atrial thrombus. A study by Kim and colleagues[43] sought to determine the accuracy of MDCT to qualitatively and quantitatively detect severe SEC or thrombus by TEE in the LAA and, in addition, to determine the ability of MDCT to characterize filling defects by separating patients with severe SEC and/or thrombus from those with lesser grades of SEC using quantitative Hounsfield unit (HU) criteria. Both imaging modalities were performed on 223 patients before PVI. For studies in which the patient was in AF, the sensitivity, specificity, positive predictive value, NPV, and accuracy were 91%, 84%, 37%, 99%, and 85%, respectively. For studies in which the presenting rhythm was not AF (sinus rhythm or atrial paced), these values were 100%, 88%, 29%, 100%, and 89%, respectively. Rhythm did not significantly affect the ability of MDCT to discern severe SEC and/or thrombus. MDCT was highly sensitive and had a very high NPV in the detection of severe LAA SEC and thrombus compared with TEE. With its high NPV, MDCT has the potential ability to effectively exclude LAA filling defects. These findings corroborate those of previous smaller studies that also showed high sensitivity in the detection of LAA thrombus.[44,45] Patients in this study were already undergoing MDCT, so there was no additional risk of radiation and contrast nephropathy beyond that for which the scan was ordered. However, with the advent of newer MDCT imaging techniques including dose modulation and prospective gated axial imaging, it will be possible to significantly reduce the radiation dose, which could expand its applicability.

Patel and colleagues[46] also assessed the diagnostic performance of 64-detector row MDCT in detecting LAA thrombus and dense nonclearing SEC as identified by TEE in patients undergoing PV isolation for treatment of AF. MDCT assessment of the LAA was performed by (1) comparison of HU densities in the LAA apex with the ascending aorta (AscAo), and (2) nonquantitative visual identification of a filling defect in the LAA. Patients with LAA thrombus or dense nonclearing SEC by TEE had significantly lower LAA/AscAo HU ratios than patients who did not (P<.001). LAA/AscAo HU cutoff ratios less than or equal to 0.75 correlated with LAA thrombus or dense nonclearing SEC by TEE, with 100% sensitivity, 72.2% specificity, 28.6% positive predictive value, and 100% NPV. In multivariate analysis, LAA/AscAo HU ratio less than or equal to 0.75 remained a robust predictor of LAA thrombus or dense nonclearing SEC by TEE (P<.001). In contrast, MDCT identification of TEE-identified LAA thrombus or dense nonclearing SEC by visual detection of LAA filling defects resulted in lower sensitivity (50%) and NPV (95.1%). Their conclusion was that current-generation MDCT successfully identifies LAA thrombus and dense nonclearing SEC with high sensitivity and moderate specificity, and that LAA/AscAo HU ratios greater than 0.75 have 100% NPV for exclusion of LAA thrombus or dense nonclearing SEC. Therefore, in patients undergoing PVI, MDCT examinations that show LAA/AscAo HU ratios greater than 0.75 may preclude the need for preprocedural TEE.

Whether MDCT alone was sufficient to exclude LAA thrombus in patients referred for catheter ablation of AF was studied by Martinez and colleagues[47] in 402 patients with symptomatic AF referred for AF ablation. In 40 patients, the LAA was underfilled, with 9 definite thrombi confirmed by TEE. Sensitivity and specificity were 100% and 92%, respectively, with an NPV of 100% and positive predictive value of 23%. Patients with LAA underfilling had substantially reduced Doppler-derived LAA emptying velocities and higher $CHADS_2$ scores (1.6 vs 1.1). No cases of LAA thrombus were observed in patients aged less than 52 years with $CHADS_2$ score less than 1. They concluded that MDCT is a sensitive (100% sensitivity) imaging modality that could be used alone, especially in patients less than 52 years of age with a $CHADS_2$ score less than 1. Incorporation of these findings could decrease the need for multiple imaging modalities and thereby reduce the cost of the procedure.

Using CT before ablation and TEE only in a subset of 1221 patients (and those who had LAA thrombus on CT), Khan and colleagues[48] showed a low incidence of LA/LAA thrombus. Nine patients had a thrombus on CT; however, on TEE, only 3 patients had an LAA thrombus before pulmonary vein antrum isolation (PVAI); of these patients, 2 had chronic AF with average ejection fraction (EF) of 48%, giving an incidence of LA or LAA thrombus in the persistent/chronic AF population of 0.4%, and 1 patient had paroxysmal atrial fibrillation (PAF) with EF 25%, giving an incidence of LA or LAA thrombus in the paroxysmal AF population of 0.14%. No patients with PAF and normal EF had LAA thrombus. Patients with LAA thrombus before PVAI had lower EF than patients without LAA thrombus (40% vs 53%, P = .007) but had similar LA size. They did not observe LA thrombus in patients with PAF with normal EF who presented for PVAI, and concluded that prescreening CT alone is likely to be sufficient in patients with PAF with normal EF, and TEE may not be needed.

ASSESSING INTRACARDIAC THROMBUS USING MRI

The data assessing MRI detection of LA and LAA thrombi are sparse. Abstract data on 110 patients undergoing two-dimensional (2D) and three-dimensional (3D) contrast and noncontrast MRI and TEE before PVI have been reported.[49] There was 100% concordance between MRI and TEE results (only 2 cases positive for thrombus). The 2D cardiac MRI (CMR) images were indeterminate in 9 cases in which 3D contrast images were most helpful in the final ruling out of LAA. They concluded that CMR offered a comparable and equally specific alternative to TEE for the complete, noninvasive evaluation of LAA thrombus in patients with AF without the obligate need for sedation, radiation, or nephrotoxicity. A study by Ohyama and colleagues[50] assessed MRI versus TEE in the detection of LAA thrombi in 50 patients with AF with a history of cardioembolic stroke. The LAA was readily visualized in all patients with MRI, and high-intensity masses in the LAA were clearly distinguishable from the LAA wall in the triple-inversion recovery sequences. In addition, thrombus could be differentiated from SEC. Concordance between detection of high-intensity mass with MRI and thrombus with TEE was high: negative MRI plus TEE in 31 patients; positive MRI plus TEE in 16 patients; and positive MRI but negative TEE in 3 patients, overall $\kappa = 0.876$ (standard error ≈ 0.068). MRI and TEE provided equivalent accuracy of LA dimension and LAA area measurements. Sizes of high-intensity masses in MRI (71.1 ± 16.3 mm^2) were consistently greater than corresponding thrombus sizes in TEE (58.3 ± 14.6 mm^2); with sizes being $\approx$23% larger with MRI than with TEE.

CT AND MRI OF CARDIAC ANATOMY

Understanding the morphologic characteristics of the LA in detail not only helps achieve a more efficient and successful ablation but may also prevent procedure-related complications. CT/MRI may facilitate AF ablation procedures by[30] (1) imaging the anatomic features of the PVs and LA before procedures, (2) assessing the anatomic relationship between the LA, esophagus, and adjacent vascular structures, (3) providing an understanding of the degree of morphologic remodeling of the PVs and LA, and (4) assisting in the detection of PV stenosis from prior procedures and identifying postprocedure complications. Electroanatomic mapping systems currently allow previously acquired CT or magnetic resonance images to be imported into the mapping systems and registered with the LA in real time. These systems help facilitate AF ablation procedures by providing detailed information about the anatomy.[51] Assessment of PV anatomy in patients before and after AF ablation using MRI has been described.[52] The results revealed (1) a close proximity between the ostia of the right PVs and the ostia of left PVs, with the mouth of the left superior pulmonary vein separated from the LA appendage by only a thin rim of tissue; (2) that PV anatomy is highly variable, with 38% of patients showing variant anatomy (23% of variants reported previously); (3) little variation in the size of the PVs within a given patient; (4) PV and LA sizes are larger in patients with AF than in controls; (5) the left PVs have a longer neck, with a greater distance between the ostium and the first branch; (6) PV ostia are oblong, with the superoinferior dimension greater than the anteroposterior dimension; and (7) RF ablation targeted immediately outside the PV ostia results in a detectable PV narrowing in 24% of PVs.

Imaging with CT or MRI preprocedurally may facilitate ablation of the PVs, especially in patients with anatomic variants. This information may be useful in selecting an appropriately sized circular mapping catheter and ascertaining that all PV orifices are evaluated during the procedure. For balloon-based procedures, this type of information is likely to be of even greater clinical importance. Another important role of MRI is its ability to provide a quantitative assessment of the location, shape, and severity of PV stenosis. However, in terms of reducing procedural time, fluoroscopy time, or improving clinical outcomes, no data exist on whether either imaging modality facilitates this. Potential advantages of MRI include the absence of potentially nephrotoxic contrast medium and absence of radiation. From a clinical standpoint, either spiral CT or MRI can be used to define PV anatomy and to screen for stenoses after ablation. With the exception of patients who have implanted devices, local expertise within a given medical institution is likely to dictate which technique is used.

RADIATION EXPOSURE DURING AF ABLATION

Catheter ablation of AF is often a complex and long procedure requiring long fluoroscopy exposure time and often preceded and followed by CT scans. An important, less easily recognized, and rarely considered potential complication of AF ablation is the delayed effect of the radiation received by the patients, including acute and subacute skin injury,[53,54] malignancy, and genetic abnormalities.[53] Radiation exposure during AF ablation has been evaluated by Lickfett and colleagues.[55] They reported: (1) markedly prolonged fluoroscopy duration, (2) greater radiation dose in the left anterior oblique projection, and (3) a lifetime risk of fatal malignancy within the range previously reported for standard supraventricular arrhythmias. However, small amounts of the patient's radiation exposure, despite the prolonged fluoroscopy durations, could be attributed to the use of very-low-frame pulsed fluoroscopy, the avoidance of magnification, and optimal adjustments of the fluoroscopy exposure rates parameters, which should be taken into consideration for every case. Because catheter ablation of AF requires significantly greater fluoroscopy duration and radiation exposure than simpler catheter ablation procedures, and especially because AF ablation procedures often need to be repeated, electrophysiologists should make every attempt to minimize radiation exposure. The increasing use of 3D mapping systems should significantly reduce fluoroscopy time and the need for biplane fluoroscopy. In addition, the use of remote navigation systems is also likely to significantly reduce radiation exposure of both the patients and the electrophysiologists performing these procedures. Performing preprocedural imaging has not been shown to reduced procedure time or fluoroscopy time for AF ablation. Although radiation dose before a procedure can be minimized by the use of CMR rather than CT in patients without a device.

IS PREPROCEDURAL TEE MANDATORY?

In several studies, the incidence of thrombi in patients undergoing PVI is low, ranging from 0.6% to 2.9%. Clinical risk factors associated with the presence of thrombus in these studies were diverse: hypertension, advanced age and cardiomyopathy,[37] $CHADS_2$ score greater than or equal to 2, and LA dilatation, but not the type of AF and rhythm at the time of TEE,[38] increased LA diameter, female sex, persistent AF and structural heart disease,[40] impaired left ventricular function and a history of congestive heart failure,[19] persistent AF, advanced age, and structural heart disease.[39] The periprocedural predictors of CVA included a $CHADS_2$ greater than or equal to 2 and a history of prior CVA.[41] These are observational studies (frequently performed in single centers) with all the inherent limitations afforded by these types of studies. The types of AF varies considerably, persistent AF occurring in 18% to 52% of patients. There is also a lack of uniformity regarding anticoagulation regimes, some centers using bridging heparin, others not. However, a unifying issue is the absence of any evidence of therapeutic anticoagulation before the procedure.

CAN THROMBI BE ACCURATELY IDENTIFIED BY CT/MRI?

Although not the gold standard, intracardiac thrombi can be effectively identified using modalities other than TEE. MDCT has been shown to be highly sensitive and has a high NPV in the detection of severe LAA SEC and thrombus compared with TEE.[43,46,47] MDCT has the potential ability to effectively exclude LAA filling defects. In addition, LAA/AscAo HU ratios greater than 0.75 show 100% NPV for exclusion of LAA thrombus or dense SEC[46] so, in patients undergoing PVI, MDCT examinations that show LAA/AscAo HU ratios greater than 0.75 may therefore preclude the need for preprocedural TEE. Martinez and colleagues[47] found that MDCT is a sensitive (100% sensitivity) imaging modality that could be used alone, especially in patients younger than 52 years with a $CHADS_2$ score less than 1. The zero incidence of LA/LAA thrombus in patients with PAF with normal EF[48] led to the suggestion that prescreening with CT is likely to be sufficient in patients with PAF with normal left ventricular function. Although observational in nature, these studies may allow the selection of a subgroup of patients in whom TEE could potentially be avoided, which is important in laboratories in which patients routinely undergo CT for assessing PV anatomy so that preprocedural scanning may serve multiple purposes and unnecessary TEE may be avoided. However, CT requires large doses of radiation, considerable time and experience are required for accurate interpretation, and it is expensive. However, it is able to accurately detect thrombi.

Although numbers are small, CMR may offer a comparable and equally specific alternative to TEE for the complete noninvasive evaluation of LAA thrombus in patients with AF[49,50] without the obligate need for sedation, radiation, or nephrotoxicity. MRI may not be suitable in a subgroup of patients who have implanted devices (eg, implantable cardioverter-defibrillator or prosthetic valve). In addition, the usefulness of MRI in patients with small thrombi or small LAA is unknown. The cost of cardiac MRI is 70% greater than TEE, precluding its routine use for thrombus detection, but, in facilities where MRI is performed for imaging of the PVs, it may become possible to exploit its potential to accurately rule out thrombus.

SUMMARY

Indications for preprocedural imaging vary and include assessing the presence of a thrombus before cannulation of the LA and delineating LA and PV anatomy either to facilitate the procedure or as a reference point to help to determine whether there are postprocedural complications. Because of the potential for various complications, it is important that these procedures are made as safe and effective as possible by combining safe procedural planning with effective therapy delivery. Predictors of thrombus formation and clinical events are variable and it seems that the need for exclusion of LA thrombus with preprocedural imaging is not necessarily determined only by the type of AF but needs to be determined on an individual-patient basis taking into account factors such as cardiovascular risks, $CHADS_2$ score, history of prior CVA, and the presence of LA dilatation and structural heart disease. The yield of LA thrombus identification with TEE among patients with paroxysmal AF who are in sinus rhythm at the time of ablation is low, particularly in patients without structural heart disease or risk factors for stroke. It is imperative that adequate anticoagulation be ensured in all patients before proceeding with ablation, but especially those in whom risk may be deemed to be low and in whom TEE may be deemed unnecessary.

To change the current approach, large randomized studies are needed to guide the selection of patients who may safely undergo ablation without TEE to exclude thrombus. For institutions routinely using CT and MRI to assess PV anatomy before procedures, the possibility of excluding intracardiac thrombi using these imaging modalities, especially in those deemed to be low risk, should be considered.

REFERENCES

1. Vidaillet H, Granada JF, Chyou PH, et al. A population-based study of mortality among patients with atrial fibrillation or flutter. Am J Med 2002;113(5):365–70.
2. Feinberg WM, Cornell ES, Nightingale SD, et al. Relationship between prothrombin activation fragment F1.2 and international normalized ratio in patients with atrial fibrillation. Stroke Prevention in Atrial Fibrillation Investigators. Stroke 1997;28(6):1101–6.
3. Falk RH. Atrial fibrillation. N Engl J Med 2001; 344(14):1067–78.
4. Wolf PA, Abbott RD, Kannel WB. Atrial fibrillation as an independent risk factor for stroke: the Framingham Study. Stroke 1991;22(8):983–8.
5. Friberg J, Buch P, Scharling H, et al. Rising rates of hospital admissions for atrial fibrillation. Epidemiology 2003;14(6):666–72.
6. Middlekauff HR, Stevenson WG, Stevenson LW. Prognostic significance of atrial fibrillation in advanced heart failure. A study of 390 patients. Circulation 1991;84(1):40–8.
7. Stevenson WG, Stevenson LW, Middlekauff HR, et al. Improving survival for patients with atrial fibrillation and advanced heart failure. J Am Coll Cardiol 1996;28(6):1458–63.
8. Stewart S, MacIntyre K, MacLeod MM, et al. Trends in hospital activity, morbidity and case fatality related to atrial fibrillation in Scotland, 1986–1996. Eur Heart J 2001;22(8):693–701.
9. Le Heuzey JY, Paziaud O, Piot O, et al. Cost of care distribution in atrial fibrillation patients: the COCAF study. Am Heart J 2004;147(1):121–6.
10. Stewart S, Murphy NF, Walker A, et al. Cost of an emerging epidemic: an economic analysis of atrial fibrillation in the UK. Heart 2004;90(3):286–92.
11. Haissaguerre M, Jais P, Shah DC, et al. Spontaneous initiation of atrial fibrillation by ectopic beats originating in the pulmonary veins. N Engl J Med 1998;339(10):659–66.
12. Pappone C, Rosanio S, Augello G, et al. Mortality, morbidity, and quality of life after circumferential pulmonary vein ablation for atrial fibrillation: outcomes from a controlled nonrandomized long-term study. J Am Coll Cardiol 2003;42(2):185–97.
13. Cappato R, Calkins H, Chen SA, et al. Worldwide survey on the methods, efficacy, and safety of catheter ablation for human atrial fibrillation. Circulation 2005;111(9):1100–5.
14. Oral H, Pappone C, Chugh A, et al. Circumferential pulmonary-vein ablation for chronic atrial fibrillation. N Engl J Med 2006;354(9):934–41.
15. Nair GM, Nery PB, Diwakaramenon S, et al. A systematic review of randomized trials comparing radiofrequency ablation with antiarrhythmic medications in patients with atrial fibrillation. J Cardiovasc Electrophysiol 2009;20(2):138–44.
16. Bertaglia E, Zoppo F, Tondo C, et al. Early complications of pulmonary vein catheter ablation for atrial fibrillation: a multicenter prospective registry on procedural safety. Heart Rhythm 2007; 4(10):1265–71.
17. Oral H, Chugh A, Ozaydin M, et al. Risk of thromboembolic events after percutaneous left atrial radiofrequency ablation of atrial fibrillation. Circulation 2006;114(8):759–65.
18. Hussein AA, Martin DO, Saliba W, et al. Radiofrequency ablation of atrial fibrillation under therapeutic international normalized ratio: a safe and efficacious periprocedural anticoagulation strategy. Heart Rhythm 2009;6(10):1425–9.
19. Puwanant S, Varr BC, Shrestha K, et al. Role of the CHADS2 score in the evaluation of thromboembolic risk in patients with atrial fibrillation undergoing transesophageal echocardiography before pulmonary vein isolation. J Am Coll Cardiol 2009;54(22): 2032–9.
20. Ren JF, Marchlinski FE, Callans DJ, et al. Increased intensity of anticoagulation may reduce risk of thrombus during atrial fibrillation ablation procedures in patients with spontaneous echo contrast. J Cardiovasc Electrophysiol 2005;16(5):474–7.
21. Wazni OM, Beheiry S, Fahmy T, et al. Atrial fibrillation ablation in patients with therapeutic international normalized ratio: comparison of strategies of anticoagulation management in the periprocedural period. Circulation 2007;116(22):2531–4.
22. Pappone C, Oral H, Santinelli V, et al. Atrio-esophageal fistula as a complication of percutaneous transcatheter ablation of atrial fibrillation. Circulation 2004;109(22):2724–6.
23. Scanavacca MI, D'Avila A, Parga J, et al. Left atrial-esophageal fistula following radiofrequency catheter ablation of atrial fibrillation. J Cardiovasc Electrophysiol 2004;15(8):960–2.

24. Sacher F, Monahan KH, Thomas SP, et al. Phrenic nerve injury after atrial fibrillation catheter ablation: characterization and outcome in a multicenter study. J Am Coll Cardiol 2006;47(12):2498–503.
25. Seward JB, Khandheria BK, Freeman WK, et al. Multiplane transesophageal echocardiography: image orientation, examination technique, anatomic correlations, and clinical applications. Mayo Clin Proc 1993;68(6):523–51.
26. Agmon Y, Khandheria BK, Gentile F, et al. Echocardiographic assessment of the left atrial appendage. J Am Coll Cardiol 1999;34(7):1867–77.
27. Pearson AC, Labovitz AJ, Tatineni S, et al. Superiority of transesophageal echocardiography in detecting cardiac source of embolism in patients with cerebral ischemia of uncertain etiology. J Am Coll Cardiol 1991;17(1):66–72.
28. Aschenberg W, Schluter M, Kremer P, et al. Transesophageal two-dimensional echocardiography for the detection of left atrial appendage thrombus. J Am Coll Cardiol 1986;7(1):163–6.
29. Zabalgoitia M, Halperin JL, Pearce LA, et al. Transesophageal echocardiographic correlates of clinical risk of thromboembolism in nonvalvular atrial fibrillation. Stroke Prevention in Atrial Fibrillation III Investigators. J Am Coll Cardiol 1998;31(7):1622–6.
30. Calkins H, Brugada J, Packer DL, et al. HRS/EHRA/ECAS expert consensus statement on catheter and surgical ablation of atrial fibrillation: recommendations for personnel, policy, procedures and follow-up. A report of the Heart Rhythm Society (HRS) Task Force on Catheter and Surgical Ablation of Atrial Fibrillation. Heart Rhythm 2007;4(6):816–61.
31. Manning WJ, Silverman DI, Katz SE, et al. Temporal dependence of the return of atrial mechanical function on the mode of cardioversion of atrial fibrillation to sinus rhythm. Am J Cardiol 1995;75(8):624–6.
32. Ellis K, Ziada KM, Vivekananthan D, et al. Transthoracic echocardiographic predictors of left atrial appendage thrombus. Am J Cardiol 2006;97(3):421–5.
33. O'Neill MD, Jais P, Hocini M, et al. Catheter ablation for atrial fibrillation. Circulation 2007;116(13):1515–23.
34. Fisher DC, Fisher EA, Budd JH, et al. The incidence of patent foramen ovale in 1,000 consecutive patients. A contrast transesophageal echocardiography study. Chest 1995;107(6):1504–9.
35. Graham LN, Melton IC, MacDonald S, et al. Value of CT localization of the fossa ovalis prior to transseptal left heart catheterization for left atrial ablation. Europace 2007;9(6):417–23.
36. Mansour M, Holmvang G, Sosnovik D, et al. Assessment of pulmonary vein anatomic variability by magnetic resonance imaging: implications for catheter ablation techniques for atrial fibrillation. J Cardiovasc Electrophysiol 2004;15(4):387–93.
37. McCready JW, Nunn L, Lambiase PD, et al. Incidence of left atrial thrombus prior to atrial fibrillation ablation: is pre-procedural transoesophageal echocardiography mandatory? Europace 2010;12(7):927–32.
38. Scherr D, Dalal D, Chilukuri K, et al. Incidence and predictors of left atrial thrombus prior to catheter ablation of atrial fibrillation. J Cardiovasc Electrophysiol 2009;20(4):379–84.
39. Yamashita E, Takamatsu H, Tada H, et al. Transesophageal echocardiography for thrombus screening prior to left atrial catheter ablation. Circ J 2010;74(6):1081–6.
40. Calvo N, Mont L, Vidal B, et al. Usefulness of transoesophageal echocardiography before circumferential pulmonary vein ablation in patients with atrial fibrillation: is it really mandatory? Europace 2011;13(4):486–91.
41. Scherr D, Sharma K, Dalal D, et al. Incidence and predictors of periprocedural cerebrovascular accident in patients undergoing catheter ablation of atrial fibrillation. J Cardiovasc Electrophysiol 2009;20(12):1357–63.
42. Bunch TJ, Crandall BG, Weiss JP, et al. Warfarin is not needed in low-risk patients following atrial fibrillation ablation procedures. J Cardiovasc Electrophysiol 2009;20(9):988–93.
43. Kim YY, Klein AL, Halliburton SS, et al. Left atrial appendage filling defects identified by multidetector computed tomography in patients undergoing radiofrequency pulmonary vein antral isolation: a comparison with transesophageal echocardiography. Am Heart J 2007;154(6):1199–205.
44. Jaber WA, White RD, Kuzmiak SA, et al. Comparison of ability to identify left atrial thrombus by three-dimensional tomography versus transesophageal echocardiography in patients with atrial fibrillation. Am J Cardiol 2004;93(4):486–9.
45. Achenbach S, Sacher D, Ropers D, et al. Electron beam computed tomography for the detection of left atrial thrombi in patients with atrial fibrillation. Heart 2004;90(12):1477–8.
46. Patel A, Au E, Donegan K, et al. Multidetector row computed tomography for identification of left atrial appendage filling defects in patients undergoing pulmonary vein isolation for treatment of atrial fibrillation: comparison with transesophageal echocardiography. Heart Rhythm 2008;5(2):253–60.
47. Martinez MW, Kirsch J, Williamson EE, et al. Utility of nongated multidetector computed tomography for detection of left atrial thrombus in patients undergoing catheter ablation of atrial fibrillation. JACC Cardiovasc Imaging 2009;2(1):69–76.
48. Khan MN, Usmani A, Noor S, et al. Low incidence of left atrial or left atrial appendage thrombus in patients with paroxysmal atrial fibrillation and normal EF who present for pulmonary vein antrum isolation procedure. J Cardiovasc Electrophysiol 2008;19(4):356–8.

49. Anreddy S, Balhan S, Yamrozik J. Is cardiovascular MRI equally as effective as TEE in evaluation of left atrial appendage thrombus in patients with atrial fibrillation undergoing pulmonary vein isolation. J Cardiovasc Magn Reson 2011;13(Suppl 1):P246.
50. Ohyama H, Hosomi N, Takahashi T, et al. Comparison of magnetic resonance imaging and transesophageal echocardiography in detection of thrombus in the left atrial appendage. Stroke 2003;34(10):2436–9.
51. Dong J, Calkins H, Solomon SB, et al. Integrated electroanatomic mapping with three-dimensional computed tomographic images for real-time guided ablations. Circulation 2006;113(2):186–94.
52. Kato R, Lickfett L, Meininger G, et al. Pulmonary vein anatomy in patients undergoing catheter ablation of atrial fibrillation: lessons learned by use of magnetic resonance imaging. Circulation 2003;107(15):2004–10.
53. Nahass GT. Fluoroscopy and the skin: implications for radiofrequency catheter ablation. Am J Cardiol 1995;76(3):174–6.
54. Nahass GT. Acute radiodermatitis after radiofrequency catheter ablation. J Am Acad Dermatol 1997;36(5 Pt 2):881–4.
55. Lickfett L, Mahesh M, Vasamreddy C, et al. Radiation exposure during catheter ablation of atrial fibrillation. Circulation 2004;110(19):3003–10.

Postablation Atrial Flutters

Aman Chugh, MD*

KEYWORDS

• Catheter ablation • Atrial flutter • Atrial fibrillation • Atrial tachycardia • Proarrhythmia

KEY POINTS

- Postablation atrial tachycardias (AT) may arise from either the left or right atrium, or from the CS.
- These tachycardias may be due to variety of mechanisms, including large or small reentrant circuits, or a focal mechanism.
- Although these tachycardias may be challenging, RF ablation is successful in approximately 90% of cases, with a low risk of complication.
- Recurrent AT after an acutely successful procedure may be due to resumption of conduction along linear lesions or emergence of a new arrhythmia substrate.
- Still, approximately 80% of patients can be rendered arrhythmia-free without the use of antiarrhythmic medications.

Patients undergoing catheter ablation of atrial fibrillation (AF) may develop organized atrial tachycardias (ATs) that may require a repeat ablation procedure. These arrhythmias usually originate from the left atrium (LA),[1] but may also arise from the coronary sinus (CS),[2] or the right atrium (RA). These postablation tachycardias differ from typical atrial flutter originating from the cavotricuspid isthmus (CTI) in many ways. Although the latter can be readily recognized by the classic appearance on the 12-lead electrocardiogram (ECG), postablation tachycardias lack an ECG signature. Typical flutter is caused by a macroreentrant circuit around the tricuspid annulus; however, there are multiple mechanisms and sites of origin responsible for postablation ATs. Radiofrequency (RF) ablation can eliminate typical flutter in virtually every patient. In contrast, mapping and ablation of postablation tachycardias is more challenging. This article discusses the various mechanisms of AT arising after AF ablation. A practical approach to mapping and ablation of these challenging arrhythmias is offered. The generic term AT is used to denote a tachycardia with any possible mechanism, as opposed to atrial flutter, which is reserved for macroreentrant tachycardias.

INCIDENCE OF POSTABLATION AT

LA reentrant AT unrelated to prior AF ablation or arrhythmia surgery is rare. However, the electrophysiologist performing catheter ablation of AF is sure to encounter organized AT during follow-up. The incidence of postablation AT depends on the ablation strategy that was used at the time of the AF procedure. If only the pulmonary veins (PVs) were targeted, for example, in patients with paroxysmal AF, the incidence of AT is about 3%.[3] The mechanism of these tachycardias is usually related to PV reconnection. When substrate ablation is performed, especially in the form of linear LA ablation, the incidence increases to 24% to 50%.[1,4] The mechanism of AT in many of these patients is macroreentry from the LA. The incidence and

Supported in part by a grant from the Leducq Transatlantic Network.
The authors have no conflicts of interest to disclose.
Division of Cardiovascular Medicine, University of Michigan, Ann Arbor, MI, USA
* Corresponding author. Cardiovascular Center, SPC 5853, 1500 East Medical Center Drive, Ann Arbor, MI 48109-5853.
E-mail address: achugh@umich.edu

http://dx.doi.org/10.1016/j.ccep.2012.06.007

the complexity of AT depend on the ablation approach during the AF procedure, and also on the underlying atrial substrate.

PREPARATION FOR THE PROCEDURE

The preparation for the AT procedure can be traced back to the initial consultation for catheter ablation of AF. During this consultation, we take the opportunity to inform our patients, especially those with persistent AF, along with their referring physicians, that there is good likelihood that they might require a repeat procedure for organized AT after the initial procedure for AF. Early recurrence of AT is common after an ablation procedure for persistent AF. If a patient develops arrhythmia recurrence within the first 3 months of the AF procedure, our practice is to perform a transthoracic cardioversion because early arrhythmias may be transient in some patients. A repeat ablation procedure is recommended to patients who develop AT after 3 months or after the transthoracic cardioversion.

Unlike the ablation procedure for typical flutter, during which catheter ablation may be performed in the arrhythmia or sinus rhythm, it is preferable to perform the procedure for postablation AT during the culprit arrhythmia. The rationale for this approach is that, in some patients, it may not be possible to induce the clinical arrhythmia, despite an aggressive induction protocol. An empiric ablation strategy in these patients is not only inefficient but may also be associated with arrhythmia recurrence and, possibly, electrical and mechanical sequelae related to extensive ablation.

For this reason, our practice is to discontinue antiarrhythmic medications when the patient develops persistent AT and a decision has been made to proceed with an AT procedure. In patients with paroxysmal AT, we recommend discontinuing antiarrhythmic medications approximately 4 weeks before the AT procedure. In the case of amiodarone, we recommend discontinuing the drug at least 2 months before the procedure. Some arrhythmias may not be inducible in patients who are still taking amiodarone, only to surface after it has been discontinued during follow-up. Rate-controlling medications should be discontinued approximately 48 hours before the procedure.

It is preferable to perform the ablation procedure while the patient is taking therapeutic doses of warfarin. This approach has been shown to be associated with a lower risk of vascular and thromboembolic complications. Given the higher risk of bleeding in patients taking dabigatran, our practice is to discontinue the drug for 36 hours before the ablation procedure. All patients presenting to the laboratory in an atrial arrhythmia undergo transesophageal echocardiography to rule out LA thrombus, irrespective of their anticoagulation status. The decision to perform transesophageal echocardiography in patients presenting in sinus rhythm should be individualized. In the absence of severe structural heart disease or atrial myopathy (which would have been discovered during the initial AF procedure), it is probably reasonable to defer transesophageal echocardiography given an extremely low risk of thrombosis, especially in the context of anticoagulation.

As alluded to earlier, it is important to be aware of the details of the prior AF procedure during preparation for the AT procedure. This information directly affects the mechanism and the complexity of the AT that will be encountered during the repeat session. If LA linear ablation were performed during the initial procedure, it is possible that the AT is caused by recovery of these lesions, which is common. Even if the AT is not related to the LA linear lesions that were deployed at the initial procedure, the operator is obligated to ensure completeness of the these lines at the end of the procedure. In contrast, if linear ablation had not been performed previously, empiric LA linear ablation, after elimination of the clinical AT, is probably not necessary.

ECG CLUES

The 12-lead ECG may be helpful in delineating the mechanism and chamber of origin of the AT. A prior study showed that the presence of an isoelectric interval between successive p-waves is consistent with a small, as opposed to a large or macroreentrant, circuit.[5] During macroreentry, there is continuous atrial activation that is responsible for the inscription of the p-wave. The diastolic interval is short, which helps explain the lack of an isoelectric interval during macroreentrant AT. For the same reason, wider p-waves are also expected during macroreentry as opposed to AT that is not caused by macroreentry. These rules may not be applicable in the setting of significant atrial scarring and conduction block, in which activation times may be long, even during focal arrhythmias.

Although most ATs after LA ablation arise from the LA or CS musculature, CTI flutter may also be encountered. Because LA ablation alters the flutter-wave morphology, the stereotypical ECG features may not be reliable in making a diagnosis of typical flutter. Nonetheless, the presence of negative flutter waves in the precordial leads suggests CTI flutter as opposed to left AT.

Negative flutter waves in the inferior leads, although less specific, may also be consistent with right atrial flutter. Isoelectric or positive p-waves throughout the precordium are consistent with an LA source. However, ECG features diagnostic of specific LA sites remain elusive.

MECHANISMS OF AT

Postablation AT may be caused by any possible mechanism, including large or macroreentrant circuits, small circuits, or a focal mechanism. In turn, a focal AT may be caused by microreentry, a triggered activity, or abnormal automaticity. It is important to delineate the mechanism of the AT before ablation because the procedural end points for AT caused by various mechanisms are different. For example, the end point for a focal AT is tachycardia termination and noninducibility. For macroreentrant circuits, the end point also includes demonstration of conduction block by strict electrophysiologic criteria.

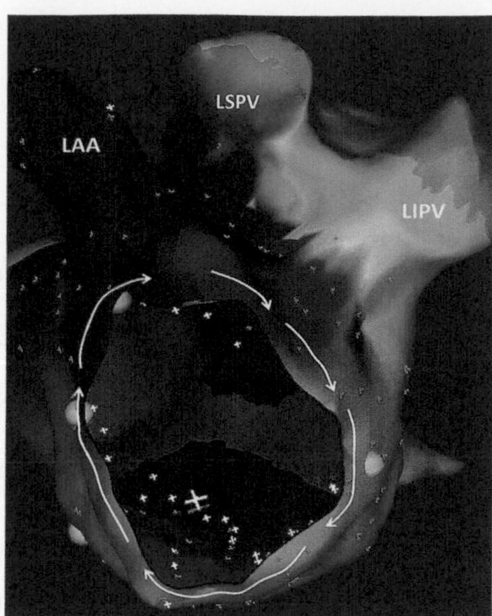

Fig. 1. Three-dimensional activation map during clockwise mitral isthmus–dependent atrial flutter. LAA, left atrial appendage; LIPV, left inferior pulmonary vein; LSPV, left superior pulmonary vein.

MAPPING AND ABLATION

Mitral Isthmus–Dependent Flutter

The most common LA macroreentrant circuit that is encountered after ablation of AF is mitral isthmus–dependent atrial flutter or perimitral reentry. Unlike typical atrial flutter during which there is counterclockwise activation around the tricuspid valve in most cases, the prevalence of counterclockwise and clockwise activation during perimitral flutter is nearly equal. The circuit is bounded by the mitral annulus and the left PVs. The criteria required to diagnose mitral isthmus–dependent atrial flutter include activation mapping, which accounts for more than 90% of the tachycardia cycle length (CL) and shows an early-meets-late pattern around the valve (**Fig. 1**); and entrainment mapping, which reveals that the postpacing interval (PPI) anywhere along the annulus approximates the tachycardia CL (within 20–30 milliseconds) (**Fig. 2**). If only entrainment mapping is used, the operator is obligated to show good return cycles from the opposite segments of the mitral annulus. For example, perimitral flutter is diagnosed if the PPIs from the lateral and septal, or anterior and inferior aspects of the mitral annulus approximate the tachycardia CL. This stipulation helps distinguish between large and small reentrant circuits (discussed later).

RF energy is delivered via an irrigated-tip ablation catheter (Thermocool, Biosense-Webster, Diamond Bar, CA) using 35 W. Although higher power settings are used in many laboratories (up to 50 W), there is probably a higher risk of steam pops and perforation with this approach. RF energy delivery is initiated at the ventricular aspect of the lateral mitral annulus and continued to the ostia of the left PVs (**Fig. 3**). If the tachycardia does not terminate despite voltage abatement or creation of local block along the isthmus, the next step is to deliver RF energy within the CS. The reason that epicardial ablation is required likely has to do with the local anatomy of the mitral isthmus. First, in about a third of cases, branches of the circumflex artery course over the epicardial isthmus.[6] The heat-sink effect of arterial flow through the circumflex may prevent adequate heating of the mitral isthmus. In addition, endocardial pouches, which are present in about 20% of patients, impede linear ablation at the mitral isthmus. Nearly all patients with pouches require epicardial ablation within the CS. In addition, the ligament of Marshall may be responsible for epicardial conduction over the isthmus. Overall, CS ablation is required in most cases either for tachycardia termination or linear block.

Before CS ablation, it is helpful to perform entrainment mapping from the distal CS to confirm that the mechanism is still perimitral flutter. Catheter ablation within the CS is commenced in the distal CS, starting at the level of the endocardial line. Use of a 3D mapping system is helpful in identifying the starting point within the CS. It is reasonable to reduce the power to 20 W during CS ablation to avoid collateral injury to the arterial system and other structures. The

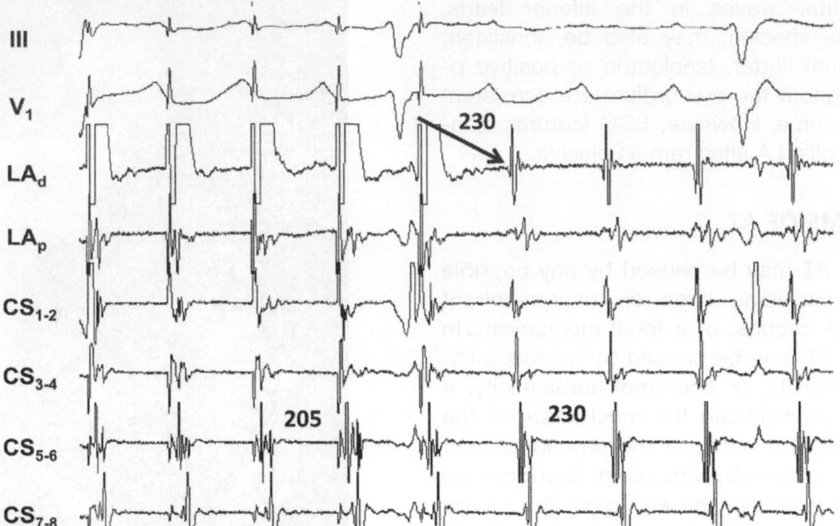

Fig. 2. Entrainment mapping from the lateral mitral annulus from the same patient as in **Fig. 1**. The postpacing interval matches the tachycardia CL, confirming the diagnosis of mitral isthmus–dependent flutter. Also shown are bipolar electrograms recorded by the distal and proximal bipoles of the left atrial (LAd and LAp) and coronary sinus (CS) catheters.

catheter is slowly withdrawn after 15 to 20 seconds, while observing the real-time impedance and temperature profiles. If the tachycardia does not terminate, the catheter is advanced again to the distal CS and the process is repeated. The incidence of arterial injury during CS ablation is high.[7] These arterial lesions are often clinically silent but occasionally present with acute myocardial infarction and life-threatening ventricular arrhythmias.

After tachycardia termination, pacing is performed to determine whether conduction block has been achieved across the mitral isthmus. It is convenient to pace the LA appendage (the ring catheter may be advanced to the base of the appendage) to check for block. In the presence of persistent conduction, CS activation precedes from the distal to the proximal electrodes. When block is achieved, there is a conduction detour, and the CS activated in a proximal-to-distal fashion (**Fig. 4**).[8]

Although it may be challenging, mitral isthmus block can be achieved in approximately 90% of cases. If the tachycardia does not terminated with

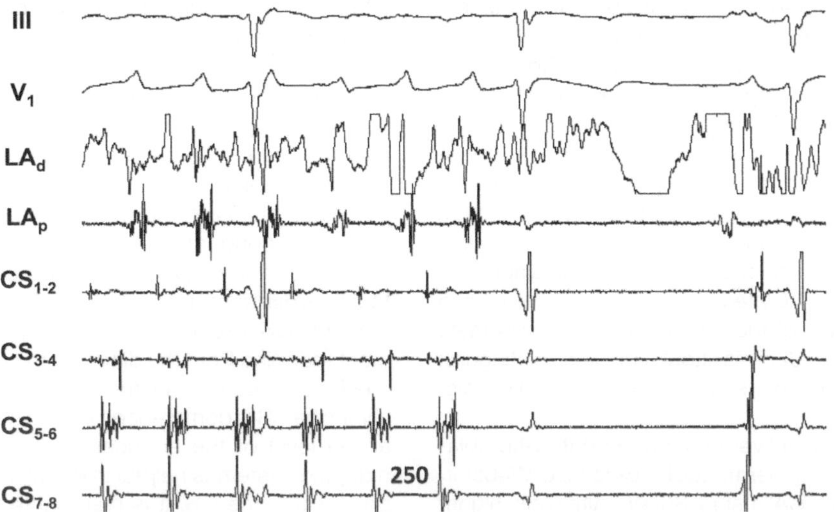

Fig. 3. Termination of perimitral flutter during endocardial RF ablation at the mitral isthmus in the same patient as in **Figs. 1** and **2**.

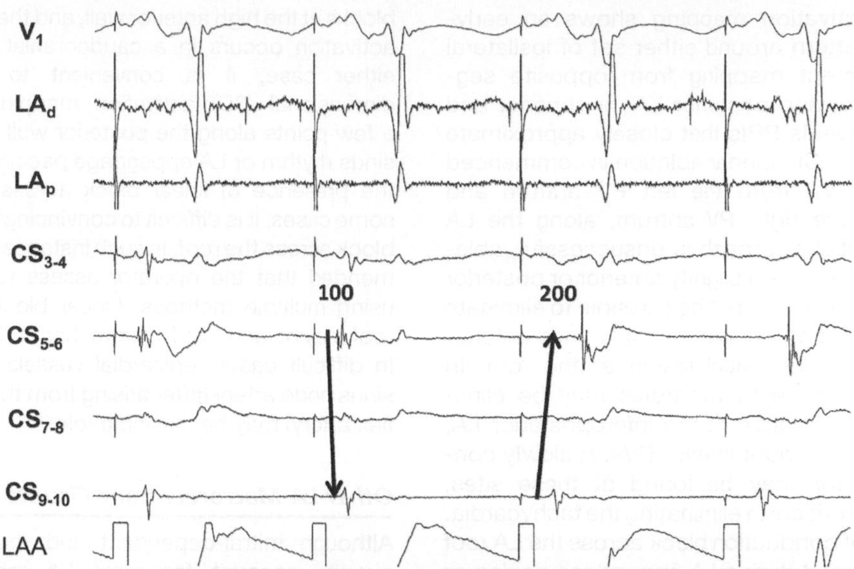

Fig. 4. Mitral isthmus block during RF energy delivery in the CS and pacing from the LAA. Note the sudden change in the activation of the CS, from distal to proximal to proximal to distal. The conduction delay also abruptly increases from 100 milliseconds to 200 milliseconds.

a lateral approach (including CS ablation), linear ablation may be performed anteriorly. In this case, linear ablation is commenced from the high anterior annulus, going over the base of the appendage, to the LA roof region, outside the left superior PV, or a longer line may be required, extending to the anterior aspect of the right superior PV. The anterior approach to perimitral reentry is not considered a first-line approach given its negative impact on LA appendage conduction and LA mechanical function.

Roof-Dependent Macroreentry

The second most common LA large reentrant circuit involves the LA roof. The wave front revolves around either the left-sided or right-sided PVs or both sets of ipsilateral PVs (double-loop reentry) (**Fig. 5**). The CS activation may be proximal to distal, or distal to proximal. The diagnostic criteria for this macroreentrant circuit are similar to those defined for perimitral reentry. In

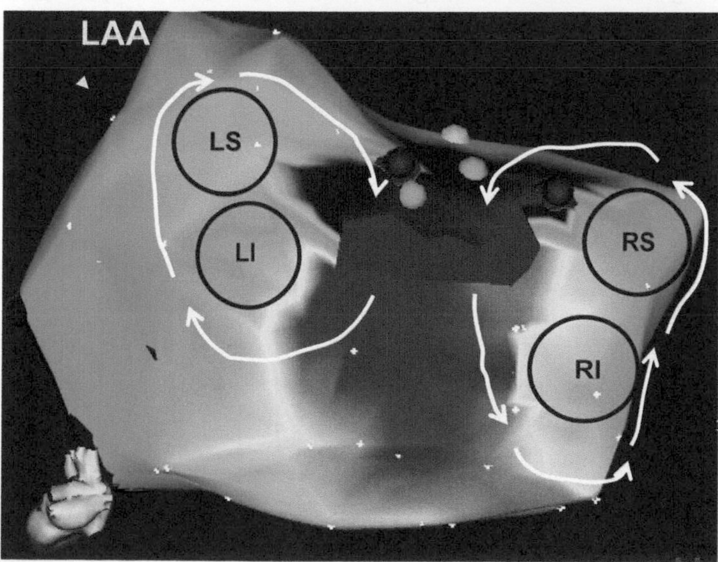

Fig. 5. Three-dimensional activation map during roof-dependent atrial flutter. There are 2 loops around the ipsilateral PV that intersect at the midposterior LA. The tachycardia was eliminated during linear ablation at the roof. LI, left inferior; LS, left superior; RI, right inferior; RS, right superior.

this case, activation mapping shows an early-meets-late pattern around either set of ipsilateral PVs. Entrainment mapping from opposite segments (anterior and posterior LA, or superior and inferior LA) reveals PPIs that closely approximate the tachycardia CL. Linear ablation is commenced (using 25–30 W) from the left PV antrum and extended to the right PV antrum, along the LA roof. If the initial approach is unsuccessful, ablation may be performed slightly anterior or posterior to the initial line. It may not be possible to eliminate these tachycardias despite multiple lines anterior or posterior to the initial lesion at the roof. In such a case, these tachycardias may be eliminated with RF ablation at the inferoposterior LA, outside the left or right inferior PVs. A slowly conducting corridor may be found at these sites, which may be critical in eliminating the tachycardia.

Presence of conduction block across the LA roof may be assessed during LA appendage pacing or during sinus rhythm. During LA appendage pacing, a corridor of double potentials should be observed across the roof (**Fig. 6**).[8] A quick method of ascertaining block across the roof is to inspect activation of the posterior LA. During LA appendage pacing in the presence of linear block, the paced wave front blocks at the anterior aspect of the roof, and, as a result, activation along the posterior LA proceeds in an ascending fashion. In the presence of conduction across the roof, activation along the posterior LA occurs in a descending fashion. An even simpler approach is to assess posterior LA activation during sinus rhythm (**Fig. 7**). After interatrial conduction across the Bachmann bundle, the wave front, in the setting of conduction block, again blocks at the high anterior wall, and the posterior LA activation occurs in a caudocranial direction. In either case, it is convenient to use three-dimensional (3D) activation mapping to collect a few points along the posterior wall during either sinus rhythm or LA appendage pacing to check for the presence of linear block across the roof. In some cases, it is difficult to convincingly show linear block across the roof. In such instances, it is recommended that the operator assess for roof block using multiple methods. Linear block across the roof may be achieved in more than 90% of patients. In difficult cases, epicardial vessels such as the sinus node artery (after arising from the left circumflex artery) may be playing a role.[9]

Other LA Macroreentrant Circuits

Although mitral-dependent and roof-dependent circuits account for most LA macroreentrant circuits, other large circuits may be encountered. One such circuit involves the anterior LA, during which the septal annulus, the right-sided PVs, and conduction block at the roof act as barriers to stabilize the arrhythmia. Linear ablation from the annulus to the right-sided PVs may terminate the tachycardia, frequently at the region of Bachmann bundle, located at the high anterior wall, outside the right superior PV. Often, the analogous portion of septal RA is involved. In such cases, linear ablation is performed from the septal aspect of the RA/superior vena cava and extended across the septal base of the RA appendage to the anterior tricuspid annulus. This circuit probably constitutes the most complex reentrant circuit that is

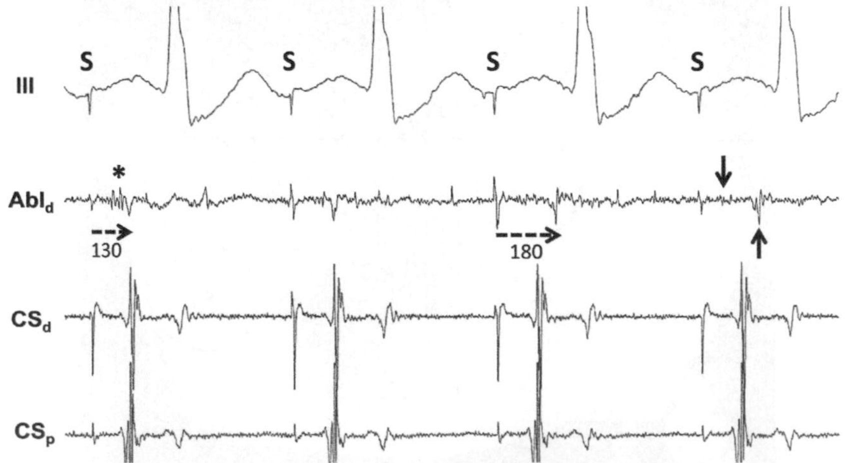

Fig. 6. Conduction block across the LA roof during RF ablation at the LA roof. During LA appendage pacing, the complex electrogram (*asterisk*) recorded by the ablation catheter (Abl) gives way to a split electrogram (*small arrows*), consistent with conduction block. The stimulus-to-electrogram interval (*dashed arrows*) also increases with the creation of conduction block. S, stimulus.

A Right Lateral

LAA
LSPV
LIPV
RSPV
RIPV

B Postero-anterior

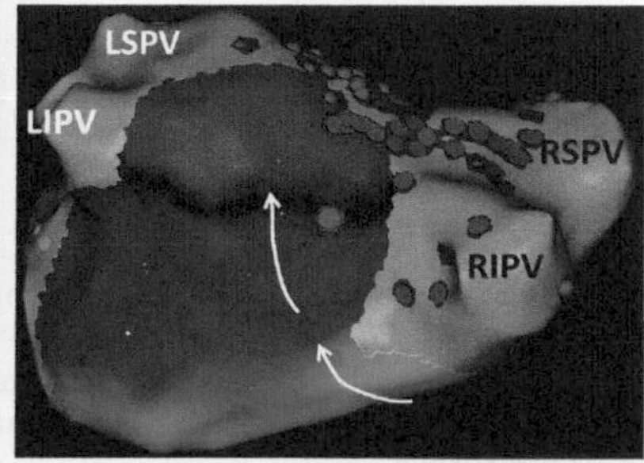

Fig. 7. Conduction block across the LA roof during sinus rhythm. (*A*) The LA breakthrough during sinus rhythm occurs at the region of the Bachmann bundle, outside the right superior pulmonary vein (RSPV). The wave front then blocks at the roof owing to conduction block. As a result, the posterior LA is activated in an ascending fashion. (*B*) Posteroanterior view. RIPV, right inferior pulmonary vein.

encountered in treatment of postablation ATs. One of the reasons that little is known about these circuits is that the area of slow conduction may reside in the epicardium, at the Bachmann bundle. Epicardial mapping may confirm this hypothesis and may obviate extensive biatrial linear endocardial ablation.

Small Reentrant Circuits

Small reentrant circuits, or localized reentry,[10] constitute an important mechanism of postablation AT. They differ from macroreentrant circuits in number of ways. First, the reentrant circuit is relegated to only 1 segment of the atrium, and the remaining portion of the atrium is activated in a passive, centrifugal fashion. For example, a common site for localized reentry after AF ablation is the lateral LA, near the ridge, bounded by the left-side PVs. In contrast with macroreentry involving the mitral annulus, during which the septal, anterior, lateral, and inferior segments are all components of the reentrant circuit, the reentrant circuit in this case is localized only to the lateral LA. Entrainment mapping reveals long return cycles, even at sites a few millimeters away from sites with excellent return cycles. This behavior is incompatible with macroreentry. Another hallmark of small circuits is the presence of very fractionated electrograms at the reentry site, accounting for much of the tachycardia CL (**Fig. 8**). This phenomenon is caused by extremely slow conduction. Interpretation of a 3D activation map during localized reentry may be challenging because of difficulty in adjudicating local activation time given the complex electrograms. Small reentrant circuits may be found virtually anywhere in the LA or RA, or even in the CS. Because of the presence of slow conduction at the critical site, these circuits are readily responsive to RF energy delivery. Tachycardia termination and noninducibility are appropriate end points for ablation of small reentrant circuits.

Focal AT After AF Ablation

It is important to be able to map and ablate focal tachycardias that arise after AF ablation. In some cases, these focal tachycardias are responsible for initiating AF. Mapping of focal AT after catheter ablation of AF is similar to mapping of focal arrhythmias in general. Activation mapping classically shows centrifugal activation from the site of origin (**Fig. 9**). However, in patients who have undergone extensive ablation or with preexisting atrial uncoupling, activation mapping may reveal nonsensical activation patterns. For this reason, it is important to clearly define the onset of the p-wave on the 12-lead ECG. The local electrogram is then compared with the p-wave onset to determine activation. If the p-wave not clearly visible, burst ventricular pacing is helpful and usually does not perturb the tachycardia, which may be the case with adenosine infusion. The initial

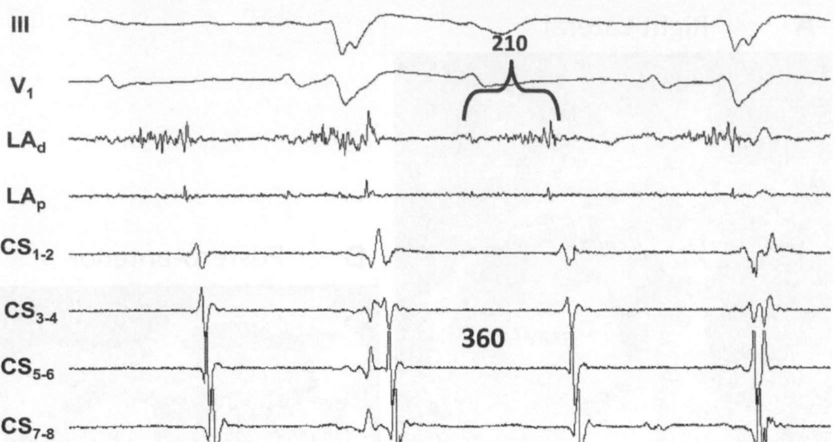

Fig. 8. Fractionated electrogram recorded from the base of the left atrial appendage, which accounts for 58% of the tachycardia CL. Mapping confirmed the presence of a small reentrant circuit emanating from the base of the LA appendage. Entrainment mapping at this site terminated the tachycardia without global capture, which confirmed that this site was critical to the maintenance of the tachycardia. RF ablation at this site rendered the tachycardia noninducible.

portion of the p-wave may also be isoelectric in multiple leads, making it challenging to define the p-wave onset.

Multiloop AT

Multiloop AT is defined as a tachycardia that requires ablation of more than 1 distinct isthmus/site for tachycardia termination. A clue to the presence of one of these challenging arrhythmias is that, despite extensive ablation over a particular isthmus, there is no change in the tachycardia CL, activation sequence, or p-wave morphology. The only clue that the tachycardia mechanism has changed is gleaned from entrainment mapping. For example, if after extensive ablation of a perimitral flutter there is no change in the tachycardia, entrainment mapping from the mitral isthmus may reveal a PPI, which had approximated the tachycardia CL before ablation, that is now long. The next step is to perform entrainment mapping at another isthmus/site. Further ablation

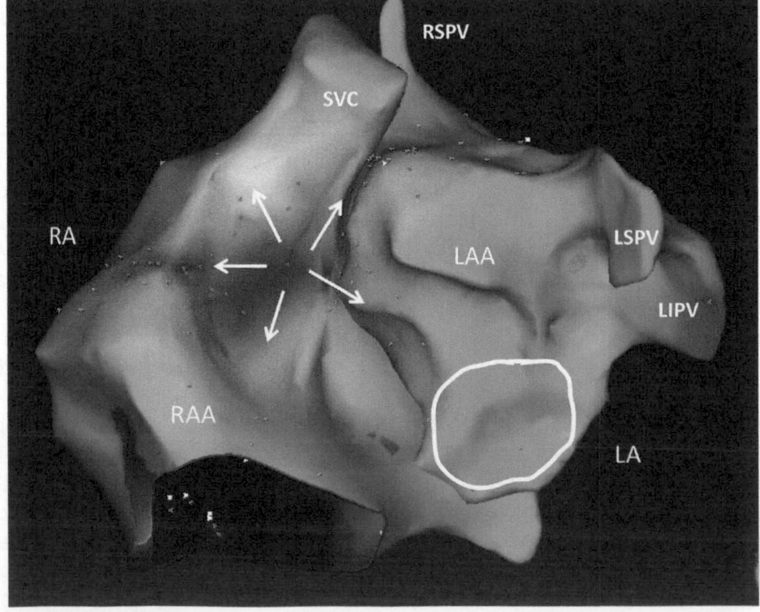

Fig. 9. Biatrial activation map during a right atrial focal tachycardia originating from the septum. Note the radial spread from the site of origin. RAA, right atrial appendage; SVC, superior vena cava.

is then guided by results of entrainment mapping. These arrhythmias are challenging because RF ablation may be required at several distinct isthmi/sites before termination. Linear block must then be confirmed at all the isthmi ablated, along with verifying PV isolation and noninducibility. Thus, multiloop tachycardias are time consuming and may be associated with a higher rate of recurrence as compared with procedures during which only 1 isthmus/site is involved.

Entrainment Versus Activation Mapping

Postablation ATs may be mapped using activation or entrainment mapping. There are advantages and disadvantages to both approaches. The main advantage of entrainment mapping that it can potentially provide the operator with the mechanistic information within a few minutes. Herein lies a pitfall. There seems to be a strong urge to start ablating immediately after a single, good PPI is obtained. However, identification of a single component of a reentrant circuit does not define the mechanism. More data, either via activation or entrainment mapping, are required to fully delineate the mechanism before delivery of RF energy. As discussed previously, defining the mechanism of the tachycardia helps determine the procedural end points. The biggest drawback to a strategy that solely uses entrainment mapping is that the pacing may alter or terminate the tachycardia, which may not be reinducible.

Activation mapping using a 3D mapping system allows the operator to visualize the circuit in 3 dimensions, and is also associated with lower fluoroscopy times. In most cases, mechanistic information can be obtained without perturbing the tachycardia. The main disadvantage of constructing a 3D activation map is that it is time consuming and that it may afford nonsensical activation patterns in patients with atrial myopathy or conduction block. In the near future, multielectrode mapping may shorten the time required to construct a high-density activation map. In practice, most clinicians use a combination of activation (either with or without[10] a 3D mapping system) and entrainment mapping.

RESULTS

The end points of tachycardia termination, linear block across the mitral isthmus and roof, reisolation of the PVs (as needed), and noninducibility can be achieved in approximately 90% of patients. However, despite this rigorous end point, approximately 25% of patients present for another procedure for arrhythmia recurrence, which is usually caused by AT and not AF. In about one-half of these patients, recurrence is caused by resumption of conduction along the mitral isthmus or roof, which speaks to the challenge of creating permanent, transmural linear lesions. In the remaining patients, recurrence is caused by development of novel small circuits that were not present during the prior AT procedure. Overall, approximately 80% of patients can be rendered arrhythmia free without the use of antiarrhythmic medications. In patients without a history of stroke or severe atrial scarring, oral anticoagulation is usually discontinued if long-term monitoring fails to reveal arrhythmia recurrence.

SAFETY CONCERNS

In a series of 173 consecutive patients undergoing 226 ablation procedures for postablation AT, serious complications arose during 2 procedures (1%). One patient developed tamponade immediately after the ablation procedure and required percutaneous drainage. In another patient, CS ablation for mitral isthmus block resulted in occlusion of the distal circumflex, which was discovered several months after the ablation procedure. Also, LA appendage isolation occurred in 5 (2%) patients. One patient required a permanent pacemaker as a result of intra-atrial dissociation. Extensive atrial uncoupling was present in these patients before the procedure.

SUMMARY

Mapping and ablation of post-AF AT is among the most challenging electrophysiologic procedures. These tachycardias may be caused by multiple mechanisms and may arise from the left or right atrium, or the CS. It is critical to define the precise mechanism before ablation because the procedural end point depends on the correct diagnosis. Using the approach described earlier, postablation ATs can be successfully ablated in approximately 90% of patients. However, a significant number of patients experience recurrence despite rigorous procedural end points.

Given the complexity of these arrhythmias, efforts should also be focused on decreasing the incidence of AT after AF ablation. One way to do this is to minimize the use of linear ablation during the AF procedure. Prospective studies are needed to identify patients who do and do not require linear ablation during a procedure for persistent AF. It is hoped that such a tailored approach will help maintain the high success rate of eliminating persistent AF,[11] and decrease the likelihood of repeat procedures for AT.

REFERENCES

1. Chugh A, Oral H, Lemola K, et al. Prevalence, mechanisms, and clinical significance of macroreentrant atrial tachycardia during and following left atrial ablation for atrial fibrillation. Heart Rhythm 2005;2:464–71.
2. Chugh A, Oral H, Good E, et al. Catheter ablation of atypical atrial flutter and atrial tachycardia within the coronary sinus after left atrial ablation for atrial fibrillation. J Am Coll Cardiol 2005;46:83–91.
3. Gerstenfeld EP, Callans DJ, Dixit S, et al. Mechanisms of organized left atrial tachycardias occurring after pulmonary vein isolation. Circulation 2004;110:1351–7.
4. Knecht S, Hocini M, Wright M, et al. Left atrial linear lesions are required for successful treatment of persistent atrial fibrillation. Eur Heart J 2008;29:2359–66.
5. Shah D, Sunthorn H, Burri H, et al. Narrow, slow-conducting isthmus dependent left atrial reentry developing after ablation for atrial fibrillation: ECG characterization and elimination by focal RF ablation. J Cardiovasc Electrophysiol 2006;17:508–15.
6. Yokokawa M, Sundaram B, Garg A, et al. Impact of mitral isthmus anatomy on the likelihood of achieving linear block in patients undergoing catheter ablation of persistent atrial fibrillation. Heart Rhythm 2011;8:1404–10.
7. Wong KC, Lim C, Sadarmin PP, et al. High incidence of acute sub-clinical circumflex artery 'injury' following mitral isthmus ablation. Eur Heart J 2011;32:1881–90.
8. Hocini M, Jais P, Sanders P, et al. Techniques, evaluation, and consequences of linear block at the left atrial roof in paroxysmal atrial fibrillation: a prospective randomized study. Circulation 2005;112:3688–96.
9. Yokokawa M, Sundaram B, Oral H, et al. The course of the sinus node artery and its impact on achieving linear block at the left atrial roof in patients with persistent atrial fibrillation Heart Rhythm 2012, in press.
10. Jais P, Matsuo S, Knecht S, et al. A deductive mapping strategy for atrial tachycardia following atrial fibrillation ablation: importance of localized reentry. J Cardiovasc Electrophysiol 2009;20:480–91.
11. Haissaguerre M, Hocini M, Sanders P, et al. Catheter ablation of long-lasting persistent atrial fibrillation: clinical outcome and mechanisms of subsequent arrhythmias. J Cardiovasc Electrophysiol 2005;16:1138–47.

Atrial Fibrillation Ablation in Obese Patients

Matthew Needleman, MD,
Hugh Calkins, MD, FACC, FHRS, FAHA*

KEYWORDS

• Atrial fibrillation • Obesity • Catheter ablation • Body mass index • Sleep apnea

KEY POINTS

- Obesity plays a strong role in the development and progression of atrial fibrillation (AF) likely through a direct effect on left atrial size.
- Obese patients have similar, if not slightly improved mortality in AF, described as the "obesity paradox."
- Catheter ablation for AF in obese patients is a reasonable option, but patients should be screened for presence of sleep apnea and counseled extensively about the likely need for longer procedure times and the possibility of repeat procedures to achieve similar success rates.
- Obese patients can be reassured that their quality of life will likely improve after successful ablation.

INTRODUCTION

Case Example

An obese 50-year-old gentleman presents for evaluation of recurrent paroxysmal atrial fibrillation (AF). He is highly symptomatic with episodic palpitations, dyspnea, and fatigue, and notes that these symptoms have been increasing in frequency. Despite routine evaluations and recommendations from his internist, he has not been able to lose weight and continues to have a body mass index (BMI) of 35 kg/m^2. His internist has screened him for both obstructive sleep apnea (OSA) and diabetes, and thus far he does not have either condition. A recent echocardiogram shows a structurally normal heart with a normal left ventricular ejection fraction, mild left atrial enlargement, and no significant valvular pathology. Noninvasive stress testing showed no evidence of myocardial ischemia. Despite therapy with flecainide and metoprolol, the patient continues to have symptomatic AF and presents to discuss additional treatment options.

This case highlights several important questions. First, what is the relationship between AF and obesity? Second, are different outcomes possible depending on the natural history of AF in obese patients or different management strategies? Finally, how do obese patients respond to and tolerate catheter ablation for AF?

As epidemic increases in both obesity and AF continue in the United States, clinicians will need to understand the associations between the two conditions and the treatment implications of their combined management. Current estimates predict that AF will be present in more than 10 million Americans in 2050.[1] Obesity also continues to be a major public health concern, and results of the National Health and Nutrition Examination Survey (NHANES) estimate the prevalence of overweight adults (BMI >25 kg/m^2) to be 68.0% and of obese adults (BMI >30 kg/m^2) to be 33.8%.[2] This contemporary review discusses the epidemiology and pathophysiology of the association between AF and obesity. It also reviews the natural history and outcomes in the obese patients with AF. Based

Dr Calkins serves as a consultant for Sanofi Aventi, Biosense Webster, Medtronic, and Atricures.
Dr Needleman has nothing to disclose.

Section of Cardiac Electrophysiology, Division of Cardiology, Johns Hopkins Medical Institutes, Sheikh Zayed Tower - Room 7125, 1800 Orleans Street, Baltimore, MD 21287, USA
* Corresponding author.
E-mail address: hcalkins@jhmi.edu

Card Electrophysiol Clin 4 (2012) 327–334
http://dx.doi.org/10.1016/j.ccep.2012.05.010
1877-9182/12/$ – see front matter

on recent advances in catheter ablation of AF, the effect of obesity on the procedure are reviewed, such as the procedural success rates, quality-of-life measures, and complication rates from the procedure in this growing population.

EPIDEMIOLOGY OF AF AND OBESITY

Multiple studies have shown that surrogate markers such as left atrial enlargement are associated with obesity,[3] and recent large studies have shown an association between obesity and new-onset AF.

Framingham Cohort Study

In a large prospective community-based observation cohort study from Framingham, Massachusetts, 5282 patients without a history of AF were evaluated and followed for a mean of 13.7 years.[4] Age-adjusted incidence rates for AF increased with increasing BMI, and for every one-unit increase in BMI, a 4% increase in AF was seen. In multivariate analysis that corrected for cardiovascular risk factors and myocardial infarction, the strong association between obesity and new-onset AF remained, but when adjusted for left atrial diameter, BMI was no longer associated with AF risk. This finding suggests that obesity increases AF risk though increasing the left atrial diameter.

Danish Study

In a large study of more than 47,000 patients from Denmark, obese men and women had an adjusted hazard ratio of 2.35 (CI, 1.70–3.25) and 1.99 (CI, 1.31–3.02) for developing AF compared with normal weight subjects.[5] The strength of this study was the large study size and large numbers of patients developing AF (553 total patients). Despite the large size, additional information such as echocardiographic left atrial size were not available. A large meta-analysis of 16 studies involving 123,249 patients was performed in obese patients.[6] In this large meta-analysis, obesity was found to increase the risk of developing AF by 49% compared with the normal population, and a linear relationship between development of AF and increases in BMI was seen.

Swedish Primary Prevention Study

Other risk factors in addition to obesity play a role in the development of AF in midlife. In the Swedish Primary Prevention study, 6903 men were evaluated during a single visit during midlife.[7] In addition to obesity, body surface area (BSA) at 20 years of age from recalled weight and height measurement and weight gain from 20 years of age to midlife were also both strongly associated with development of AF. Although no echocardiographic evidence was available in this study, the authors suggest that this may be related to left atrial size. This theory that larger men with large BSA have higher rates of AF has biologic plausibility. Rats have infrequent atrial fibrillation, whereas larger mammals such as horses have a significant AF burden, suggesting that an animal's size is an important determinant in the development of AF.[8]

Olmsted County, Minnesota Study

Obesity has also been shown to have a significant effect on the progression of and development of AF. In a longitudinal cohort study of Olmsted County, Minnesota, identified 3248 patients with paroxysmal AF who where then followed for progression to permanent AF.[9] BMI, left atrial size, and progression of AF were then analyzed over a median follow-up of 5.1 years. After adjusting for age and sex, BMI had a significant effect on progression of AF (hazard ratio [HR], 1.54; CI, 1.2–2.0). In the subset of patients who had echocardiographic data, left atrial volume incrementally added to the progression of AF, but did not weaken the BMI association with progression to permanent AF. This study shows that both BMI and increased left atrial size are independent predictors of progression to permanent AF.

Women's Health Study

Another interesting study evaluated short- and long-term changes in BMI as part of the Women's Health Study and correlated these with development of new-onset AF.[10] Overall, the authors found a linear relationship, with a 4.7% increase in risk for new-onset AF development per kg/m^2 of BMI over the mean follow-up of 12.9 years, similar to findings of previous studies. The most novel part of this study was that in women younger than 60 years, short-term elevations in BMI seen over the first 60 months of the study had a 41% adjusted increase of developing AF compared with those who maintained a nonobese BMI (<30 kg/m^2). The investigators estimated that short-term increase in BMI was directly attributable to 18.3% of incident AF development, even after adjusting for markers of inflammation. This study suggests that on a population level, a weight control strategy may reduce the societal burden of AF.

Niigata Preventive Medicine Study

Many patients with obesity have a concurrent metabolic syndrome, with increased blood pressure, high fasting glucose, dyslipidemia, and abdominal adiposity as evidenced by increased waist circumference. In a prospective observational cohort study of more than 28,000 patients, the obesity component of the metabolic syndrome had a hazard ratio of 1.64 for the development of AF at 4.5 years, second only to the elevated blood pressure component as an AF risk factor.[11]

The Reasons for Geographic and Racial Differences in Stroke and Atherosclerosis Risk in Communities Studies

Results of the Reasons for Geographic and Racial Differences in Stroke (REGARDS) study, a large population-based study to oversample African American adults from the southern United States, showed that each additional component of the metabolic syndrome increased the risk of AF development in a linear fashion.[12] In addition to BMI alone, this study showed that waist circumference was also a strong predictor of AF development, with an odds ratio of 1.17 when adjusted for age, gender, race, education, income, physical activity, smoking, and nonsteroidal antiinflammatory drug use in this large cohort of more than 30,000 patients. In another large study looking at multiple risk factors for development of AF from the Atherosclerosis Risk in Communities (ARIC) study, obesity was again the second leading risk factor for AF development, secondary to hypertension.[13] Despite having higher rates of hypertension and obesity, African Americans seemed to have lower rates of AF compared with whites, suggesting a yet unexplained genetic difference in this group. This study concluded that, overall, 56.5% of AF cases could be attributed to at least one risk factor that was potentially preventable.

PATHOPHYSIOLOGY OF AF IN OBESE PATIENTS

Although the epidemiologic association between AF and obesity has been well described, the pathophysiology of this association is less clear. A relationship seems to exist among obesity, inflammation, and AF development. C-reactive protein (CRP) has been shown to be elevated in patients with metabolic syndrome[14] and also in those with AF.[15] Postablation elevated CRP elevations also help to explain early recurrences of AF after successful ablation.[16] In addition, high levels of adiponectin, an adipocyte-derived plasma protein, have been found in patients with persistent AF, suggesting that obesity plays a direct inflammatory role in AF.[17]

Pericardial adipose tissue has also been shown to have a direct effect on development of AF. The volume of pericardial fat tissue was highly associated with paroxysmal and persistent AF independent of traditional risk factors, including BMI.[18,19] Pericardial fat has also been associated with poorer outcomes after AF ablation.[20] Chang and colleagues[21] showed that patients with metabolic syndrome undergoing catheter ablation for AF had a higher incidence of shorter complex fractional atrial electrogram intervals and a higher incidence of nonpulmonary vein origins of AF. The authors suggest that more fat infiltration in the left atrium may interfere with left atrial conduction and contribute to these findings. In addition, ganglionated plexuses are frequently found in adipose tissue. These ganglionated plexuses are frequently associated with initiation and maintenance of AF, and ablation of these areas provide incremental value over pulmonary vein isolation.[22]

Because the posterior wall of the left atrium is located near central adipose tissue, this epicardial adipose tissue likely affects the initiation and maintenance of AF though both inflammatory and direct infiltrative effects of the fat.[23] The direct effect of this adipose tissue is to induce atrial tachyarrhythmias though paracrine effects of adipocytokines and other inflammatory markers. The left atrium then responds by producing fibrosis and fatty infiltration that provide the substrate for maintaining AF. This complex cascade of events provides multiple potential options for therapeutic approaches to reduce the effects of obesity on AF.

RATE CONTROL, RHYTHM CONTROL, AND MORTALITY OF OBESE PATIENTS WITH AF

Although the incidence of AF is higher in patients with obesity, its influence on outcomes in these patients has also been described. A post hoc analysis was performed using available BMI data from the Atrial Fibrillation Follow-up Investigation of Rhythm Management (AFFIRM) study.[24] Although BMI data were unavailable for 1542 patients, the remaining patients were classified as having normal BMIs (18.5–25 kg/m^2), overweight BMIs (25–30 kg/m^2), and obese BMIs (>30 kg/m^2). More than 74.4% of all patients were overweight or obese. Overall, the overweight and obese patients were younger but had a higher prevalence of hypertension, myocardial infarction, congestive heart failure, diabetes, and coronary artery disease. The overweight and obese patients had larger left atrial size and were more likely to be undergoing medical therapy for hyperlipidemia and hypertension. Using normal BMI as a reference, patients in the overweight and obese groups were less likely to experience death, cardiovascular death, or the combined end point. The HR for the overweight group was 0.64 (95% CI, 0.48–0.84) and was 0.80 (95% CI, 0.68–0.93) for the obese group.

Another post hoc analysis from the AFFIRM trial found similar results with regard to a reduced mortality in both the overweight and obese patients.[25] This analysis also showed that the obese patients had higher resting heart rates and were more poorly controlled with the rate-control strategy at 1 year. The rhythm-control strategy showed no significant differences in achieving sinus rhythm between the overweight and obese groups compared with the normal weight groups. Both analyses suggest multiple pathophysiologic reasons for this apparent "obesity paradox," including the possibility of malnutrition and cardiac cachexia in the normal weight subjects. The most important message from both these studies is that treatment strategies do not significantly differ for obese and normal weight subjects, but that rate control may be more difficult in obese patients.

OUTCOMES OF CATHETER ABLATION FOR AF IN OBESE PATIENTS

As catheter ablation techniques continue to improve and ablation becomes a more established treatment for patients with symptomatic AF,[26,27] several studies have evaluated outcomes in catheter ablation for AF in obese patients. This section reviews the four prospective studies on this subject, and highlights the conflicting results.

Mayo Clinic Study

The first published study investigated 523 patients with highly symptomatic AF undergoing catheter ablation at the Mayo Clinic.[28] These patients were enrolled between 2000 and 2005 and followed through October 2006; 82% of patients were classified as either overweight or obese. These patients tended to be younger, had more-advanced AF (persistent or permanent), and had more hypertension, diabetes, structural heart disease, sleep apnea, and left atrial enlargement. Over the mean follow-up period of 12 months, 72% of patients were free from AF and did not require antiarrhythmic drugs. In the overweight and obese groups, the freedom from AF off antiarrhythmic drugs was 72% and 70%, respectively, and no statistically significant difference was seen. Although overall outcomes were not statistically different, more patients in the higher BMI group had to undergo repeat procedures, and 48% of these patients had atrial flutter as the presenting rhythm for the second procedure. On multivariate analysis, the only significant variable for AF recurrence was preprocedure AF duration. Quality of life was significantly lower in the higher BMI groups at baseline as assessed using the SF-36 questionnaire. After ablation at 3 and 12 months, all BMI groups had a significant increase in quality of life, but the higher BMI group continued to have the lowest scores. No statistically significant differences were seen in complication rates, but increases in procedure times and the radiation dose were seen in the higher BMI groups.

University of Michigan Study

The next study evaluating outcomes from catheter ablation for AF in obese subjects was published from University of Michigan group.[29] Between July 2005 and June 2006, 324 consecutive patients undergoing catheter ablation were evaluated and stratified as normal weight, overweight, and obese. At a mean duration of 7 months, the patients with OSA had a significant reduction in success off antiarrhythmic drugs compared with those without OSA (41% vs. 63%, respectively; $P = .02$). With respect to BMI, on univariate analysis, each one-unit increase in BMI was associated with a 5% increase in the recurrence of AF after a single ablation procedure. On multivariate analysis after adjustment for age; gender; type and duration of AF; left atrial size; and left ventricular ejection fraction, BMI as a continuous variable or as classified in groups as overweight or obese did not prove to be significant. No statistically significant complications were seen between groups and no difference was seen in procedure times, but obese patients had higher fluoroscopy doses and more radiofrequency applications than normal weight patients. In summary, although OSA was in independent predictor of lower success after a single catheter ablation procedure for AF, overweight and obese BMIs were not independent predictors of lower success rates.

European Study

A recent study from Europe also evaluated the impact BMI has on catheter ablation for AF.[30] This study included 226 consecutive patients with highly symptomatic drug-refractory AF who underwent catheter ablation. Of this group, 63.3 patients were overweight or obese. Of these, more were likely to be younger, have hypertension, have increased left atrial diameter, and have increased markers of inflammation compared with normal weight subjects. After a mean follow-up of 432 days, 58% of patients were in sinus rhythm without antiarrhythmic medications. Although not statistically significant, a trend was seen toward higher AF recurrence in the obese and overweight groups. The mean procedure time was longer in the obese subjects, and radiation exposure was also significantly higher in the obese and overweight subjects. No significant differences in complications were seen between the groups.

Johns Hopkins Study

Another prospective study from the Johns Hopkins group showed significantly different results.[31] In this study, 109 consecutive patients were followed for a mean duration of 11 months. All patients underwent screening with the Berlin questionnaire for OSA and all underwent catheter ablation for AF. Of all patients, 69% had clinical success as defined by at least a 90% reduction in AF burden after a 3-month blanking period. On univariate analysis, persistent AF, elevated BMI, and OSA were all risk factors for failure after catheter ablation for AF. On multivariate analysis though, only BMI was an independent predictor of failure after catheter ablation for AF. As a continuous variable, each unit increase in BMI increased the probability of procedural failure by 11%. When evaluated by groups, the odds ratio of procedural failure was 3.28 (95% CI, 0.93–11.6; $P = .06$) in overweight patients and 3.84 (95% CI, 1.04–14.27; $P = .04$) in obese patients. Although no significant differences were seen in procedural times or fluoroscopy times in all groups, all four major complications occurred in the overweight or obese patients, whereas no complications occurred in the normal weight patients. Two patients had hypotension, likely caused by a protamine reaction; one patient had an arteriovenous fistula that was managed conservatively; and a final patient had cardiac tamponade treated with a pericardial drain.

Analysis of Mayo Clinic, University of Michigan, European, and Johns Hopkins Studies

What is the explanation for the desperate results among these four studies? First, two of the studies did not include OSA, and the Michigan group only evaluated a small number of patients with a sleep study. Thus, the effects of concurrent OSA in these studies could not be fully evaluated. Because sleep studies are expensive and time-consuming, a simple validated test such as the Berlin questionnaire[32] may provide additional information about OSA in patients with obesity. Another major difference in these studies is that the Mayo group included repeat procedures in their overall success rates, whereas the other groups only evaluated the initial procedure. All groups showed elevated radiation doses in the obese groups, but the Hopkins group reported fluoroscopy instead, which may also help explain this difference. Finally, with regard to complications, all groups had low complication rates and defined major complications slightly differently. The European group did not specify the types of complications, and the Mayo Clinic group did not include vascular complications. In both the Michigan and Hopkins groups, vascular complications seemed to occur in the overweight and obese groups but not in the normal weight groups.

Additional Studies

Additional studies have confirmed the importance of BMI in AF recurrence after catheter ablation. In a case-control study of patients undergoing catheter ablation for AF, a weight of more than 200 lb was a significant predictor of very late recurrence.[33] In another study, 72 patients with paroxysmal or persistent AF underwent ablation and after a mean duration of 12.5 months, 61% remained in sinus rhythm without antiarrhythmic medications.[34] On univariate analysis, BMI, left atrial dimension, and markers of inflammation were all associated with recurrent AF. On multivariate analysis, however, hypertension and left atrial diameter were significant, whereas BMI was not. Another study evaluated 186 patients with drug-refractory AF who underwent catheter ablation.[35] In this study's multivariate analysis, predictors of late recurrence of AF included the overweight/obese group, with an odds ration of 4.71 (95% CI, 1.71–12.98; P .003), which was the strongest predictor in the study. Taken together, these studies suggest that overweight and obese patients have more recurrence of AF after catheter ablation for AF.

QUALITY OF LIFE AFTER CATHETER ABLATION IN OBESE PATIENTS

Additional studies have investigated how catheter ablation for the treatment of symptomatic AF affects quality of life. In a large prospective study by Wokhlu and colleagues,[36] 502 patients with symptomatic AF underwent catheter ablation and were followed for a median duration of 3.1 years. Overall, mean scores before the first or last ablation were similar, but scores at 3 months, 1 year, and 24 months after the last ablation were all significantly higher. In multivariate analysis, obesity predicted a 6.8-point decrease in SF-36 score improvement. Complications such as cardiac tamponade, in-hospital stroke/transient ischemic attack, and pulmonary vein stenosis did not have a long-term impact on quality of life in this study.

Another study by Mohanty and colleagues[37] specifically examining the effect of BMI on quality of life after catheter ablation for AF enrolled 660 patients classified as normal weight (BMI <25 kg/m^2) or as overweight or obese (BMI >25 kg/m^2). Quality-of-life surveys were completed for all patients before and 12 months after ablation using four questionnaires, including the SF-36 form, Beck Depression Inventory, Hospital Anxiety and Depression Scale, and State-Trait Anxiety Inventory. Of the patients enrolled in the study, 21% were normal weight and 79% were overweight or obese. The overweight and obese patients had a higher prevalence of hyperlipidemia, hypertension, diabetes, coronary artery disease, and larger left atrial diameters at baseline. Given the higher prevalence of comorbidities, the overweight and obese patients had lower quality-of-life scores at baseline. After the follow-up period, 64% of patients in the normal weight group (after 1.3 procedures) and 63% of patients in the overweight/obese group (after 1.4 procedures) were AF-free, a difference that was not statistically significant. Although no significant improvement was seen in the normal weight patients' quality of life at 1 year, one was seen in the high BMI groups' quality of life scores. When the subgroup of successful ablations were evaluated, the change in quality of life in the overweight and obese subjects continued to be statistically significant, whereas only a nonsignificant trend toward improved quality of life was seen in the normal weight subjects.

The differences in quality of life after catheter ablation for AF are complex. The study by Mohanty and colleagues[37] describes no significant benefit in the normal weight group, and the investigators suggest that this difference compared with overweight and obese patients may be related to an older population and a lower percentage of paroxysmal patients who are both typically less symptomatic. The authors also suggest that their administration of questionnaires by mail allowed patients to be more honest instead of attempting to please health care providers who may have asked the questions. The authors also suggest that their results are similar to those of Wokhlu and colleagues,[36] in that patients with higher baseline quality-of-life scores (the normal weight subjects) experience less benefit.

ADDITIONAL CONSIDERATIONS AND COMPLICATIONS OF CATHETER ABLATION IN OBESE PATIENTS

In large studies evaluating major complications from catheter ablation for arrhythmias, overweight and obese patients do not have worse outcomes. In a study of 1676 consecutive ablation procedures, major complication rates for AF procedures were found to be 5.2%.[38] On multivariate analysis, an obese BMI was not found to be a major predictor of complications from catheter ablation. In a study specifically evaluating catheter ablation of AF, BMI was not found to be a major predictor of complications.[39]

Although BMI has not been shown to increase complications during catheter ablation for AF, other procedural factors have important implications when making treatment decisions. Some studies have evaluated fluoroscopic time and have shown no difference regarding BMI, but the actual radiation administered to obese patients may be higher given the automatic exposure control adjusted to patient attenuation. A study to specifically evaluate radiation dose in patients undergoing catheter ablation was performed in 85 patients who were stratified as normal weight, overweight, and obese.[40] In this study, no statistically significant procedural or fluoroscopic time differences were seen. The major finding of this study was that the effective radiation dose was 15.2 mSv in normal weight subjects, 26.9 mSv in overweight subjects, and 39.0 mSv in obese subjects. These findings were statistically significant, and when the lifetime attributable risk of developing cancer was calculated, it was significantly higher in the overweight and obese subjects.

Undiagnosed left atrial thrombus before catheter ablation for AF could potentially be catastrophic. Tang and colleagues[41] evaluated 433 consecutive patients with nonvalvular AF undergoing catheter ablation for AF with preoperative transesophageal echocardiogram and found 26 patients with left atrial or left atrial appendage thrombus. Patients with thrombus were found to have a significantly higher BMI. The incidence of left atrial thrombus was 10.6% in the group with a BMI greater then 27 kg/m^2 and 3.0% in patients with a BMI of less than 27 kg/m^2. After considering the typical risk factors for stroke and the classification of atrial fibrillation, BMI was the third strongest predictor of left atrial thrombus, with a odds ratio of 4.02 (95% CI, 1.19–13.55; *P* = .025).

SUMMARY

Patients such as the one presented in the case example will continue to increase in frequency as the obesity epidemic continues. What can one tell obese patients with symptomatic AF who have failed antiarrhythmic medications and are interested in discussing catheter ablation? They can be told that obesity plays a strong role in the development and progression of AF, likely mediated through a direct effect on left atrial size. Despite the increased burden of AF in the obese population, patients have similar, if not slightly improved mortality, described as the "obesity paradox." Catheter ablation for AF in obese patients is a reasonable option, but patients like the one presented should be screened for sleep apnea and counseled extensively about the likely need for longer procedure times and the possibility of repeat procedures to achieve similar success rates. Patients can be reassured that their quality of life will likely improve after successful ablation. Although no statistically significant increases in procedural complications have occurred in obese subjects, patients should be counseled about the increased radiation dose and the higher incidence of left atrial thrombus preablation.

REFERENCES

1. Miyasaka Y, Barnes ME, Gersh BJ, et al. Secular trends in the incidence of atrial fibrillation in Olmsted County, Minnesota, 1980 to 2000, and implications on the projections for future prevalence. Circulation 2006;114:119–25.
2. Flegal KM, Carroll MD, Ogden CL, et al. Prevalence and trends in obesity among US adults, 1999–2008. JAMA 2010;303(3):235–41.
3. Pritchett AM, Jacobsen SJ, Mahoney DW, et al. Left atrial volume as an index of left atrial size: a population-based study. J Am Coll Cardiol 2003;41:1036–43.
4. Wang TJ, Parise H, Levy D, et al. Obesity and the risk of new-onset atrial fibrillation. JAMA 2004;292: 2471–7.
5. Frost L, Hune LJ, Vestergaard P. Overweight and obesity as risk factors for atrial fibrillation or flutter: the Danish diet, cancer, and Health Study. Am J Med 2005;118:489–95.
6. Wanahita N, Messerli FH, Bangalore S, et al. Atrial Fibrillation and obesity-results of a meta-analysis. Am Heart J 2008;155:310–5.
7. Rosengren A, Jauptman PJ, Lappas G, et al. Big med and atrial fibrillation: effects of body size and weight gain on risk of atrial fibrillation in men. Eur Heart J 2009;30:1113–20.
8. Meijler FL. Comparative aspects of the dual role of the human atrioventricular node. Br Heart J 1986; 55:286–90.
9. Tsang TSM, Barnes ME, Miyasaka Y, et al. Obesity as a risk factor for the progression of paroxysmal to permanent atrial fibrillation: a longitudinal cohort study of 21 years. Eur Heart J 2008;29:2227–33.
10. Tedrow UB, Conen D, Ridker PM, et al. The long- and short-term impact of elevated body mass index on the risk of new atrial fibrillation. J Am Coll Cardiol 2010;55:2319–27.
11. Watanabe H, Tanabe N, Watanabe T, et al. Metabolic syndrome and risk of development of atrial fibrillation: the Niigata preventive medicine study. Circulation 2008;117:1255–60.
12. Tanner RM, Barber U, Carson AP, et al. Association of the metabolic syndrome with atrial fibrillation among United States adults (from the Reasons for Geographic and Racial Differences in Stroke [REGARDS] study). Am J Cardiol 2011;108:227–32.
13. Huxley RR, Lopez FL, Folsom AR, et al. Absolute and attributable risks of atrial fibrillation in relation to optimal and borderline risk factors. Circulation 2011;123:1501–8.
14. Ridker PM, Buring JE, Cook NR, et al. C-reactive protein, the metabolic syndrome, and risk of incident cardiovascular events: an 8 year-follow-up of 14 719 initially healthy American women. Circulation 2003; 107:391–7.
15. Chung MK, Martin DO, Sprecher D, et al. C-Reactive protein elevation in patients with atrial arrhythmias: inflammatory mechanisms and persistence of atrial fibrillation. Circulation 2001;103:2886–91.
16. McCabe JM, Smith LM, Tseng ZH, et al. Protracted CRP elevation after atrial fibrillation ablation. Pacing Clin Electrophysiol 2008;31:1146–51.
17. Shimano M, Shibata R, Tsuji Y, et al. Circulating adiponectin levels in patients with atrial fibrillation. Circ J 2008;72:1120–4.
18. Al Chekakie MO, Welles CC, Metoyer R, et al. Pericardial fat is independently associated with human atrial fibrillation. J Am Coll Cardiol 2010;56:784–8.
19. Thanassoulis G, Massaro JM, O'Donnell CJ, et al. Pericardial fat is associated with prevalent atrial fibrillation: the Framingham heart study. Circ Arrhythm Electrophysiol 2010;3:345–50.
20. Wong CX, Abed HS, Molaee P, et al. Pericardial fat is associated with atrial fibrillation severity and ablation outcome. J Am Coll Cardiol 2011;57:1745–51.
21. Chang SL, Tuan TC, Tai CT, et al. Comparison of outcome in catheter ablation of atrial fibrillation in patients with versus without the metabolic syndrome. Am J Cardiol 2009;103:67–72.
22. Nakagawa H, Scherlag BJ, Patterson E, et al. Pathophysiologic basis of autonomic ganglionated plexus ablation in patients with atrial fibrillation. Heart Rhythm 2009;6:S26–34.
23. Lin YK, Chen YJ, Chen SA. Potential atrial arrhythmogenicity of adipocytes: Implications for the genesis of atrial fibrillation. Med Hypotheses 2010; 74:1026–9.
24. Badheka AO, Rathod A, Kizilbash MA, et al. Influence of obesity on outcomes in atrial fibrillation: yet another obesity paradox. Am J Med 2010;123:646–51.
25. Ardestani A, Hoffman HJ, Cooper HA. Obesity and outcomes among patients with established atrial fibrillation. Am J Cardiol 2010;106:369–73.
26. Fuster V, Ryden LE, Cannom DS, et al. ACC/AHA/ESC 2006 Guidelines for the Management of Patients with Atrial Fibrillation: a report of the American College of Cardiology/American Heart Association Task Force on Practice Guidelines and the European Society of Cardiology Committee for Practice Guidelines (Writing Committee to Revise the 2001 Guidelines for the Management of Patients With Atrial

Fibrillation): developed in collaboration with the European Heart Rhythm Association and the Heart Rhythm Society. Circulation 2006;114:e257–354.
27. Calkins H, Brugada J, Packer DL, et al. HRS/EHRA/ECAS expert Consensus Statement on catheter and surgical ablation of atrial fibrillation: recommendations for personnel, policy, procedures and follow-up. A report of the Heart Rhythm Society (HRS) Task Force on catheter and surgical ablation of atrial fibrillation. Heart Rhythm 2007;4:816–61.
28. Cha YM, Friedman PA, Asirvatham SJ, et al. Catheter ablation for atrial fibrillation in patients with obesity. Circulation 2008;117:2583–90.
29. Jongnarangsin K, Chugh A, Good F, et al. Body mass index, obstructive sleep apnea, and outcomes of catheter ablation. J Cardiovasc Electrophysiol 2008;19:668–72.
30. Letsas KP, Siklody CH, Korantzopoulos P, et al. The impact of body mass index on the efficacy and safety of catheter ablation of atrial fibrillation. Int J Cardiol, in press. doi:10.1016/j.ijcard.2011.06.092.
31. Chilukuri K, Dalal D, Gadrey S, et al. A prospective study evaluating the role of obesity and obstructive sleep apnea for outcomes after catheter ablation of atrial fibrillation. J Cardiovasc Electrophysiol 2010;21:521–5.
32. Gami AS, Pressman G, Caples SM, et al. Association of atrial fibrillation and obstructive sleep apnea. Circulation 2004;110:364–7.
33. Mainigi SK, Sauer WH, Cooper JM, et al. Incidence and predictors of very late recurrence of atrial fibrillation after ablation. J Cardiovasc Electrophysiol 2007;18:69–74.
34. Letsas KP, Weber R, Burkle G, et al. Pre-ablative predictors of atrial fibrillation recurrence following pulmonary vein isolation: the potential role of inflammation. Europace 2009;11:158–63.
35. Cai L, Yin Y, Ling Z, et-al. Predictors of late recurrence of atrial fibrillation after catheter ablation. Int J Cardiol, in press. doi:10.1016/j.ijcard.2011.06.094.
36. Wokhlu A, Monahan KH, Hodge DO, et al. Long-term quality of life after ablation of atrial fibrillation. J Am Coll Cardiol 2010;55:2308–16.
37. Mohanty S, Mohanty P, Di Biase L, et al. Influence of body mass index on quality of life in atrial fibrillation patients undergoing catheter ablation. Heart Rhythm 2011;8:1847–52.
38. Bohen M, Stevenson WG, Tedro UB, et al. Incidence and predictors of major complications from contemporary catheter ablation to treat cardiac arrhythmias. Heart Rhythm 2011;8:1661–6.
39. Hoyt H, Bhonsale A, Chilukuri K, et al. Complications arising from catheter ablation of atrial fibrillation: temporal trends and predictors. Heart Rhythm 2011;8:1869–74.
40. Ector J, Dragusin O, Adriaenssens B, et al. Obesity is a major determinant of radiation dose in patients undergoing pulmonary vein isolation for atrial fibrillation. J Am Coll Cardiol 2007;50:234–7.
41. Tang RB, Liu XH, Kalifa J, et al. Body mass index and risk of left atrial thrombus in patients with atrial fibrillation. Am J Cardiol 2009;104:1699–703.

Ablation of Persistent Atrial Fibrillation
AF Termination is the End Point

Ashok J. Shah, MD, Shinsuke Miyazaki, MD, Amir S. Jadidi, MD, Xingpeng Liu, MD, Daniel Scherr, MD, Patrizio Pascale, MD, Laurent Roten, MD, Yuki Komatsu, MD, Stephen B. Wilton, MD, Michala E. Pedersen, MD, Sebastien Knecht, MD, Nicolas Derval, MD, Frederic Sacher, MD, Meleze Hocini, MD, Michel Haïssaguerre, MD, Pierre Jais, MD*

KEYWORDS

• Persistent atrial fibrillation • Catheter ablation • Atrial fibrillation termination • End point

KEY POINTS

- Several different persistent atrial fibrillation (AF) ablation strategies exist, with suboptimal acute and long-term clinical outcomes.
- Acute AF termination predicts long-term clinical outcome, but intraprocedural AF termination is difficult to attain as an end point of persistent AF ablation and necessitates extensive left atrial and often biatrial ablation.
- Stepwise ablation of persistent AF including pulmonary venous isolation, defragmentation, and linear ablation involves extensive biatrial ablation with higher AF termination rates than for any other strategy.
- Intraprocedural AF termination is favored by short duration of continuous AF (<2 years) and long baseline AF cycle length (>140 milliseconds).
- Studies in which AF termination did not predict long-term clinical success did not adopt a stepwise ablation approach, or had a long duration of continuous AF ($\geq$2 years) and/or short baseline AF cycle length (<130 milliseconds).

INTRODUCTION

Catheter ablation strategies have had limited clinical success in patients with persistent or long-standing persistent atrial fibrillation (AF) when compared with their paroxysmal counterparts.[1] The existence of different ablation strategies for persistent AF in the centers performing them and the vast variability in their success rates suggest that the mechanisms underlying the initiation and maintenance of persistent AF are not limited to 1 or 2 structures as in paroxysmal AF, but are more varied and sporadic.[2] Several alternative mechanisms perhaps are partly related to the significant remodeling instilled by the arrhythmia on the atria in terms of its structural and electrophysiologic properties. Although pulmonary vein isolation (PVI) continues to remain the fundamental step, strategies involving electrogram-guided biatrial substrate modification and/or linear lesions,

Conflicts of interest: None.
Disclosures: None.

Hôpital Haut Leveque and Université Bordeaux II, Bordeaux, France
* Corresponding author. Hôpital Cardiologique du Haut-Lévêque, 33604 Bordeaux-Pessac, France.
E-mail address: pierre.jais@chu-bordeaux.fr

Card Electrophysiol Clin 4 (2012) 335–342
http://dx.doi.org/10.1016/j.ccep.2012.05.005
1877-9182/12/$ – see front matter

targeted at interrupting self-sustaining reentrant wavefronts or focal sources and creating barriers in the path of propagation of wavelets, have been incorporated into ablation therapy for persistent and long-standing persistent AF in an attempt to improve outcomes.[3,4] Although an integrated approach combining all the strategies leads to higher rates of intraprocedural arrhythmia termination in persistent AF patients than for any isolated strategy or their other combinations, the extensive nature of biatrial ablation and a substantially high rate of recurrence of organized arrhythmia[4] make the approach debatable. Consequently there is an absence of consensus, and the search for an ideal ablation strategy in persistent AF continues.

This article reviews the literature on various techniques in the ablation of persistent AF, with the aim of highlighting the role of intraprocedural arrhythmia termination, defined as conversion to sinus rhythm or intermediate atrial tachycardia, in the predictability of arrhythmia recurrence. Because arrhythmia termination is not observed universally as a procedural end point, only those studies wherein it has been specifically reported, and its predictive role in arrhythmia recurrence is considered, are described (**Table 1**).

STEPWISE ABLATION APPROACH

Strategy

The stepwise ablation of long-standing persistent AF is a sequential approach including PVI, electrogram-based left atrial ablation, linear ablations at the roof and the left mitral isthmus, and discretionary right atrial ablation (superior vena cava, appendage, right septum, intercaval or cavotricuspid isthmus lines). The effect of ablation is assessed by measuring any increment in AF cycle length in the appendages at the end of each step. Another important feature is the procedural end point. Termination of AF to sinus rhythm or intermediate atrial tachycardia(s) during ablation beyond the step of PVI is the preferred procedural end point and is considered as successful termination of the arrhythmia. Patients who remain in AF after all key anatomic regions are ablated may be cardioverted at the end of the procedure. On the other hand, if AF termination occurs early during the stepwise procedure, the subsequent rhythm could be a major deciding factor in the deployment of the linear lesions.

Acute Termination and Postablation Arrhythmia

The stepwise ablation approach is associated with acute arrhythmia termination rates ranging from 47% to 87%.[3–8]

In the pioneer report,[3] 87% (52 of 60) of patients achieved AF termination during ablation. Early arrhythmia recurrence during the first week after ablation (paroxysmal AF in 6 patients, sustained AF in 2, and atrial tachycardia [AT] in 4) was more commonly observed in the group of patients without AF termination: 4 of 8 (50%) versus 8 of 52 (15%), respectively ($P = .04$; Fisher's exact test). In addition, sustained arrhythmia was more common in the subgroup of patients without acute AF termination: 3 of 4 versus 1 of 8 ($P = .066$; Fisher's exact test). Delayed arrhythmia recurrence was observed in nearly half of the patients. Organized AT was its predominant form, documented in 24 patients. Almost all the patients with late recurrence were subjected to repeat ablation procedure, including 4 patients who underwent the ablation procedure three times.

Rostock and colleagues[5] observed acute termination rates of 77% (68 of 88 patients). A second ablation procedure was required for recurrent AF/AT in the majority (54 of 88 patients). Only 11 patients required a third ablation procedure. Patients with acute termination predominantly had AT(s) as recurrent arrhythmia(s) (83%), whereas those without mainly presented with recurrent AF (85%).

Lin and colleagues[6] observed acute AF termination in 47% (14 of 30) of patients at the index procedure. Recurrence of arrhythmia observed in 5 of 14 (36%) patients occurred equally between its types (AF and AT). All 5 patients underwent repeat ablation procedure, with one requiring it twice.

In a prospective study involving 153 consecutive patients who underwent catheter ablation of persistent AF using a stepwise approach with the procedural end point being AF termination, O'Neill and colleagues[7] reported acute termination rates of 85% (130 of 153 patients). Seventy-nine patients underwent repeat procedures: 64 of 130 in the termination group (6 AF, 58 AT) and 15 in the nontermination group (9 AF, 7 AT). The predominance of AF in the nontermination group and of AT in the termination group was striking.

Recently, Rostock and colleagues[8] reported their experience in a large series of 395 patients with persistent AF (mean duration 16 months) undergoing de novo catheter ablation using the stepwise approach. Procedural termination of AF was achieved in 259 (66%) patients, of whom 39 (15%) terminated directly from AF to sinus rhythm and 220 (85%) to an intermediate AT. Median follow-up time was 26 (range 15–39) months in 108 patients (27%) without recurrences after a single procedure, and 24 (range 9–52) months in 287 patients (73%) with recurrence of arrhythmias. All but 2 patients with AT recurrences reached the end point of procedural AF termination during index ablation.

Table 1
Comparison of acute termination rates and their impact on clinical success after persistent AF ablation

Investigators[Ref.]	Year	N	Duration of Follow-Up (mo)	Acute AF Termination Rate (%)	Determination of Clinical Recurrence	Acute AF Termination Predicted or Associated with Absence of Recurrence
Stepwise Approach						
Haïssaguerre et al[3]	2005	60	11 ± 6	57 (87)	Objective	Yes (1/57 vs 2/3)
Rostock et al[5]	2008	88	20 ± 4	68 (77)	Objective	Yes
Lin et al[6]	2009	30	19 ± 11	14 (47)	Subjective	Yes
O'Neill et al[7]	2009	153	32 ± 11	130 (85)	Objective	Yes
Hocini et al[4]	2010	148	22 ± 9	104 (70)	Objective	Yes
Rostock et al[8]	2011	395	27 ± 7	259 (66)	Objective	Yes
Pulmonary Vein Isolation + Lines + Defractionation/Focal Ablation						
Li et al[9]	2008	92	12 ± 11	32 (35)	Objective	Yes
Fiala et al[10]	2008	135	25 ± 14	67 (50)	Subjective	Yes
Pulmonary Vein Isolation + Defractionation						
Estner et al[11]	2008	35	19 ± 12	23 (66)	Objective	No
Oral et al[12]	2009	50	10 ± 3	9 (18)	Objective	No
Pulmonary Vein Isolation + Lines						
Elayi et al[14]	2008	47	17 ± 2	6 (13)	Objective	No
Lin et al[6]	2009	30	19 ± 11	05 (17)	Subjective	No
Pulmonary Vein Antral Isolation + Defractionation						
Elayi et al[14]	2008	49	16 ± 1	36 (74)	Objective	No
Elayi et al[15]	2010	306	25 ± 7	178 (58)	Objective	No
Defractionation Only						
Nademanee et al[16]	2004	64	12	58 (91)	Objective	Yes
Oral et al[17]	2007	100	14 ± 7	16 (16)	Objective	No
Oral et al[18]	2008	85	16 ± 7	20 (24)	Objective	Yes (17/19 vs 36/66)
Pulmonary Vein Isolation Only						
Oral et al[12]	2009	69	10 ± 3	19 (28)	Objective	No
Pulmonary Vein Antral Isolation Only						
Elayi et al[14]	2008	48	16 ± 1	18 (44)	Objective	No

Extended Clinical Success

Haïssaguerre and colleagues[3] reported sinus rhythm after multiple procedures in 57 (95%) patients at the end of 11 ± 6, months including 4 patients on antiarrhythmic drugs. Among 3 patients with recurrent AF or AT, 2 patients belonged to the group of patients who failed to attain acute arrhythmia termination during the index ablation procedure. Anticoagulation was discontinued in 49 patients and continued in 11 patients, including the patient with persistent electrical disconnection of the left atrial appendage. No patient sustained any form of thromboembolic event during follow-up. Acute termination observed during the index or subsequent procedure was associated with clinical success on follow-up (recurrent AF in 1 of 57 patients with acute termination vs 2 of 3 without acute termination, $P = .001$).

Rostock and colleagues[5] reported sinus rhythm after multiple procedures in 71 (81%) patients at the end of mean follow-up of 20 ± 4 months, and observed failure to terminate AF by ablation during the 2 procedures as a strong predictor for recurrence of AF. All 12 patients in whom AF was not terminated during the index and redo procedures demonstrated recurrence of chronic AF. These patients were characterized by larger left atrial diameter (54 ± 5 mm vs 48 ± 7 mm; $P = .005$), a marginally impaired left ventricular function (50% ± 14% vs 58% ± 12%; $P = .048$), a longer duration of chronic AF (44 ± 49 months vs 17 ± 21 months; $P = .001$), and a significantly shorter baseline AF cycle length (124 ± 4 vs 146 ± 4 milliseconds; $P = .001$) than the patients with AF termination. Furthermore, all but one of these patients had a structural heart disease (dilated cardiomyopathy, congestive heart failure, coronary artery disease, and hypertensive heart disease).

Lin and colleagues[6] reported sinus rhythm after multiple procedures in 25 (83%) of 30 patients at a mean follow-up of 10 ± 7 months. On multivariate analysis, the procedural AF termination predicted ($P = .016$) longer sustenance of sinus rhythm after a single procedure (70%). Repeat procedures were required in significantly more patients without than with procedural AF termination ($P = .04$). The latter analysis included some patients who were not subjected to electrogram-based ablation. Of note, the arrhythmia monitoring on follow-up was symptom guided.

At the completion of minimum 12 months after last ablation, O'Neill and colleagues[7] reported sinus rhythm in 95% of 130 patients in whom AF was terminated compared with 52% of 23 in whom AF could not be terminated after multiple procedures. A lower incidence of recurrent AF was observed in patients in whom AF was terminated during the index procedure, compared with those who had not (5% vs 39%; $P = .0001$, mean follow-up 32 + 11 months).

In the largest series of patients undergoing stepwise ablation for persistent AF reported so far, Rostock and colleagues[8] observed that after a follow-up of 27 ± 7 months, 108 (27%) patients were free of arrhythmia recurrences with a single procedure. However, after 2.3 ± 0.6 procedures, 312 (79%) patients were free of arrhythmia, with concomitant antiarrhythmic treatment in 15%. Female gender, duration of persistent AF, and congestive heart failure were predictive of the clinical outcome after first ablation. However, the strongest predictors for single-procedure success were longer baseline AF cycle length and procedural AF termination. In addition, procedural AF termination during the index procedure also predicted a favorable outcome after the last procedure, thereby emerging as a predictor of overall clinical success.

PVI + DEFRACTIONATION + LINES ± FOCAL-SOURCE ABLATION

Strategy

Similarly to the steps of the stepwise approach, Li and colleagues[9] undertook circumferential pulmonary vein (PV) ablation guided by a 3-dimensional (3D) electroanatomic system with the end points of continuous circular lesions, and electrical PVI followed by ablation of complex fractionated left atrial electrograms until AF was terminated or fractionation was eliminated. If typical atrial flutter was documented before the procedure, or a macro-reentrant AT spontaneously occurred during ablation, the critical isthmus responsible was identified and ablated.

Fiala and colleagues[10] described their experience of stepwise ablation in 135 patients with persistent AF including 100 patients with long-standing persistent AF. The ablation strategy consisted of ipsilateral antral PVI followed by left atrial linear and focal ablation aimed at successive elimination of potential reentry circuits, rotors, and focal sources. The regions exhibiting fractionated electrograms were targeted as a part of the linear ablation and if the fractionation was still present after completion of the linear ablation, they were selectively targeted by the successive focal ablation.

Acute Termination and Postablation Arrhythmia

Li and colleagues[9] reported acute termination of AF during ablation in 35% (32 of 92) patients without the use of antiarrhythmic drugs. Atrial arrhythmias recurred in 49% (45 of 92) patients during early follow-up and were managed medically for a period of 10 to 12 weeks postablation. Ablation was not repeated to determine the predictors of early recurrence and delayed cure after a single procedure.

Fiala and colleagues[10] reported procedural AF termination in 38 (38%) of 100 patients with long-lasting AF and 29 (83%) of 35 patients with short-lasting persistent AF. The arrhythmia terminated into AT in 45 (67%) patients. Repeat ablation was performed in 43 (43%) and 9 (26%) patients with long-lasting persistent and short-lasting persistent AF, respectively.

Extended Clinical Success

Li and colleagues[9] reported 58% (53 of 92 patients followed for 12 ± 11 months, ≤25 months) clinical success after a single ablation procedure. AF termination ($P = .01$) and LA size ($P = .03$) were significantly related to clinical cure despite early recurrences such that AF termination emerged as the only independent predictor of delayed clinical cure (odds ratio 1.47; 95% confidence interval 1.05–1.87; $P = .02$).

Fiala and colleagues[10] reported that during the follow-up period of 26 ± 14 and 25 ± 14 months since the last ablation procedure, 87 (87%) and 31 (89%) patients with long-lasting persistent and short-lasting persistent AF, respectively, remained free of the arrhythmia recurrence. Of these patients, 66 (66%) and 28 (80%) in each respective group were free of antiarrhythmic drugs. The ability to restore sinus rhythm by ablation was associated with favorable clinical outcome in the group of long-lasting persistent AF.

PVI + DEFRACTIONATION

Strategy

Using a combination of PVI and defractionation techniques, Estner and colleagues[11] and Oral and colleagues[12] have studied acute procedural termination of AF as a predictor of long-term clinical success in persistent AF. PVs were circumferentially isolated at the antral level with the end point of complete electrical isolation; this was followed by ablation of areas with complex fractionated atrial electrograms with an end point of complete elimination of fractionated electrogram or conversion of AF to sinus rhythm/organized AT. Cardioversion was attempted otherwise. Linear lesions were deployed to transect the circuit of macroreentrant tachycardia if it occurred during the course of ablation.

Acute Termination and Postablation Arrhythmia

Estner and colleagues[11] found that among 35 patients ablated using a combination of PVI and defractionation, 23 (66%) patients achieved acute termination of AF (sinus rhythm in 8 and organized AT in 15). Nine patients required a second ablation procedure for recurrent arrhythmia over 19 ± 12 months.

Oral and colleagues[12] reported acute termination in 9 (18%) of 50 patients undergoing antral PVI followed by defractionation. Arrhythmia recurred in 17 (34%) patients, predominantly as AF, during a mean follow-up of 7 ± 2 months.

Extended Clinical Success

Estner and colleagues[11] reported 74% clinical cure rate at mean follow-up of 19 ± 12 months postablation using the PVI + defractionation combination approach. However, the long-term outcome was not statistically different between the acute termination and nontermination groups.

Oral and colleagues[12] reported sinus rhythm in 18 (36%) patients at the end of 10 ± 3 months following the index procedure and in 30 (60%) patients at the end of 9 ± 4 months after the last procedure, off antiarrhythmic drugs. Acute termination did not predict extended clinical success.

PVI + LINEAR ABLATION

Strategy

Lin and colleagues[6] undertook circumferential PVI combined with at least 2 left atrial linear lesions (anterior roof line and the lateral mitral isthmus line) guided by a 3D electroanatomic system to study the outcomes of this combined approach in persistent AF and compare it with the procedure that also added defractionation. Voltage abatement of more than 50%, and not the bidirectional block, was the end point of left atrial linear ablation.

Acute Termination and Postablation Arrhythmia

Lin and colleagues[6] reported acute termination in 6 (20%) of 30 patients. Recurrence of AF was observed in 15 patients (50%, paroxysmal in 6 and persistent in 9) and recurrence of AT was observed in 3 patients (10%). Patients underwent up to 4 repeat procedures, including additional defractionation in 3 patients.

Extended Clinical Success

At a mean follow-up of 27 ± 9 months after the last procedure, 20 (66%) patients were in sinus rhythm including 2 patients on concomitant drug therapy. PVI combined with linear ablation without defractionation did not predict clinical success.

PV ANTRAL ISOLATION ± DEFRACTIONATION/ LINEAR ABLATION

Kanj and colleagues[13] described PV antral isolation (combined PV and posterior left atrial isolation), and Elayi and colleagues[14] compared the procedural and clinical outcomes between PV antral isolation alone, PV antral isolation combined with defractionation, and PVI combined with linear ablation. Acute termination was not reported to be predictive of clinical success in any of these strategies. Elayi and colleagues[15] later reported absence of an influential role of acute termination of AF from combined PV antral isolation and defractionation in predicting long-term clinical success in a large series of patients. This topic is covered in more detail in an article by Natale and colleagues elsewhere in this issue.

DEFRACTIONATION ALONE

Strategy

Nademanee and colleagues[16] undertook 3D electroanatomic system–guided widespread substrate ablation using a biatrial defractionation approach in 64 persistent AF patients. Bipolar voltage 0.15 mV or more filtered at 30 to 500 Hz was considered as a low-amplitude signal. Complex fractionation was defined as an electrogram composed of 2 or more deflections and/or perturbation of the baseline with continuous activation present over a 10-second recording period. Very rapid atrial activity (cycle length ≤120 ms averaged over a 10-second recording period) was also targeted. Elimination of fractionated signal or acute arrhythmia termination was the preferred end point of ablation.

Oral and colleagues[17] also reported the clinical outcomes of persistent AF ablation using the left atrial defragmentation strategy and the end points described above. The same investigators evaluated the impact of right atrial defragmentation besides left atrial defractionation in long-lasting persistent AF in a randomized manner.[18]

Acute Termination and Postablation Arrhythmia

Nademanee and colleagues[16] reported acute termination of AF in 58 (91%) patients including 18 (28%) who required concomitant ibutilide treatment. Arrhythmia recurrence necessitated repeat ablation in 19 (30%) patients.

Oral and colleagues[17] observed acute termination of AF in 16 (16%) patients during left atrial defragmentation. During 14 ± 7 months of follow-up after a single ablation procedure, 67% patients continued to experience atrial arrhythmia, predominantly AF. A second ablation procedure was required in 44% of patients.

In a randomized trial evaluating the outcomes of biatrial defragmentation, Oral and colleagues[18] reported acute arrhythmia termination in 20 (24%) of 85 patients. Repeat ablation procedure was required in 26 (31%) patients, predominantly for AF.

Extended Clinical Success

Nademanee and colleagues[16] reported arrhythmia-free 1-year survival in 56 (88%) patients after 2 procedures. Immediate arrhythmia termination translated into sustained clinical success.

Oral and colleagues[17] reported arrhythmia-free survival in 57% patients at 13 ± 7 months after the last ablation procedure, and observed no relationship between the acute termination of AF during ablation and long-term freedom from recurrent AF.

In the biatrial defragmentation study, Oral and colleagues[18] reported freedom from arrhythmia at 16 ± 7 months after the final procedure in a significantly higher number of patients experiencing procedural AF termination (89% vs 55%, $P = .006$) than otherwise, thereby associating acute termination with better clinical success at the given follow-up.

PVI ALONE

Strategy

Oral and colleagues[12] studied the role of acute termination of persistent AF after circumferential PVI alone in the prediction of long-term clinical success. PVs were isolated at the antral level with a circular decapolar mapping catheter under 3D electroanatomic guidance. Electrical PVI was the desired end point, which was attained in all patients.

Acute Termination and Postablation Arrhythmia

Acute termination was reported in 19 (28%) of 69 patients.[12] At a mean follow-up of 10 ± 3 months after a single procedure, 35 (51%) patients had recurrence, predominantly in the form of AF. Up to 3 repeat procedures were performed, which included additional defractionation at the discretion of the operator.

Extended Clinical Success

At a mean follow-up of 9 ± 4 months after the last procedure, 49 (70%) patients were in sinus rhythm. Acute AF termination did not predict the clinical success after PVI alone.

DISCUSSION

Just as the search for an ideal persistent AF ablation procedure is far from over, so too is the quest for an ideal procedural end point. Nevertheless, the evidence from the current literature is favoring the need for a composite of extensive index catheter ablation and at least one repeat procedure in the majority of long-lasting persistent AF patients to eliminate organized ATs arising therefrom.

Although acute AF termination is desirable, not all the ablation strategies concur around it as an end point. Considering that extensive ablation performed during the index procedure or cumulatively over several procedures is mandatory for the acute elimination of persistent AF, it would be difficult to compare acute termination as an end point between 2 strategies with different extents of biatrial ablation. Elayi and colleagues[15] did not observe acute termination predictive of clinical success after pulmonary antral isolation combined with complex atrial defragmentation. However, linear lesions were not undertaken in their population, with relatively longer duration of long-lasting persistent AF and shorter baseline AF cycle length compared with the population wherein acute termination predicted clinical success (**Table 2**).[7,8] Thus,

Table 2
Comparison of reports evaluating acute termination of persistent AF as a predictor of clinical success

	Investigators,[Ref.] Year		
Parameter	**Elayi et al,[15] 2010**	**O'Neill et al,[7] 2009**	**Rostock et al,[8] 2011**
N	306	153	395
Ablation strategy	Pulmonary vein isolation + defractionation	Stepwise	Stepwise
Linear ablation	No	Yes	Yes
Mean duration of sustained AF (mo)	>25	22	16
Mean baseline AF cycle length (ms)	<130	>150	>150
Acute termination predicted clinical success	No	Yes	Yes

the disparity in the observations between these investigators could by also be attributed to the difference in the clinical arrhythmia characteristics of the populations under consideration. These differences could be considered substantial because the parameters such as the duration of uninterrupted persistent AF and its baseline cycle length have been reported as the best predictors of acute AF termination during a stepwise approach.[7] Of note, Elayi and colleagues[15] observed a significant difference in the mean preablation AF cycle length between the groups with and without acute termination during ablation (128 ± 21 milliseconds in patients with AF termination versus 104 ± 18 milliseconds in patients without AF termination; $P = .036$).

The evidence favoring acute termination as an end point predominantly emerges from a strategy that combines PVI with defractionation and linear ablation because each of the 2 steps subsequent to PVI significantly contributes to arrhythmia termination. Therefore, all the reports a describing stepwise ablation approach in persistent AF consistently observe acute arrhythmia termination as an important predictor of, or strongly associated with, the clinical success. Although Li and colleagues[9] and Fiala and colleagues[10] described their approaches of ablating AF differently from the stepwise approach, the strategies are very similar, barring some alteration in the order of the steps undertaken during ablation. In concurrence with the outcomes of the stepwise approach, both groups concluded that acute arrhythmia termination predicts or is favorably associated with extended clinical success in persistent AF.

Combinations such as PVI + defractionation[11,12] and PVI + linear ablation[6,14] could be considered as relatively less extensive ablation approaches than the stepwise approach or the approach that combines all 3 of its steps in any order. Consequently, limited ablation from any of these less extensive combination strategies could be held responsible for substantially low rates (below 20%) (see **Table 1**) of acute AF termination that failed to affect the overall clinical success.

When isolated approaches are considered, the extensive defractionation-only approach recommended by Nademanee and colleagues[16] failed to reproduce their clinical outcomes, including acute termination rates from other centers. However, the acute termination achieved during defractionation was associated with better clinical success.[16,18] This finding could be attributed to the extensive nature of the defractionation strategy described by Nademanee and colleagues, which is absent when PVI-alone is undertaken. Oral and colleagues[12] made an intriguing observation in another interesting study, where 19 of 69 patients achieved sinus rhythm after antral PVI-alone and another 9 of 50 patients did so after additional defractionation. Acute termination was associated with clinical success after a single procedure, although PVI-alone did not affect such significant association (sinus rhythm in 15 of 19 patients with acute termination versus 31 of 50 patients without acute termination, $P = .2$).

SUMMARY

Acute termination is a predictor of sustained clinical success when it is achieved after extensive biatrial substrate ablation through defragmentation and linear lesions in addition to PVI. Moreover, the acute arrhythmia termination rates are favorably influenced in the presence of persistent AF of less than 2 years with relatively long baseline AF cycle length (>140 milliseconds). In less favorable situations, intraprocedural termination of the

clinical arrhythmia is difficult, necessitating further development to improve the ensuing clinical outcome.

REFERENCES

1. Weerasooriya R, Khairy P, Litalien J, et al. Catheter ablation for atrial fibrillation: are results maintained at 5 years of follow-up? J Am Coll Cardiol 2011;57(2):160–6.
2. Brooks AG, Stiles MK, Laborderie J, et al. Outcomes of long-standing persistent atrial fibrillation ablation: a systematic review. Heart Rhythm 2010;7(6):835–46.
3. Haïssaguerre M, Hocini M, Sanders P, et al. Catheter ablation of long-lasting persistent atrial fibrillation: clinical outcome and mechanisms of subsequent arrhythmias. J Cardiovasc Electrophysiol 2005; 16(11):1138–47.
4. Hocini M, Nault I, Wright M, et al. Disparate evolution of right and left atrial rate during ablation of long-lasting persistent atrial fibrillation. J Am Coll Cardiol 2010;55(10):1007–16.
5. Rostock T, Steven D, Hoffman B, et al. Chronic atrial fibrillation is a biatrial arrhythmia. Data from catheter ablation of chronic atrial fibrillation aiming arrhythmia termination using a sequential ablation approach. Circ Arrhythm Electrophysiol 2008;1:344–53.
6. Lin YJ, Tai CT, Chang SL, et al. Efficacy of additional ablation of complex fractionated atrial electrograms for catheter ablation of nonparoxysmal atrial ibrillation. J Cardiovasc Electrophysiol 2009;20(6):607–15.
7. O'Neill MD, Wright M, Knecht S, et al. Long-term follow-up of persistent atrial fibrillation ablation using termination as a procedural endpoint. Eur Heart J 2009;30:1105–12.
8. Rostock T, Salukhe TV, Steven D, et al. Long-term single- and multiple-procedure outcome and predictors of success after catheter ablation for persistent atrial fibrillation. Heart Rhythm 2011;8(9): 1391–7.
9. Li XP, Dong JZ, Liu XP, et al. Predictive value of early recurrence and delayed cure after catheter ablation for patients with chronic atrial fibrillation. Circ J 2008; 72:1125–9.
10. Fiala M, Chovancik J, Nevralova R, et al. Termination of long-lasting persistent versus short-lasting persistent and paroxysmal atrial fibrillation by ablation. Pacing Clin Electrophysiol 2008;31:985–97.
11. Estner HL, Hessling G, Ndrepepa G, et al. Acute effects and long-term outcome of pulmonary vein isolation in combination with electrogram-guided substrate ablation for persistent atrial fibrillation. Am J Cardiol 2008;101:332–7.
12. Oral H, Chugh A, Yoshida K, et al. A randomized assessment of the incremental role of ablation of complex fractionated atrial electrograms after antral pulmonary vein isolation for long-lasting persistent atrial fibrillation. J Am Coll Cardiol 2009;53:782–9.
13. Kanj MH, Wazni OM, Natale A. How to do circular mapping catheter-guided pulmonary vein antrum isolation: the Cleveland Clinic approach. Heart Rhythm 2006;3:866–9.
14. Elayi CS, Verma A, Di Biase L, et al. Ablation for longstanding permanent atrial fibrillation: results from a randomized study comparing three different strategies. Heart Rhythm 2008;5:1658–64.
15. Elayi CS, Di Biase L, Barrett C, et al. Atrial fibrillation termination as a procedural endpoint during ablation in long-standing persistent atrial fibrillation. Heart Rhythm 2010;7:1216–23.
16. Nademanee K, McKenzie J, Kosar E, et al. A new approach for catheter ablation of atrial fibrillation: mapping of the electrophysiologic substrate. J Am Coll Cardiol 2004;43:2044–53.
17. Oral H, Chugh A, Good E, et al. Radiofrequency catheter ablation of chronic atrial fibrillation guided by complex electrograms. Circulation 2007;115: 2606–12.
18. Oral H, Chugh A, Good E, et al. Randomized evaluation of right atrial ablation after left atrial of complex fractionated atrial electrograms for long-lasting persistent atrial fibrillation. Circ Arrhythm Electrophysiol 2008;1:6–13.

Ablation for Atrial Fibrillation
Termination of Atrial Fibrillation is Not the End Point

Pasquale Santangeli, MD[a,b], Luigi Di Biase, MD, PhD, FHRS[a,b], Amin Al-Ahmad, MD, FHRS[c], Rodney Horton, MD[a], J. David Burkhardt, MD[a], Javier E. Sanchez, MD[a], Rong Bai, MD, FHRS[a,d], Agnes Pump, MD[a,e], Sanghamitra Mohanty, MD[a], Andrea Natale, MD, FHRS, FESC[a,c,f,g,h,*]

KEYWORDS

- Pulmonary vein isolation • Nonparoxysmal atrial fibrillation • Catheter ablation
- Procedural end point

KEY POINTS

- Termination of atrial fibrillation (AF) represents an unreliable procedural end point during ablation of nonparoxysmal AF.
- Periprocedural termination of AF lacks adequate sensitivity and specificity in predicting long-term freedom from recurrent arrhythmia after catheter ablation of nonparoxysmal AF.

INTRODUCTION

Radiofrequency catheter ablation of atrial fibrillation (AF) is an established treatment in patients with symptomatic drug-refractory AF, with benefits extending toward reduction of symptoms, hospitalizations, and improved quality of life.[1–4] Over the last years, intense research has been directed toward the discovery and validation of electrophysiologic and anatomic targets fundamental for triggering and maintaining the arrhythmia.[5–9] Above all, pulmonary veins have a dominant role in AF, and focal discharges from these structures have been implicated in the initiation of AF.[10] Based on these findings, empiric isolation of the pulmonary veins has been performed with the highest procedural success in patients with paroxysmal AF, in whom spontaneous pulmonary vein firing is frequently the only trigger for AF paroxysms.[3,5] As a consequence, achieving durable pulmonary vein isolation is the main procedural end point for catheter ablation of paroxysmal AF,[3,4,11] and extending the ablation lesions beyond the pulmonary vein antra does not improve the procedural success in this setting.[11–13] In these patients, periprocedural termination of AF is obviously not an end point, given the nature of the arrhythmia that is, by definition, self terminating.

Patients with AF of longer duration, such as those with persistent and long-standing persistent

[a] Texas Cardiac Arrhythmia Institute, St David's Medical Center, 3000 North I-35, Suite 720, Austin, TX 78705, USA; [b] University of Foggia, Foggia, Italy; [c] Division of Cardiology, Stanford University, 300 Pasteur Dr MC 5319, A260, Stanford, CA 94305, USA; [d] Department of Internal Medicine, Tong-Ji Hospital, Tong-Ji Medical College, Huazhong University of Science and Technology, Wuhan, People's Republic of China; [e] Faculty of Medicine, Heart Institute, University of Pecs, Pecs, Hungary; [f] Case Western Reserve University, Cleveland, OH, USA; [g] Interventional Electrophysiology, Scripps Clinic, San Diego, CA, USA; [h] EP Services, California Pacific Medical Center, San Francisco, CA, USA
* Corresponding author.
E-mail address: dr.natale@gmail.com

Card Electrophysiol Clin 4 (2012) 343–352
http://dx.doi.org/10.1016/j.ccep.2012.06.005

AF, require the targeting of additional sites for successful ablation, including the entire left atrial posterior wall, and complex fractionated atrial electrograms (CFAE).[14,15] In these patients, periprocedural AF termination has been suggested as an end point, although its reliability in predicting long-term success is controversial.[14,16–30] From a pathophysiological perspective, the rationale underlying periprocedural AF termination is obscure, given the lack of precise knowledge regarding the substrate(s) and circuit(s) underlying AF. In this regard, terminating AF during ablation is, most of the time, a mere play of chance that may erratically occur at any point during the procedure, including mapping.[31]

Subjective definitions of AF termination within the published studies, ranging from conversion to atrial tachycardia,[14,19,20,28,29] atrial flutter,[21,25–27] or directly to sinus rhythm,[17,18,22,23,32] together with biased reporting of long-term outcomes, with the arbitrary exclusion of atrial tachycardias among procedural failures when assessing the predictive value of AF termination in some studies,[19,24] further affect the methodological validity and clinical reliability of AF termination as a procedural end point.

This article provides quantitative evidence against the appropriateness of considering AF termination as a reliable procedural end point.

TERMINATION OF AF AS A PROCEDURAL END POINT: SCOPE OF THE PROBLEM

The controversy on whether AF termination should be considered a procedural end point during catheter ablation of nonparoxysmal AF has essentially arisen after the finding by some investigators of a statistically significant association between periprocedural AF termination and long-term freedom from recurrent arrhythmia.[24,29] In this regard, it is important to remember that statistical association does not necessarily imply causal association; this concept, well recognized and extensively studied in epidemiologic science,[33] is frequently disregarded in clinical science.

Notwithstanding, to be considered a procedural end point AF termination should have high sensitivity and specificity in predicting the long-term arrhythmia-free survival. Furthermore, a causal relationship between achievement of AF termination and long-term freedom from recurrent arrhythmia should be demonstrated. For instance, increasing rates of periprocedural AF termination should be paralleled by equivalent improvements in long-term arrhythmia-free survival within published studies. Of note, none of the aforementioned points hold true for periprocedural AF termination, and here the authors discuss why.

EVIDENCE FROM STUDIES SPECIFICALLY ASSESSING THE VALUE OF AF TERMINATION AS A PROCEDURAL END POINT

Thus far, 2 studies have been specifically designed to evaluate the role of periprocedural AF termination as an end point during catheter ablation of nonparoxysmal AF.[16,24] O'Neill and colleagues[24] from the Bordeaux group reported the long-term follow-up of ablated persistent AF using termination as a procedural end point. Overall, 153 patients with persistent AF (mean duration 22 months) were included, and the stepwise ablation approach was used in such patients with the desired procedural end point being AF termination, defined as direct conversion to sinus rhythm or to any intermediate atrial tachycardia or flutter.[24] The procedural end point was achieved in 130 (85%) patients, and was associated with a lower recurrence rate of AF at a median follow-up of 34 months (log-rank $P<.001$) but with a significantly higher recurrence of atrial tachycardia (log-rank $P = .02$), compared with patients not achieving the end point. Putting together these results, periprocedural AF termination was not associated with a better total arrhythmia (ie, AF plus atrial tachycardia)-free survival at follow-up when compared with patients who did not achieve the end point (log-rank $P = .5$).

Similar results were found by the authors' group in a subsequent study.[16] A total of 306 patients with long-standing persistent AF (mean duration 26 months) underwent pulmonary vein antrum isolation plus CFAE ablation. Direct periprocedural conversion to sinus rhythm occurred only in 6 (2%) patients, with 172 (56%) organizing into an intermediate atrial tachycardia. After a mean follow-up of 25 $\pm$ 6.9 months, 306 (69%) patients remained in sinus rhythm, without statistical difference between patients who achieved periprocedural AF termination and those who did not achieve the end point. Similarly to the study by O'Neill and colleagues,[24] periprocedural AF termination predicted the predominant mode of recurrence (ie, atrial tachycardia, $P = .022$).[16]

In conclusion, data from 2 large studies specifically designed to evaluate the role of periprocedural AF termination as an end point during catheter ablation of nonparoxysmal AF consistently support the notion that AF termination does not predict long-term freedom from any atrial arrhythmia recurrence (ie, AF or atrial tachycardia/flutter) (**Fig. 1**), although it seems to predict the mode of recurrence.

The lack of reliability of AF termination in predicting arrhythmia-free survival is also consistent with other published series on catheter

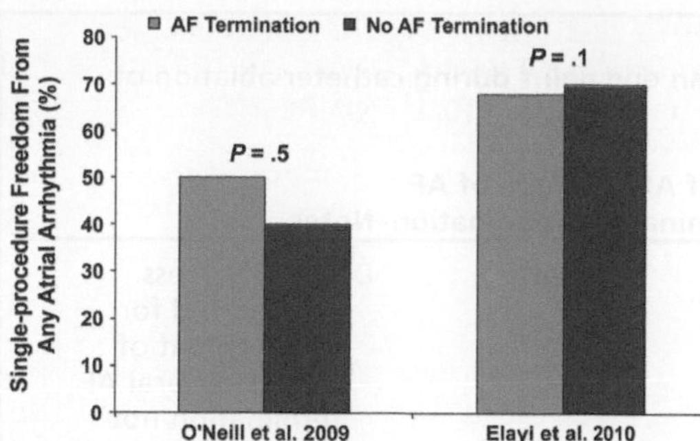

Fig. 1. Lack of association between periprocedural AF termination and long-term freedom from recurrent arrhythmia (AF or atrial tachycardia/flutter) in studies specifically evaluating the role of AF termination as a procedural end point.[16,24]

ablation of nonparoxysmal AF, as discussed in the following section.

SYSTEMATIC REVIEW OF THE AVAILABLE EVIDENCE

To fully evaluate the role of periprocedural AF termination as an end point during catheter ablation of nonparoxysmal AF, the authors systematically reviewed the available evidence on this topic.

Search Strategy and Study Selection for Analysis

An extensive literature search on PubMed, CENTRAL, BioMedCentral, Cardiosource, clinicaltrials.gov, and ISI Web of Science was performed (January 1980 to December 2011). Search keywords included "atrial fibrillation AND," "radiofrequency catheter ablation," "ablation," "catheter ablation," "termination," "atrial fibrillation termination," "long-term success," "success," "persistent atrial fibrillation," "long-standing persistent atrial fibrillation," "chronic atrial fibrillation". Proceedings from the annual American Heart Association (AHA), American College of Cardiology (ACC), European Society of Cardiology (ESC), Heart Rhythm Society (HRS), and Europace meetings for the past 5 years, and scientific societies' Web sites were also manually searched. Studies were included if they specifically assessed the long-term success of catheter ablation of nonparoxysmal AF according to the achievement of periprocedural termination of AF during the index procedure. Data were gathered regarding study inclusion criteria, the total number of patients included, the ablation strategy adopted, the number of patients in whom periprocedural AF termination was achieved, the long-term single-procedure success rate (defined as freedom from any atrial arrhythmia), the success rates separately in patients achieving periprocedural AF termination and in those not achieving the end point.

Data Analysis

To quantitatively establish the value of periprocedural termination of AF as an end point, a pooled analysis of the accuracy of AF termination in predicting long-term freedom from recurrent arrhythmia was performed. To this aim, the single-procedure freedom from any recurrent arrhythmia (AF or atrial tachycardia/flutter) was extracted separately in patients in whom periprocedural AF termination was achieved and in those not achieving the end point, and a calculation of sensitivity, specificity, false-negative rates, and false-positive rates was obtained. A Forest plot of sensitivity and specificity for each individual study, with their 95% confidence interval (CI), was constructed.

Pooled analysis of accuracy data was performed by means of a hierarchical summary receiving-operating characteristic (HS-ROC) model, as described by Rutter and Gatsonis.[30] In brief, the HS-ROC assumes that there is an underlying ROC curve in each included study, with parameters of diagnostic accuracy assumed to have normal distributions, as in conventional random-effects meta-analysis. The HS-ROC model returns a summary curve for the model, a summary value of sensitivity and specificity (displayed as a summary operating point), and a 95% confidence region for the summary operating point. Individual study weight was given based on effective study sample size. Analyses were performed using the STATA 11.2 software package (Stata Corporation, College Station, TX, USA).

AF Termination as a Procedural End Point: Sensitivity and Specificity in Predicting Outcomes

Systematic search permitted the retrieval of 16 studies meeting prespecified inclusion criteria (**Table 1**). Three were randomized controlled trials evaluating different ablation techniques for nonparoxysmal AF[14,25,27]; the remaining 13 studies were observational series (mostly single center) assessing the outcomes and predictors of success of catheter ablation of nonparoxysmal AF.[16–24,26,28,29,32] The ablation strategies adopted in these studies were highly heterogeneous, and included pulmonary vein antrum isolation only,[14,27] CFAE ablation only,[25,26,32] and a combination of pulmonary vein antrum isolation plus CFAE with or without linear ablation.[14,16–18,21–23,27]

Table 1
Studies evaluating termination of atrial fibrillation as an end point during catheter ablation of nonparoxysmal AF

Authors[Ref.]	Year	No. of Patients	RCT	Ablation Technique	% of AF Termination	Type of AF Termination	Notes
Nademanee et al[32]	2004	64	No	CFAE only	91	SR	Detailed success rates sorted for achievement of periprocedural AF termination not reported
Haissaguerre et al[19]	2005	60	No	Stepwise	87	SR, AT/AFL	AF recurrences at long term sorted for achievement of acute AF termination unclear
Oral et al[26]	2007	100	No	PVI only	16	SR, AT/AFL	Detailed success rates sorted for achievement of periprocedural AF termination not reported
Rostock et al[29]	2008	88	No	Stepwise	77	SR, AT/AFL	—
Fiala et al[18]	2008	135	No	PVI + Linear ablation + CFAE	50	SR	—
Oral et al[25]	2008	85	Yes	CFAE only	24	SR, AT/AFL	—
Li et al[21]	2008	92	No	PVI + Linear ablation + CFAE	35	SR, AT/AFL	AF recurrences at long term sorted for achievement of acute AF termination unclear
Elayi et al[14]	2008	144	Yes	CPVA + Linear ablation vs PVAI only vs PVAI + CFAE	44	SR, AT/AFL	—
Estner et al[17]	2008	35	No	PVI + CFAE	23	SR	—
O'Neill et al[24]	2009	153	No	Stepwise	85	SR, AT/AFL	—
Lin et al[22]	2009	60	No	PVI + Linear ablation	33	SR	—
Lo et al[23]	2009	85	No	Stepwise	54	SR	39% of patients had paroxysmal AF
Oral et al[27]	2009	119	Yes	PVI + CFAE vs PVI only	24	SR, AT/AFL	—
Elayi et al[16]	2010	306	No	PVAI + CFAE	58	SR, AT/AFL	—
Hocini et al[20]	2010	148	No	Stepwise	86	SR, AT/AFL	—
Rostock et al[28]	2011	292	No	Stepwise	70	SR, AT/AFL	Included the 292/395 patients in whom the multivariable Cox regression analysis was performed

Abbreviations: AF, atrial fibrillation; AT/AFL, intermediate atrial tachycardia/flutter; CFAE, complex fractionated electrograms; PVI, pulmonary vein isolation; PVAI, pulmonary vein antrum isolation; RCT, randomized controlled trial; SR, sinus rhythm.

Six studies specifically evaluated the stepwise ablation approach, which sequentially includes pulmonary vein antrum isolation, linear ablation across the roof of the left atrium between the left and right upper pulmonary veins and at the mitral isthmus, ablation at the inferior left atrium toward the coronary sinus and the base of the left atrial appendage, and left atrial ablation guided by CFAE mapping.[19,20,22,24,28,29] Definition of periprocedural AF termination was also heterogeneous between included studies, and ranged from conversion to sinus rhythm (5 studies),[17,18,22,23,32] to direct conversion to sinus rhythm or transition to any intermediate atrial tachycardia or flutter (11 studies).[14,16,19,20,24–29]

Overall, a total of 1966 patients were included in the analysis, with 1118 (57%) achieving periprocedural AF termination. Single-procedure success rates at follow-up sorted by achievement of AF termination during the index procedure were reported in 14 studies[14,16–24,26–29]; 2 studies reported only detailed data for the association between early recurrences (ranging from 1 week to 1 month after the procedure) and periprocedural AF termination.[19,21] After a mean follow-up of 18 $\pm$ 9 months, 957 (48%) patients remained free from recurrent arrhythmia (AF or atrial tachycardia) after a single procedure. A significant heterogeneity between studies in the accuracy of AF termination in predicting long-term freedom from recurrent arrhythmia was found, with a sensitivity ranging from 22%[17] to 97%,[20,29] and a specificity ranging from 20%[24] to 89% (**Fig. 2**).[25] At pooled analysis, periprocedural AF termination predicted single-procedure arrhythmia-free survival with a sensitivity of 70% (95% CI 54%–83%) and a specificity of 58% (95% CI 43%–72%) (see **Fig. 2**).

These figures account for a pooled rate of false-positive results (ie, patients with periprocedural AF termination and recurrent arrhythmia at follow-up) of 42%, and for a pooled rate of false-negative results (ie, patients without periprocedural AF termination remaining free from recurrent arrhythmia at follow-up) of 30%.

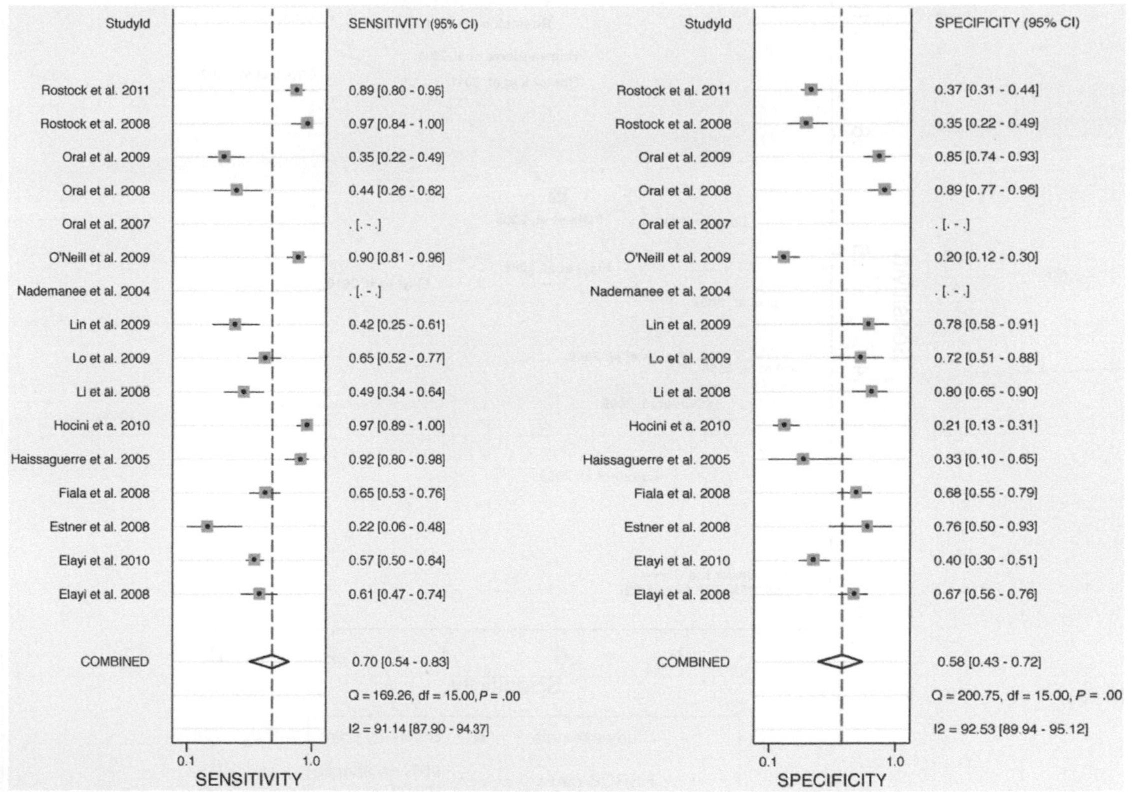

Fig. 2. Forest plot showing the individual and pooled of sensitivity (*left panel*) and specificity (*right panel*) of periprocedural AF termination in predicting single-procedure long-term freedom from recurrent arrhythmia (atrial fibrillation or atrial tachycardia/flutter). Square boxes denote either sensitivity (*left panel*) or specificity (*right panel*). Horizontal lines represent 95% confidence intervals (CI). Overall, periprocedural AF termination predicted long-term freedom from recurrent arrhythmia after a single procedure with a sensitivity of 70% (95% CI 54%–83%) and a specificity of 58% (95% CI 43%–72%).

At pooled HS-ROC analysis, the area under the curve of the diagnostic accuracy of AF termination in predicting long-term single-procedure success was 0.68 (95% CI 0.64–0.72) (**Fig. 3**).

In conclusion, an analysis of the available evidence does not support AF termination as a procedural end point during catheter ablation of nonparoxysmal AF, because of the lack of adequate sensitivity and specificity for predicting long-term procedural success. It is indeed estimable that nearly 1 in every 2 patients achieving such an end point will experience arrhythmia recurrence after the index procedure, and about 1 in every 3 patients not achieving periprocedural AF termination will remain free from recurrent arrhythmia.

Of note, the present analysis might even overestimate the value of AF termination in predicting procedural outcomes, because it was based only on studies in which the predictive value of such an end point has been specifically assessed and reported. In this regard the presence of bias in favor of AF termination may play a role attributable to the well-known tendency of investigators (and Journals) to report selectively (and publish) only studies showing positive associations.[34,35]

AF Termination as a Procedural End Point: From Association to Causation

The nonequivalence of statistical association and causation has long been recognized,[33] but this error of interpretation remains common. While the results of a statistical test of association may reflect a true relationship between the tested variables, it should always be considered that the findings might, in fact, be due to an alternative explanation. Chance, bias, and confounding are well known to produce false results, leading researchers to believe and conclude the existence of a given association when, actually, it does not exist. This section discusses the role of each confounding factor in the believed (or claimed) relationship between periprocedural AF termination and long-term freedom from recurrent arrhythmias.

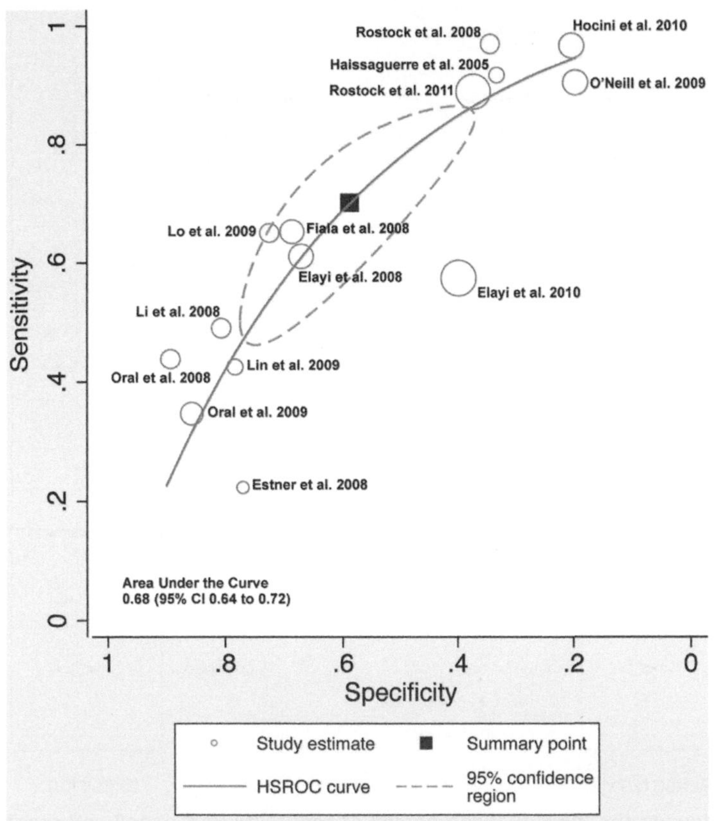

Fig. 3. Hierarchical summary receiver-operating characteristics curve (HS-ROC) showing the individual (*circles*) and pooled (*red square*: summary point) sensitivity and specificity of periprocedural AF termination in predicting long-term single-procedure freedom from recurrent arrhythmia. The dimension of each circle denotes the weight from study sample size. The summary area under the curve was 0.68, further supporting the unreliability of AF termination as a procedural end point.

Chance

The sample size in clinical studies on catheter ablation of AF is generally inadequate, with a consequent lack of power to detect real differences between subgroups. In this setting, chance alone should be always considered as a possible explanation to any reported finding, especially when the study sample size is relatively small. Of note, none of the 16 studies reviewed here performed a formal calculation of the sample size and statistical power,[14,16–29,32] which clearly affects the methodological validity of the reported findings, especially considering that statistics were widely used in these studies to test different investigators' hypotheses and draw conclusions.

The authors performed a retrospective calculation of the power of the studies, reporting a statistically significant association between AF termination and long-term freedom from recurrent arrhythmias (**Fig. 4**). Disturbingly, out of the 11 studies reporting such an association,[18–25,28,29,32] only 6 (54%) had a power of 80% or more,[18,20,23,25,28,29] with only 3 (27%) having a power of at least 90%.[18,28,29] In situations like this there is significant risk that the reported findings might be falsely positive, especially when the probability to define statistical significance is set to the classic value of .05.[36] A common way to detect false-positive statistical association is to rely on effect sizes (ie, CI) rather than only on *P* values, a method that the authors have used and recommended in several previous studies,[37,38] with strong methodological rationale.[39]

Chance might therefore play a prominent role in the reported association between periprocedural AF termination and long-term freedom from recurrent arrhythmias, and there is a concrete risk that such an association might be falsely positive, because most studies were underpowered in addressing the issue.

Bias

None of the studies that focused on periprocedural AF termination clarified whether investigators assessing the long-term freedom from arrhythmia recurrence were blinded to the baseline procedural results.[14,16–29,32] Although recurrent arrhythmia is relatively unaffected by detection bias, because of objective ways of outcomes assessment (eg, electrocardiographic monitoring), lack of blindness might introduce bias in studies reporting long-term freedom from recurrent arrhythmia separately for AF and atrial tachycardia/flutter recurrence.[24] In these settings, the arbitrary disaggregation of outcomes further affect the reliability of the findings, and often the usual level of statistical significance (ie, *P* value <.05) becomes ineffective for

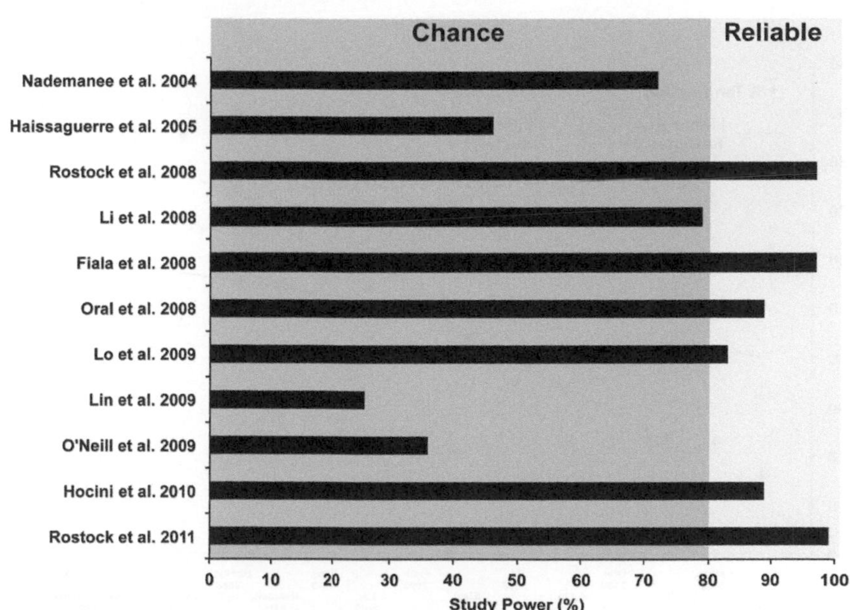

Fig. 4. Indirect calculation of the statistical power of studies reporting an association between periprocedural AF termination and long-term outcome after catheter ablation of nonparoxysmal AF. The great majority of such studies was significantly underpowered, which increases the likelihood of false statistical associations. Chance = study results may be due to play of chance; Reliable = study results are reliable. In the study by Nademanee and colleagues,[32] the power calculation was based on the assumption of detecting a 50% difference in the long-term freedom from AF after a single procedure in the 2 groups (AF termination versus no AF termination).

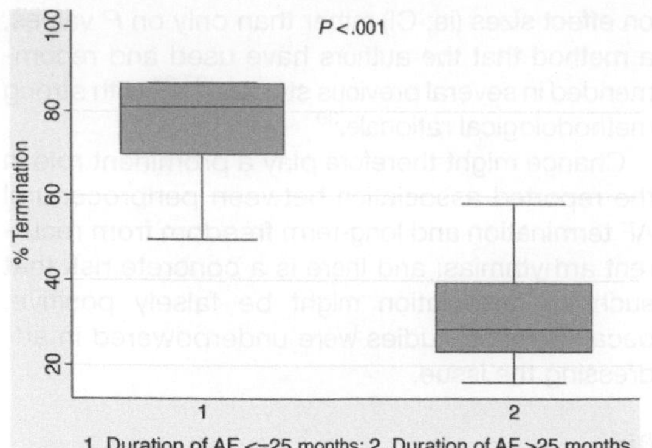

Fig. 5. Example of undetected confounding. The box plot shows the percentage of periprocedural AF termination plotted against the duration of AF in included studies (dichotomized at a value of 25 months). Studies reporting the highest rate of periprocedural AF termination were also those enrolling patients with shorter duration of persistent AF, who are more likely to achieve acute AF termination and experience better long-term outcome. In this case, serious undetected confounding might invalidate the association between periprocedural AF termination and long-term outcome.

ruling out chance as an explanation for the reported findings.

Furthermore, because most patients might actually present with both atrial tachycardia/flutter and AF, it is unclear how the investigators classified such cases, and lack of blindness might have introduced bias attributing more (or less) long-term recurrences of AF or atrial tachycardia/flutter according to the achievement of periprocedural AF termination.

Confounding

A thorough analysis of the available evidence also suggests that unmeasured confounders might have spuriously produced an association between periprocedural AF termination and long-term outcomes. For instance, type and duration of AF are well-known predictors of long-term freedom from recurrent arrhythmia.[40,41] Among patients with nonparoxysmal AF, both the chance of conversion to sinus rhythm and the risk of AF recurrence are tightly linked to the duration of AF, with patients presenting with chronic AF having less chance of conversion to sinus rhythm and the highest chance of recurrence after conversion.

If the duration of persistent AF is plotted against the rate of periprocedural AF termination within the included studies, it appears clear that studies reporting a high rate of AF termination were also those including patients with a shorter duration of persistent AF (**Fig. 5**). Such patients are also those experiencing the better long-term outcomes, and the association between periprocedural AF termination and long-term success might merely reflect

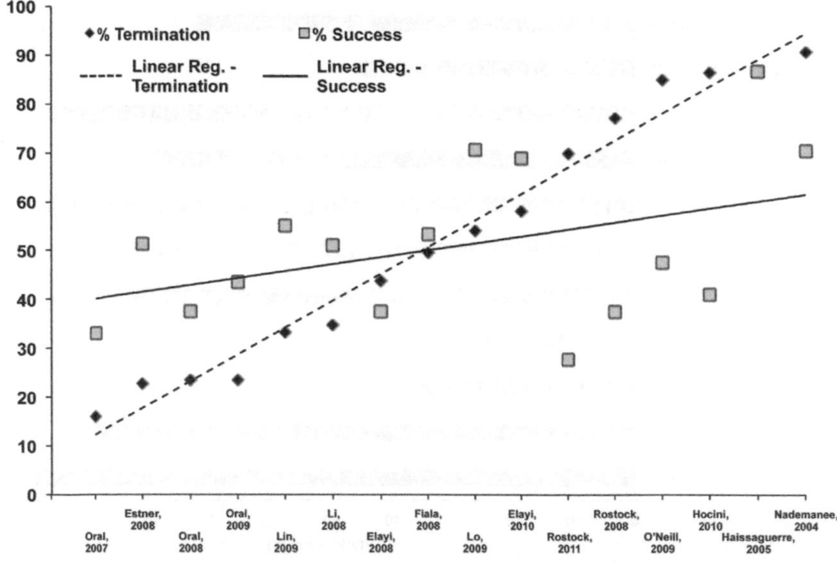

Fig. 6. Evidence that the association between acute AF termination and long-term procedural outcome is not causal. The rates (*y-axis*) of acute AF termination (*black lozenges*) and single-procedure success (*gray boxes*) are sequentially displayed for each included study (*x-axis*). Linear regression (Reg.) has been performed for both the acute AF termination (*dashed line*) and procedural success (*continuous line*). The plot shows that increasing rates of AF termination are not paralleled by an equal increase of procedural success, suggesting that acute AF termination is not independently associated with better procedural outcome.

an association between shorter duration of AF and better long-term outcome after catheter ablation.

The lack of parallel increase in success rates with increasing rates of periprocedural AF termination within included studies (**Fig. 6**) further supports the notion that the reported association is certainly not causal, and likely spurious.

SUMMARY

Periprocedural termination of AF lacks adequate sensitivity and specificity in predicting long-term freedom from recurrent arrhythmia after catheter ablation of nonparoxysmal AF. It is indeed expected that nearly half of patients achieving the end point will experience arrhythmia recurrence, whereas one-third of patients not achieving such an end point will maintain sinus rhythm at long-term follow-up. Available evidence is also affected by major methodological limitations, and false associations that arise from play of chance, built-in biases, and unmeasured confounders cannot be definitely excluded.

In conclusion, AF termination represents an unreliable procedural end point during ablation of nonparoxysmal AF.

REFERENCES

1. Jais P, Cauchemez B, Macle L, et al. Catheter ablation versus antiarrhythmic drugs for atrial fibrillation: the A4 study. Circulation 2008;118(24):2498–505.
2. Wann LS, Curtis AB, January CT, et al. 2011 ACCF/AHA/HRS focused update on the management of patients with atrial fibrillation (Updating the 2006 Guideline): a report of the American College of Cardiology Foundation/American Heart Association Task Force on Practice Guidelines. Heart Rhythm 2011;8(1):157–76.
3. Wazni OM, Marrouche NF, Martin DO, et al. Radiofrequency ablation vs antiarrhythmic drugs as first-line treatment of symptomatic atrial fibrillation: a randomized trial. JAMA 2005;293(21):2634–40.
4. Wilber DJ, Pappone C, Neuzil P, et al. Comparison of antiarrhythmic drug therapy and radiofrequency catheter ablation in patients with paroxysmal atrial fibrillation: a randomized controlled trial. JAMA 2010;303(4):333–40.
5. Marrouche NF, Martin DO, Wazni O, et al. Phased-array intracardiac echocardiography monitoring during pulmonary vein isolation in patients with atrial fibrillation: impact on outcome and complications. Circulation 2003;107(21):2710–6.
6. Nakagawa H, Scherlag BJ, Lockwood DJ, et al. Localization of left atrial autonomic ganglionated plexuses using endocardial and epicardial high frequency stimulation in patients with atrial fibrillation. Heart Rhythm 2005;2005(6):S10.
7. Oral H, Scharf C, Chugh A, et al. Catheter ablation for paroxysmal atrial fibrillation: segmental pulmonary vein ostial ablation versus left atrial ablation. Circulation 2003;108(19):2355–60.
8. Pachon MJ, Pachon ME, Lobo TJ, et al. A new treatment for atrial fibrillation based on spectral analysis to guide the catheter RF-ablation. Europace 2004;6(6):590–601.
9. Pappone C, Santinelli V, Manguso F, et al. Pulmonary vein denervation enhances long-term benefit after circumferential ablation for paroxysmal atrial fibrillation. Circulation 2004;109(3):327–34.
10. Haissaguerre M, Jais P, Shah DC, et al. Spontaneous initiation of atrial fibrillation by ectopic beats originating in the pulmonary veins. N Engl J Med 1998;339(10):659–66.
11. Di Biase L, Elayi CS, Fahmy TS, et al. Atrial fibrillation ablation strategies for paroxysmal patients: randomized comparison between different techniques. Circ Arrhythm Electrophysiol 2009;2(2):113–9.
12. Hayward RM, Upadhyay GA, Mela T, et al. Pulmonary vein isolation with complex fractionated atrial electrogram ablation for paroxysmal and nonparoxysmal atrial fibrillation: a meta-analysis. Heart Rhythm 2011;8(7):994–1000.
13. Li WJ, Bai YY, Zhang HY, et al. Additional ablation of complex fractionated atrial electrograms after pulmonary vein isolation in patients with atrial fibrillation: a meta-analysis. Circ Arrhythm Electrophysiol 2011;4(2):143–8.
14. Elayi CS, Verma A, Di Biase L, et al. Ablation for longstanding permanent atrial fibrillation: results from a randomized study comparing three different strategies. Heart Rhythm 2008;5(12):1658–64.
15. Haissaguerre M, Sanders P, Hocini M, et al. Catheter ablation of long-lasting persistent atrial fibrillation: critical structures for termination. J Cardiovasc Electrophysiol 2005;16(11):1125–37.
16. Elayi CS, Di Biase L, Barrett C, et al. Atrial fibrillation termination as a procedural endpoint during ablation in long-standing persistent atrial fibrillation. Heart Rhythm 2010;7(9):1216–23.
17. Estner HL, Hessling G, Ndrepepa G, et al. Acute effects and long-term outcome of pulmonary vein isolation in combination with electrogram-guided substrate ablation for persistent atrial fibrillation. Am J Cardiol 2008;101(3):332–7.
18. Fiala M, Chovancik J, Nevralova R, et al. Termination of long-lasting persistent versus short-lasting persistent and paroxysmal atrial fibrillation by ablation. Pacing Clin Electrophysiol 2008;31(8):985–97.
19. Haissaguerre M, Hocini M, Sanders P, et al. Catheter ablation of long-lasting persistent atrial fibrillation: clinical outcome and mechanisms of subsequent

arrhythmias. J Cardiovasc Electrophysiol 2005; 16(11):1138–47.

20. Hocini M, Nault I, Wright M, et al. Disparate evolution of right and left atrial rate during ablation of long-lasting persistent atrial fibrillation. J Am Coll Cardiol 2010;55(10):1007–16.
21. Li XP, Dong JZ, Liu XP, et al. Predictive value of early recurrence and delayed cure after catheter ablation for patients with chronic atrial fibrillation. Circ J 2008; 72(7):1125–9.
22. Lin YJ, Tai CT, Chang SL, et al. Efficacy of additional ablation of complex fractionated atrial electrograms for catheter ablation of nonparoxysmal atrial fibrillation. J Cardiovasc Electrophysiol 2009;20(6):607–15.
23. Lo LW, Tai CT, Lin YJ, et al. Predicting factors for atrial fibrillation acute termination during catheter ablation procedures: implications for catheter ablation strategy and long-term outcome. Heart Rhythm 2009;6(3):311–8.
24. O'Neill MD, Wright M, Knecht S, et al. Long-term follow-up of persistent atrial fibrillation ablation using termination as a procedural endpoint. Eur Heart J 2009;30(9):1105–12.
25. Oral H, Chugh A, Good E, et al. Randomized evaluation of right atrial ablation after left atrial ablation of complex fractionated atrial electrograms for long-lasting persistent atrial fibrillation. Circ Arrhythm Electrophysiol 2008;1(1):6–13.
26. Oral H, Chugh A, Good E, et al. Radiofrequency catheter ablation of chronic atrial fibrillation guided by complex electrograms. Circulation 2007; 115(20):2606–12.
27. Oral H, Chugh A, Yoshida K, et al. A randomized assessment of the incremental role of ablation of complex fractionated atrial electrograms after antral pulmonary vein isolation for long-lasting persistent atrial fibrillation. J Am Coll Cardiol 2009;53(9):782–9.
28. Rostock T, Salukhe TV, Steven D, et al. Long-term single- and multiple-procedure outcome and predictors of success after catheter ablation for persistent atrial fibrillation. Heart Rhythm 2011;8(9):1391–7.
29. Rostock T, Steven D, Hoffmann B, et al. Chronic atrial fibrillation is a biatrial arrhythmia: data from catheter ablation of chronic atrial fibrillation aiming arrhythmia termination using a sequential ablation approach. Circ Arrhythm Electrophysiol 2008;1(5): 344–53.
30. Rutter CM, Gatsonis CA. A hierarchical regression approach to meta-analysis of diagnostic test accuracy evaluations. Stat Med 2001;20(19):2865–84.
31. Tzou WS, Saghy L, Lin D. Termination of persistent atrial fibrillation during left atrial mapping. J Cardiovasc Electrophysiol 2011;22(10):1171–3.
32. Nademanee K, McKenzie J, Kosar E, et al. A new approach for catheter ablation of atrial fibrillation: mapping of the electrophysiologic substrate. J Am Coll Cardiol 2004;43(11):2044–53.
33. Hill AB. The environment and disease: association or causation? Proc R Soc Med 1965;58:295–300.
34. Easterbrook PJ, Berlin JA, Gopalan R, et al. Publication bias in clinical research. Lancet 1991; 337(8746):867–72.
35. Chan AW, Hrobjartsson A, Haahr MT, et al. Empirical evidence for selective reporting of outcomes in randomized trials: comparison of protocols to published articles. JAMA 2004;291(20):2457–65.
36. Royall RM. The effect of sample size on the meaning of significance tests. Am Stat 1986;40(4):313–5.
37. Santangeli P, Pelargonio G, Dello Russo A, et al. Gender differences in clinical outcome and primary prevention defibrillator benefit in patients with severe left ventricular dysfunction: a systematic review and meta-analysis. Heart Rhythm 2010;7(7): 876–82.
38. Santangeli P, Di Biase L, Dello Russo A, et al. Meta-analysis: age and effectiveness of prophylactic implantable cardioverter-defibrillators. Ann Intern Med 2010;153(9):592–9.
39. Matthews JN, Altman DG. Statistics notes. Interaction 2: compare effect sizes not P values. BMJ 1996;313(7060):808.
40. Bhargava M, Di Biase L, Mohanty P, et al. Impact of type of atrial fibrillation and repeat catheter ablation on long-term freedom from atrial fibrillation: results from a multicenter study. Heart Rhythm 2009;6(10): 1403–12.
41. Weerasooriya R, Khairy P, Litalien J, et al. Catheter ablation for atrial fibrillation: are results maintained at 5 years of follow-up? J Am Coll Cardiol 2011; 57(2):160–6.

Atrial Fibrillation Ablation Strategy: "Ready Made" or "Tailored"?

Hamid Ghanbari, MD, MPH, Hakan Oral, MD*

KEYWORDS

• Ablation • Pulmonary vein • Trigger • Linear lesion • Atrial fibrillation

KEY POINTS

- Catheter ablation has evolved as an effective treatment modality to eliminate atrial fibrillation (AF); however, despite marked advances, ablation strategies continue to evolve due to the complex and multifactorial nature of AF.
- A standardized and primarily an anatomic ablation strategy may not be sufficient to eliminate all mechanisms of AF operative in a given patient.
- The tailored ablation strategy can eliminate specific triggers and drivers of AF operative in a particular patient so that unnecessary, extensive ablation is avoided.
- The tailored ablation strategy is limited by the accuracy and sensitivity of methods used in identifying specific mechanisms of AF.
- Further improvements in outcomes of catheter ablation of AF largely depend on better understanding and identification of the drivers that are critical to perpetuation of AF.

Atrial fibrillation (AF) is the most prevalent arrhythmia leading to hospital admissions.[1] It has been estimated that the number of patients diagnosed with AF will increase to more than 15 million by 2050.[2] AF is associated with an increase in the risk of stroke, congestive heart failure, and overall mortality.[3–5] Catheter ablation has evolved as an effective treatment modality to eliminate AF over the last decade and has been widely adopted. Despite marked advances, ablation strategies continue to evolve due to the complex and multifactorial nature of AF.[6] It still remains to be determined whether a fixed anatomic ablation strategy or a guided ablation strategy tailored to the specific mechanisms operative is the most appropriate choice. Notwithstanding, these 2 fundamental strategies do not need to be mutually exclusive, and a hybrid approach can also be considered.

MECHANISMS OF AF

A complex interplay between the triggers and substrate is important in initiation and perpetuation of AF.[7] Several mechanisms have been proposed to play a critical role in the genesis of AF and may coexist in the same patient.[8]

Pulmonary Vein (Thoracic Vein) Arrhythmogenicity

Premature depolarizations originating from the pulmonary vein (PV) and other thoracic veins, such as the coronary sinus, ligament of Marshall, and superior and inferior venae cavae, have been demonstrated to initiate AF. Subsequently, rapid repetitive discharges, intermittent PV tachycardias, and their interplay with a left atrial substrate and other thoracic veins were recognized to play a critical role in perpetuation of AF.[9] A recent histoembryologic study demonstrated that most of the posterior left atrium and myocardial sleeves in the PVs share a common embryologic origin and possess similar histologic characteristics, suggesting that posterior left atrium and antrum of the PVs are likely to be as arrhythmogenic as the tubular portion of

Division of Cardiovascular Medicine, University of Michigan, Ann Arbor, MI, USA
* Corresponding author. CVC, SPC 5853, 1500 East Medical Center Drive, Ann Arbor, MI 48109-5853.
E-mail address: oralh@umich.edu

Card Electrophysiol Clin 4 (2012) 353–361
http://dx.doi.org/10.1016/j.ccep.2012.05.007
1877-9182/12/$ – see front matter

the PVs consistent with the observations from clinical studies.[10]

High-Frequency Sources: Rotors

High-frequency sources may initiate spiral waves (rotors), which later may lead to wavebreak and fibrillatory conduction as they encounter structural and functional heterogeneities in the atrial tissue particularly at high activation rates.[11,12] Although rotors have been reproducibly demonstrated in experimental studies using optical mapping techniques and also in simulation models, a challenge has been how best to identify the rotors in real time in the human atria. Although post hoc analysis of electrograms recorded during AF in the human heart has demonstrated the presence of frequency gradients as well as a spatial relationship between sites of termination of AF during ablation and sites of highest frequency, real-time mapping of rotors remains a major challenge during catheter ablation of AF.[13]

Multiple Wavelet Theory

Based on a computational model, multiple wavelets changing in direction and number were proposed to explain perpetuation of AF. Both sites of fixed and functional block were thought to play a role in facilitating these reentrant wavelets, particularly at sites of anatomic boundaries and fibrosis.[11,12,14]

Autonomic Dysregulation

The interactive atrial neural network innervates the atria and interconnects the ganglionated plexi that play an important role in autonomic regulation.[15] A parasympathetic dominance shortens the effective refractory period of the atrial tissue and increases automaticity and triggered activity. Increased parasympathetic activity has been demonstrated to facilitate inducibility and sustainability of AF.[16,17]

ANATOMIC ABLATION

PV Isolation

PV isolation (PVI) is usually the essential first step during catheter ablation of AF. Several approaches have been performed to isolate the PVs. As the arrhythmogenic potential of the PV antrum is recognized, techniques of circumferential PVI have largely replaced the initial techniques of segmental ostial PVI and focal ostial PV ablation. Antral PVI or wide-area circumferential ablation can be successfully performed based on anatomic landmarks around the PV antrum often with the guidance of a 3-dimensional navigation system. However, it is critically important to confirm complete electrical isolation of the PVs. Entrance and exit block are the endpoints of PVI. Recent studies suggest that it may be important to assess dormant PV conduction during adenosine infusion. Clinical studies are underway to determine whether dormant PV conduction is associated with clinical recurrences of AF after PVI.[18] An exception to anatomic PVI is a focal ablation strategy that targets a single PV fascicle or isolation of a single PV in a patient with clearly documented focal atrial tachycardia or fibrillation whose AF terminates during ablation and is rendered noninducible after focal ablation.

Antral PVI is highly effective in eliminating paroxysmal AF; however, it has modest efficacy in patients with persistent AF. Antral PVI eliminates PV arrhythmogenicity and also some of the non-PV triggers of AF that may arise from the posterior left atrium or antrum of the PVs. Antral PVI may also result in debulking of the left atrium and may reduce the wavelength available to harbor a reentrant circuit. Another potential effect of antral PVI may include ablation of ganglionated plexi. It also is possible that antral PVI eliminates some, if not most, of the high-frequency drivers of AF that are thought to have anchor points around the antrum of the PVs.

Linear Ablation

Linear lesions usually include a roof line connecting the left and right superior PVs and a mitral line connecting the mitral annulus to the inferior PVs (**Fig. 1**). Other possible linear ablation (LA) sites include lesions across the anterior left atrium and along the septum.[19] Addition of linear lesions is intended to modify the arrhythmogenic LA substrate and atrial macroreentrant circuits involved in maintenance of AF. Bidirectional block across the linear lesions should be confirmed to minimize the risk of proarrhythmia due to macro- or microreentrant atrial flutters that use gaps along the ablation lines.[20–22] Addition of linear lesions after antral PVI has been reported to improve the probability of maintaining sinus rhythm particularly in patients with persistent AF, despite an increase in the incidence of recurrent atrial flutter, which often prompts a repeat ablation.[23] In a prior study, in patients with persistent AF who had AF ablation, only 20% undergoing PVI alone remained in sinus rhythm compared with 69% following PVI combined ablation at the roof and mitral isthmus.[21] An anatomic approach using circumferential PV ablation (CPVA) with adjunctive roof and mitral isthmus ablation can significantly reduce the AF burden at 12-month follow-up.[24] In another study,

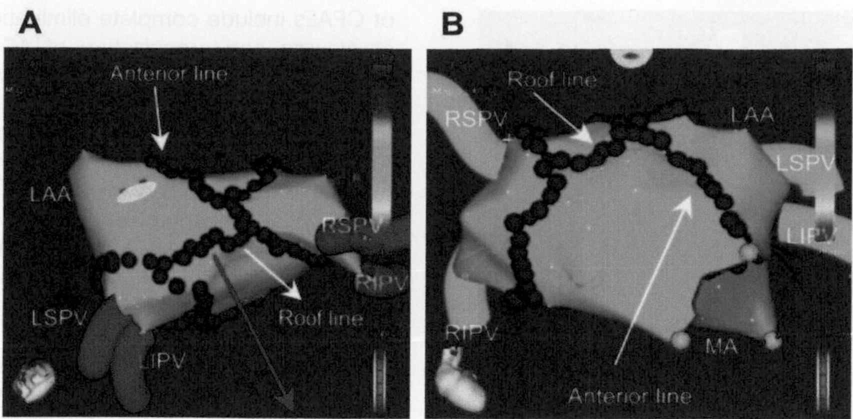

Fig. 1. Anatomic ablation. Shown are cranial (*A*) and anterior-posterior projections (*B*) of an electroanatomic map illustrating ablation lines created to encircle left- and right-sided PVs 1 to 2 cm from their ostia. Additional ablation lines guided by local electrograms were created in roof and anterior left atrium (*A, B*). LAA, left atrial appendage; LI, left inferior; LS, left superior; MA, mitral annulus; PV, pulmonary vein; RI, right inferior; RM, right middle; RS, right superior. (*From* Oral H, Chugh A, Lemola K, et al. Noninducibility of atrial fibrillation as an end point of left atrial circumferential ablation for paroxysmal atrial fibrillation: a randomized study. Circulation 2004;110(18):2797–801; with permission.)

which sought noninducibility of AF as the procedural endpoint, adjunctive LA after PVI was associated with freedom from AF in 91% of patients with paroxysmal AF.[25] These findings suggest that LA in addition to targeting triggers may substantially modify the left atrial substrate and promote maintenance of sinus rhythm after AF ablation. Most atrial tachycardias after LA result from gaps in the ablation lines and can often be successfully ablated.[26,27]

Ablation of Cavotricuspid Isthmus

Cavotricuspid isthmus dependent atrial flutter (CTI-AFL) is common in patients with AF.[28,29] In patients with AF who have either a history of typical AFL or an inducible episode of typical AFL during an electrophysiologic study, ablation of CTI is the preferred approach.[30] However, prophylactic CTI ablation in patients with no clinical evidence of typical AFL appears to add no incremental benefit.[31]

TAILORED ABLATION APPROACH

Because the pathogenesis of AF is multifactorial and complex, a standardized and primarily an anatomic ablation strategy may not be sufficient to eliminate all mechanisms of AF operative in a given patient, whereas it may be more than necessary and may lead to a compromise in left atrial transport function due to excessive ablation and an increase in the risk of complications in other patients. Therefore, key to the success of a tailored ablation strategy is accurate identification of all drivers of AF and making sure they have been effectively eliminated.

In a prior study, a tailored ablation strategy was used in 153 consecutive patients with symptomatic, paroxysmal AF. All PVs were mapped and PV tachycardias were identified and eliminated using partial or complete PVI. If AF was still inducible after elimination of all PV tachycardias, left atrial mapping was performed to identify and ablate sites of complex electrograms or sites with electrograms faster than those in the coronary sinus. Additional ablation was also performed in the coronary sinus and/or superior vena cava to target complex or rapid electrograms until AF became noninducible or until target sites were eliminated (**Fig. 2**). During a mean follow-up of 11 ± 4 months, 77% of patients were free from AF and/or atrial flutter without antiarrhythmic drug therapy.[32]

Complex Fractionated Atrial Electrogram

Complex fractionated atrial electrograms (CFAEs) have often been targeted to eliminate drivers of AF with or without concomitant PVI. CFAEs are defined as atrial electrograms with a short cycle length (≤120 ms) and continuous electrical activity or fractionation (**Fig. 3**).[33] Although our understanding of mechanism of CFAEs continues to evolve, CFAEs have been suggested to indicate areas of slow conduction, wavefront collision, conduction block or pivot points for reentrant circuits, or high-frequency sources (rotors). CFAEs may also indicate sites of ganglionated plexi

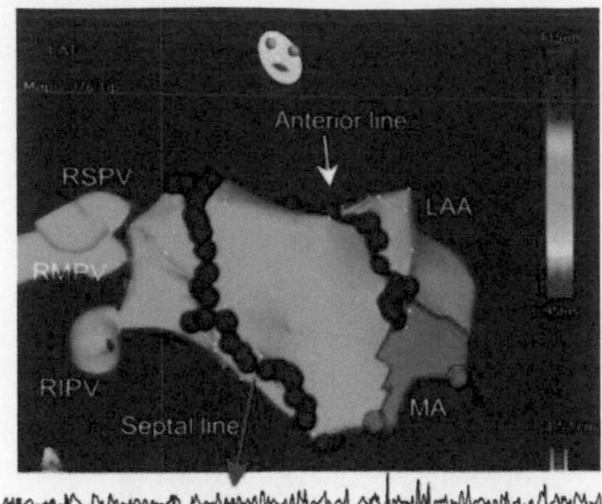

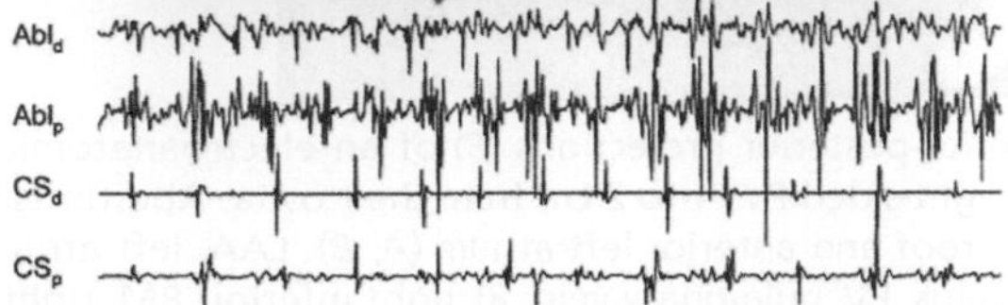

Fig. 2. Examples of complex fractionated atrial electrograms (CFAEs): CFAEs are characterized by fractionation, continuous electrical activity or a short cycle length. LAA, left atrial appendage; LI, left inferior; LS, left superior; MA, mitral annulus; PV, pulmonary vein; RI, right inferior; RM, right middle; RS, right superior. (*From* Oral H, Chugh A, Lemola K, et al. Noninducibility of atrial fibrillation as an end point of left atrial circumferential ablation for paroxysmal atrial fibrillation: a randomized study. Circulation 2004;110(18):2797–801; with permission.)

(AF nests); however, it also is possible that CFAEs are recorded at sites of anisotropic conduction or summation of electrograms from multiple layers of overlapping myocardial fibers with different fiber orientation.[8,34–37] End points for ablation at sites of CFAEs include complete elimination of CFAEs or slowing and organization of AF to an atrial tachycardia or directly to sinus rhythm.[32,33,38]

In a prior study, ablation of CFAEs without routine isolation of PVs was reported to eliminate AF in 90% of patients with paroxysmal or persistent AF at 1-year follow-up (**Fig. 4**).[33] In another study, 119 consecutive patients with long-standing persistent AF were randomized to antral PVI alone or antral PVI and ablation of CFAEs. After up to 2 hours of additional ablation of CFAEs, the probability of maintain sinus rhythm was similar between the 2 groups regardless of whether CFAEs were ablated after antral PVI. However, AF was terminated in a minority of patients during ablation of CFAEs in that study.[39]

In a meta-analysis of 7 controlled trials with a total of 622 patients, ablation of CFAES in conjunction with PVI was found to be associated with a higher likelihood of maintaining sinus rhythm in patients with nonparoxysmal AF, but not in those with paroxysmal AF.[40] However, CFAEs were identified using variable criteria among these studies.[41]

Stepwise Ablation

The stepwise approach incorporates several strategies in a sequential fashion.[38,42] After PVI first, CFAEs and sites of frequency gradients are targeted, followed by LA along the left atrial roof and mitral isthmus. Non-PV focal triggers of AF that may originate from the superior vena cava, coronary sinus, or right atrium are also targeted as necessary.[43] In a prior study, after extensive

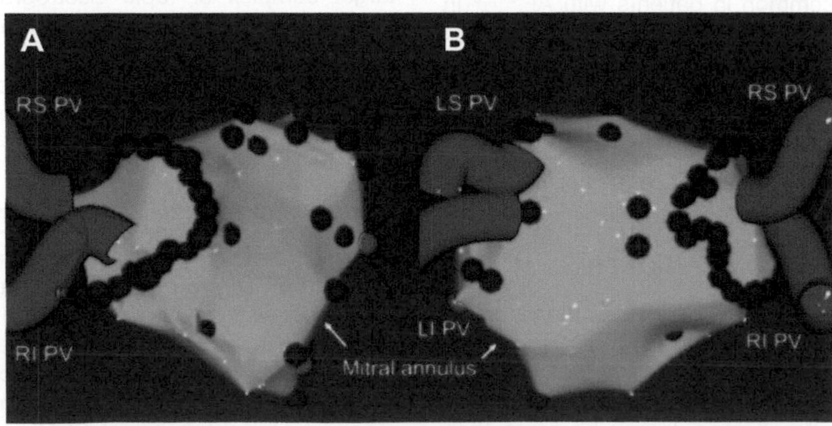

Fig. 3. Tailored ablation. After encircling of the righ-sided PVs to eliminate PV tachycardias, left atrial ablation was performed to target CFAEs. Shown are the right anterior oblique (*A*) and posteroanterior (*B*) projections of the 3-dimentional left atrial geometry. Red tags indicate sites of radiofrequency energy applications. LAA, left atrial appendage; LI, left inferior; LS, left superior; MA, mitral annulus; PV, pulmonary vein; RI, right inferior; RM, right middle; RS, right superior. (*From* Oral H, Chugh A, Good E, et al. A tailored approach to catheter ablation of paroxysmal atrial fibrillation. Circulation 2006;113(15):1824–31; with permission.)

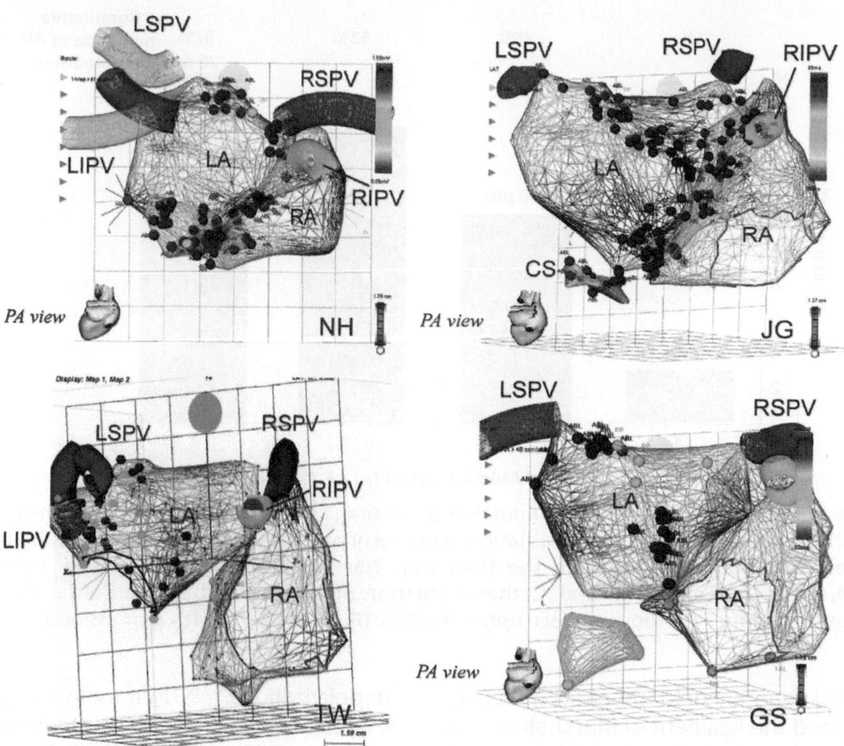

Fig. 4. Ablation of CFAEs. Shown are posteroanterior projections of sites of CFAE ablation that resulted in termination of AF in 4 different patients. LAA, left atrial appendage; LI, left inferior; LS, left superior; MA, mitral annulus; PV, pulmonary vein; RI, right inferior; RM, right middle; RS, right superior. (*From* Nademanee K, McKenzie J, Kosar E, et al. A new approach for catheter ablation of atrial fibrillation: mapping of the electrophysiologic substrate. J Am Coll Cardiol 2004;43(11):2044–53; with permission.)

left and right atrial ablation, AF was terminated in 87% of the patients, and more than 90% of patients with long-standing persistent AF were reported to have remained in sinus rhythm at 1-year follow-up; however, multiple procedures often for atrial flutter or atrial tachycardia were necessary.[38] Despite extensive ablation and a subsequent delay in left atrial conduction, recovery of left atrial transport function was eventually observed in most patients.[44] Although detailed mapping of complex electrograms after PVI is an integral part of stepwise ablation strategy, linear lesions were necessary in more than 80% of the patients to terminate AF (**Fig. 5**). Stepwise ablation strategy is highly effective in eliminating AF; however, it is effort intense and requires detailed mapping with a long procedure duration and extensive atrial ablation. Repeat procedures due to proarrhythmia are often necessary.

Spectral Mapping

Sites of high dominant frequency (DF) have been suggested to represent rotors as critical drivers of AF.[45,46] These sites typically show rapid periodicity but lack significant fractionation.[46] However, sites adjacent to areas of maximal periodicity often display the greatest fractionation, which may explain the efficacy of CFAE ablation.[46] In paroxysmal AF, the DF sites are more prevalent within the PVs, whereas in permanent AF, the DF sites commonly exist within the left atrium.[47] In a prior study, ablation at DF sites resulted in significant prolongation of the AF cycle length and termination of AF.[47] Moreover, a significant reduction in DF after ablation is associated with a higher probability of maintaining sinus rhythm in both paroxysmal and persistent AF patients.[48,49] Currently, there are several limitations of DF maping as an ablation strategy. These factors include lack of high-resolution mapping to precisely locate DF sites, real-time analysis of DF, and spatiotemporal stability of DF sites.[41]

Non-PV Foci

Although the PVs are a dominant source of premature and repetitive depolarizations responsible for initiation of AF,[9,50] non-PV ectopic activity can trigger AF.[50–54] Most non-PV triggers of AF are located in the superior vena cava, crista terminalis, coronary sinus, left atrial free wall, left atrial

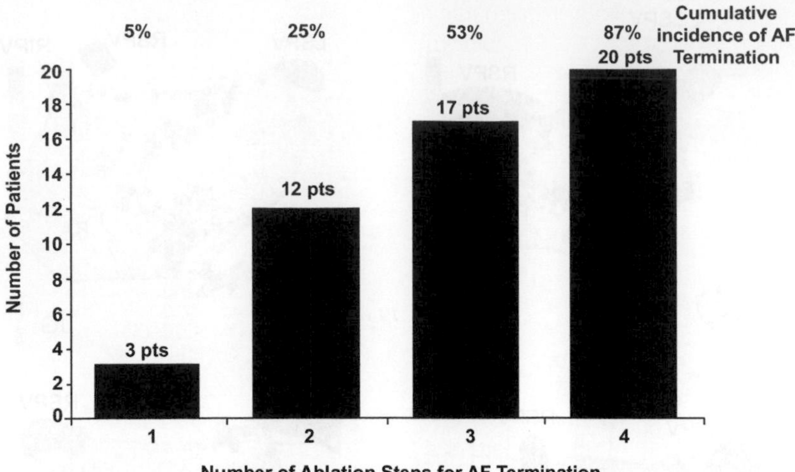

Fig. 5. Stepwise ablation. The number and cumulative percentage of patients terminating with each step of ablation. Of note, the first 3 steps (PVI, atrial ablation, and coronary sinus/superior vena cava ablation) were performed in a randomized order, although the final step was linear ablation in all cases. (*Reproduced from* Haissaguerre M, Hocini M, Sanders P, et al. Catheter ablation of long-lasting persistent atrial fibrillation: critical structures for termination. J Cardiovasc Electrophysiol 2005;16(11):1125–37; with permission.)

appendage, and ligament of Marshall.[54] The superior vena cava and the ligament of Marshall usually account for initiation of AF in less than 5%– to 10% of patients with AF.[52] The coronary sinus may play a more complex role in the initiation and perpetuation of AF.[55] Bursts of focal rapid repetitive activity have been identified in the coronary sinus in 3% of patients with paroxysmal or persistent AF.[56] Epicardial and endocardial ablation along and in the coronary sinus in patients with paroxysmal or persistent AF who remained in AF after PVI can lead to termination of AF in up to 35% of the patients.[57] Sources within the right atrium also may be important in the pathogenesis of AF in a small portion of patients. Using a stepwise ablation strategy in patients with persistent AF, only 3% of the patients had termination of AF with right atrial ablation.[43] These observations suggest that the non-PV sources may play a critical role in a small proportion of patients with AF, and a tailored ablation strategy would be helpful in looking for these non-PV triggers of AF.

Autonomic Ganglionated Plexi

Ganglionic plexi (GP) are a complex cluster of sympathetic and parasympathetic neurons, which supply the autonomic innervation of the LA.[58] Most GP are located above the LA and in fat pads at the superior vena cava aorta, and the PV-LA junctions and ablation of these sites can effectively denervate the LA.[59] An increase in parasympathetic activity may shorten the atrial refractory period and facilitate triggered activity and premature depolarizations.[60,61] In a meta-analysis of 6 trials evaluating the role of GP ablation in AF, early recurrence was significantly higher after GP ablation alone compared with PVI. Freedom from AF recurrence was significantly improved by additional GP ablation when compared with PVI or maze procedure. However, GP ablation alone was associated with an increase in AF recurrence compared with PVI alone.[62] The precise location of GP can be mapped using high-frequency stimulation as well as by monitoring the changes due to autonomic effects on the heart during radio frequency (RF) ablation.[63] Future studies are necessary to determine the specific role of mapping and targeting of GP in patients undergoing catheter ablation of AF. The procedural end point for this strategy should be lack of inducible vagal reflexes.[61] There is clinical evidence that complete vagal denervation during CPVA significantly reduces recurrence of AF at 1-year follow-up.[64] However, at this point, it is not quite clear whether favorable effects seen are related to substrate modification of the LA or solely due to ablation of GP.[19]

SUMMARY

One of the advantages of the tailored ablation strategy is elimination of specific triggers and drivers of AF operative in a particular patient so that unnecessary, extensive ablation is avoided and all potential mechanisms of AF regardless of the anatomic location have been eliminated. However, the challenges and limitations of a tailored ablation strategy include the accuracy and sensitivity of identifying specific mechanism of AF. To date, no approach has been confirmed to have sufficient sensitivity and specificity to identify drivers of AF particularly those in the atrial substrate. On the other hand, anatomic approach offers a standardized approach targeting most common mechanisms of AF. Although effective in most patients, anatomic approach may not be sufficient to eliminate all potential mechanisms of AF and may be more than necessary in other patients.

As the parameters and tools to identify drivers of AF beyond PVs continue to evolve, a practical approach may be to start with an anatomic ablation strategy and tailor ablation to eliminate the residual drivers of AF after PVI, particularly in patients with persistent AF. Further improvements in outcomes of catheter ablation of AF and strategies such as tailored ablation will largely depend on better understanding and thereby better identification of the drivers that are critical to perpetuation of AF.

REFERENCES

1. Go AS, Hylek EM, Phillips KA, et al. Prevalence of diagnosed atrial fibrillation in adults: national implications for rhythm management and stroke prevention: the AnTicoagulation and Risk Factors in Atrial Fibrillation (ATRIA) Study. JAMA 2001;285(18):2370–5.
2. Miyasaka Y, Barnes ME, Gersh BJ, et al. Secular trends in incidence of atrial fibrillation in Olmsted County, Minnesota, 1980 to 2000, and implications on the projections for future prevalence. Circulation 2006;114(2):119–25.
3. Benjamin EJ, Wolf PA, D'Agostino RB, et al. Impact of atrial fibrillation on the risk of death: the Framingham Heart Study. Circulation 1998;98(10):946–52.
4. Wang TJ, Larson MG, Levy D, et al. Temporal relations of atrial fibrillation and congestive heart failure and their joint influence on mortality: the Framingham Heart Study. Circulation 2003;107(23):2920–5.
5. Wolf PA, Abbott RD, Kannel WB. Atrial fibrillation as an independent risk factor for stroke: the Framingham Study. Stroke 1991;22(8):983–8.
6. Ghanbari H, Schmidt M, Machado C, et al. Ablation strategies for atrial fibrillation. Expert Rev Cardiovasc Ther 2009;7(9):1091–101.
7. Allessie MA, Boyden PA, Camm AJ, et al. Pathophysiology and prevention of atrial fibrillation. Circulation 2001;103(5):769–77.
8. Konings KT, Kirchhof CJ, Smeets JR, et al. High-density mapping of electrically induced atrial fibrillation in humans. Circulation 1994;89(4):1665–80.
9. Haissaguerre M, Jais P, Shah DC, et al. Spontaneous initiation of atrial fibrillation by ectopic beats originating in the pulmonary veins. N Engl J Med 1998;339(10):659–66.
10. Oral H, Ozaydin M, Tada H, et al. Mechanistic significance of intermittent pulmonary vein tachycardia in patients with atrial fibrillation. J Cardiovasc Electrophysiol 2002;13(7):645–50.
11. Savelieva I, Camm J. Update on atrial fibrillation: part I. Clin Cardiol 2008;31(2):55–62.
12. Jalife J. Rotors and spiral waves in atrial fibrillation. J Cardiovasc Electrophysiol 2003;14(7):776–80.
13. Stiles MK, Brooks AG, Kuklik P, et al. High-density mapping of atrial fibrillation in humans: relationship between high-frequency activation and electrogram fractionation. J Cardiovasc Electrophysiol 2008;19(12):1245–53.
14. Moe GK, Abildskov JA. Atrial fibrillation as a self-sustaining arrhythmia independent of focal discharge. Am Heart J 1959;58(1):59–70.
15. Hou Y, Scherlag BJ, Lin J, et al. Interactive atrial neural network: determining the connections between ganglionated plexi. Heart Rhythm 2007;4(1):56–63.
16. Po SS, Scherlag BJ, Yamanashi WS, et al. Experimental model for paroxysmal atrial fibrillation arising at the pulmonary vein-atrial junctions. Heart Rhythm 2006;3(2):201–8.
17. Bettoni M, Zimmermann M. Autonomic tone variations before the onset of paroxysmal atrial fibrillation. Circulation 2002;105(23):2753–9.
18. Macle L, Khairy P, Verma A, et al. Adenosine following pulmonary vein isolation to target dormant conduction elimination (ADVICE): methods and rationale. Can J Cardiol 2012;28(2):184–90.
19. Wright M, Haissaguerre M, Knecht S, et al. State of the art: catheter ablation of atrial fibrillation. J Cardiovasc Electrophysiol 2008;19(6):583–92.
20. Hocini M, Jais P, Sanders P, et al. Techniques, evaluation, and consequences of linear block at the left atrial roof in paroxysmal atrial fibrillation: a prospective randomized study. Circulation 2005;112(24):3688–96.
21. Willems S, Klemm H, Rostock T, et al. Substrate modification combined with pulmonary vein isolation improves outcome of catheter ablation in patients with persistent atrial fibrillation: a prospective randomized comparison. Eur Heart J 2006;27(23):2871–8.
22. Jais P, Hocini M, Hsu LF, et al. Technique and results of linear ablation at the mitral isthmus. Circulation 2004;110(19):2996–3002.
23. Gaita F, Caponi D, Scaglione M, et al. Long-term clinical results of 2 different ablation strategies in patients with paroxysmal and persistent atrial fibrillation. Circ Arrhythm Electrophysiol 2008;1(4):269–75.
24. Kottkamp H, Tanner H, Kobza R, et al. Time courses and quantitative analysis of atrial fibrillation episode

number and duration after circular plus linear left atrial lesions: trigger elimination or substrate modification: early or delayed cure? J Am Coll Cardiol 2004;44(4):869–77.

25. Jais P, Hocini M, Sanders P, et al. Long-term evaluation of atrial fibrillation ablation guided by noninducibility. Heart Rhythm 2006;3(2):140–5.
26. Mesas CE, Pappone C, Lang CC, et al. Left atrial tachycardia after circumferential pulmonary vein ablation for atrial fibrillation: electroanatomic characterization and treatment. J Am Coll Cardiol 2004;44(5):1071–9.
27. Chugh A, Oral H, Lemola K, et al. Prevalence, mechanisms, and clinical significance of macroreentrant atrial tachycardia during and following left atrial ablation for atrial fibrillation. Heart Rhythm 2005;2(5):464–71.
28. Waldo AL. Pathogenesis of atrial flutter. J Cardiovasc Electrophysiol 1998;9(Suppl 8):S18–25.
29. Waldo AL, Feld GK. Inter-relationships of atrial fibrillation and atrial flutter mechanisms and clinical implications. J Am Coll Cardiol 2008;51(8):779–86.
30. Scharf C, Veerareddy S, Ozaydin M, et al. Clinical significance of inducible atrial flutter during pulmonary vein isolation in patients with atrial fibrillation. J Am Coll Cardiol 2004;43(11):2057–62.
31. Pontoppidan J, Nielsen JC, Poulsen SH, et al. Prophylactic cavotricuspid isthmus block during atrial fibrillation ablation in patients without atrial flutter: a randomised controlled trial. Heart 2009;95(12):994–9.
32. Oral H, Chugh A, Good E, et al. A tailored approach to catheter ablation of paroxysmal atrial fibrillation. Circulation 2006;113(15):1824–31.
33. Nademanee K, McKenzie J, Kosar E, et al. A new approach for catheter ablation of atrial fibrillation: mapping of the electrophysiologic substrate. J Am Coll Cardiol 2004;43(11):2044–53.
34. Cosio FG, Palacios J, Vidal JM, et al. Electrophysiologic studies in atrial fibrillation. Slow conduction of premature impulses: a possible manifestation of the background for reentry. Am J Cardiol 1983;51(1):122–30.
35. Ohe T, Matsuhisa M, Kamakura S, et al. Relation between the widening of the fragmented atrial activity zone and atrial fibrillation. Am J Cardiol 1983;52(10):1219–22.
36. Verma A, Novak P, Macle L, et al. A prospective, multicenter evaluation of ablating complex fractionated electrograms (CFEs) during atrial fibrillation (AF) identified by an automated mapping algorithm: acute effects on AF and efficacy as an adjuvant strategy. Heart Rhythm 2008;5(2):198–205.
37. Narayan SM, Wright M, Derval N, et al. Classifying fractionated electrograms in human atrial fibrillation using monophasic action potentials and activation mapping: evidence for localized drivers, rate acceleration, and nonlocal signal etiologies. Heart Rhythm 2011;8(2):244–53.
38. Haissaguerre M, Hocini M, Sanders P, et al. Catheter ablation of long-lasting persistent atrial fibrillation: clinical outcome and mechanisms of subsequent arrhythmias. J Cardiovasc Electrophysiol 2005;16(11):1138–47.
39. Oral H, Chugh A, Yoshida K, et al. A randomized assessment of the incremental role of ablation of complex fractionated atrial electrograms after antral pulmonary vein isolation for long-lasting persistent atrial fibrillation. J Am Coll Cardiol 2009;53(9):782–9.
40. Li WJ, Bai YY, Zhang HY, et al. Additional ablation of complex fractionated atrial electrograms after pulmonary vein isolation in patients with atrial fibrillation: a meta-analysis. Circ Arrhythm Electrophysiol 2011;4(2):143–8.
41. Latchamsetty R, Morady F. Complex fractionated atrial electrograms: a worthwhile target for ablation of atrial fibrillation? Circ Arrhythm Electrophysiol 2011;4(2):117–8.
42. O'Neill MD, Jais P, Takahashi Y, et al. The stepwise ablation approach for chronic atrial fibrillation–evidence for a cumulative effect. J Interv Card Electrophysiol 2006;16(3):153–67.
43. Haissaguerre M, Hocini M, Sanders P, et al. Catheter ablation of long-lasting persistent atrial fibrillation: critical structures for termination. J Cardiovasc Electrophysiol 2005;16(11):1125–37.
44. Takahashi Y, O'Neill MD, Hocini M, et al. Effects of stepwise ablation of chronic atrial fibrillation on atrial electrical and mechanical properties. J Am Coll Cardiol 2007;49(12):1306–14.
45. Chang SH, Ulfarsson M, Chugh A, et al. Time- and frequency-domain characteristics of atrial electrograms during sinus rhythm and atrial fibrillation. J Cardiovasc Electrophysiol 2011;22(8):851–7.
46. Kalifa J, Tanaka K, Zaitsev AV, et al. Mechanisms of wave fractionation at boundaries of high-frequency excitation in the posterior left atrium of the isolated sheep heart during atrial fibrillation. Circulation 2006;113(5):626–33.
47. Sanders P, Berenfeld O, Hocini M, et al. Spectral analysis identifies sites of high-frequency activity maintaining atrial fibrillation in humans. Circulation 2005;112(6):789–97.
48. Atienza F, Almendral J, Jalife J, et al. Real-time dominant frequency mapping and ablation of dominant frequency sites in atrial fibrillation with left-to-right frequency gradients predicts long-term maintenance of sinus rhythm. Heart Rhythm 2009;6(1):33–40.
49. Yoshida K, Chugh A, Good E, et al. A critical decrease in dominant frequency and clinical outcome after catheter ablation of persistent atrial fibrillation. Heart Rhythm 2009;7(3):295–302.
50. Chen SA, Hsieh MH, Tai CT, et al. Initiation of atrial fibrillation by ectopic beats originating from the pulmonary

veins: electrophysiological characteristics, pharmacological responses, and effects of radiofrequency ablation. Circulation 1999;100(18):1879–86.
51. Tsai CF, Tai CT, Hsieh MH, et al. Initiation of atrial fibrillation by ectopic beats originating from the superior vena cava: electrophysiological characteristics and results of radiofrequency ablation. Circulation 2000; 102(1):67–74.
52. Lin WS, Tai CT, Hsieh MH, et al. Catheter ablation of paroxysmal atrial fibrillation initiated by non-pulmonary vein ectopy. Circulation 2003;107(25): 3176–83.
53. Haissaguerre M, Hocini M, Sanders P, et al. Localized sources maintaining atrial fibrillation organized by prior ablation. Circulation 2006;113(5):616–25.
54. Higa S, Tai CT, Chen SA. Catheter ablation of atrial fibrillation originating from extrapulmonary vein areas: Taipei approach. Heart Rhythm 2006;3(11): 1386–90.
55. Oral H. Atrial fibrillation: mechanisms, features, and management. In: Zipes DP, Jalife J, editors. Cardac electrophysiology: from cell to bedside. Philadelphia: Saunders; 2008. p. 577–88.
56. Knecht S, O'Neill MD, Matsuo S, et al. Focal arrhythmia confined within the coronary sinus and maintaining atrial fibrillation. J Cardiovasc Electrophysiol 2007;18(11):1140–6.
57. Haissaguerre M, Hocini M, Takahashi Y, et al. Impact of catheter ablation of the coronary sinus on paroxysmal or persistent atrial fibrillation. J Cardiovasc Electrophysiol 2007;18(4):378–86.
58. Armour JA, Murphy DA, Yuan BX, et al. Gross and microscopic anatomy of the human intrinsic cardiac nervous system. Anat Rec 1997;247(2):289–98.
59. Chiou CW, Eble JN, Zipes DP. Efferent vagal innervation of the canine atria and sinus and atrioventricular nodes. The third fat pad. Circulation 1997; 95(11):2573–84.
60. Takahashi Y, Jais P, Hocini M, et al. Shortening of fibrillatory cycle length in the pulmonary vein during vagal excitation. J Am Coll Cardiol 2006; 47(4):774–80.
61. Scherlag BJ, Yamanashi W, Patel U, et al. Autonomically induced conversion of pulmonary vein focal firing into atrial fibrillation. J Am Coll Cardiol 2005; 45(11):1878–86.
62. Zhou Q, Hou Y, Yang S. A meta-analysis of the comparative efficacy of ablation for atrial fibrillation with and without ablation of the ganglionated plexi. Pacing Clin Electrophysiol 2011;34(12):1687–94.
63. Lemery R, Birnie D, Tang AS, et al. Feasibility study of endocardial mapping of ganglionated plexuses during catheter ablation of atrial fibrillation. Heart Rhythm 2006;3(4):387–96.
64. Pappone C, Santinelli V, Manguso F, et al. Pulmonary vein denervation enhances long-term benefit after circumferential ablation for paroxysmal atrial fibrillation. Circulation 2004;109(3):327–34.

Anticoagulation Issues in Patients with AF

Antonio Rossillo, MD, Andrea Corrado, MD, Paolo China, MD, Michela Madalosso, MD, Sakis Themistoclakis, MD*

KEYWORDS

• Atrial fibrillation • Anticoagulation • Stroke • Bleeding • Catheter ablation

KEY POINTS

- The evaluation of the risk of stroke for individual patients with atrial fibrillation (AF) is a crucial factor in the decision to provide anticoagulation therapy.
- Novel oral anticoagulants, as compared with warfarin, are associated with a lower or similar rate of stroke and systemic embolism and a lower rate of hemorrhagic stroke. These drugs are administered at a fixed dose, have a shorter pick action and half-life, and do not require international normalized ratio monitoring.
- After a successful AF ablation, oral anticoagulation therapy discontinuation seems to be feasible in patients with a $CHADS_2$ score greater than or equal to 2 and normal left atrial function. However, larger prospective randomized trials are needed to confirm the safety of this strategy.

Atrial fibrillation (AF) is the most common sustained cardiac arrhythmia, with a prevalence between 0.9% and 2.5% in the general population and an increasing incidence with age. This arrhythmia is associated with a 6-fold increased risk of a thromboembolic (TE) event compared with patients in sinus rhythm[1] and accounts for about 1.5% of all strokes in people aged 50 to 59 years and almost 25% of strokes in people aged 80 to 89 years.

TE events generally result from left atrium thrombi, the left atrial appendage (LAA) being the most common source of thrombus formation, with an incidence of 91% in patients with nonvalvular AF. The pathogenesis of LAA thrombi has not been fully elucidated but the relative stasis of the blood within the appendage, caused by its anatomy and altered function during AF, is thought to play a major role.

RISK STRATIFICATION FOR STROKE AND THROMBOEMBOLISM

The risk of TE events in AF is not homogeneous; various clinical features have been identified to help stratify the risk into high-, moderate-, and low-risk categories. The risk increases in the presence of valvular heart disease, such as rheumatic mitral stenosis or prosthetic cardiac valves. In patients with nonvalvular AF, age is an important determinant of ischemic stroke, increasing the relative risk (RR) of stroke in AF by 1.4 in each decade of advanced age. Previous stroke or transient ischemic attack (TIA) (RR 2.5), diabetes (RR 1.7), history of hypertension (RR 1.6), and heart failure (RR 1.4) also contribute, as do vascular disease, left atrium enlargement, left ventricular dysfunction, and the female gender.[2]

Several TE risk-stratification protocols have been proposed in the past years based on the

Cardiovascular Department, Ospedale dell'Angelo, Mestre-Venice, Italy
* Corresponding author. Cardiovascular Department, Ospedale dell'Angelo, Via Paccagnella 11, 30174 Mestre- Venice, Italy.
E-mail address: themistoclakis@yahoo.it

Card Electrophysiol Clin 4 (2012) 363–373
http://dx.doi.org/10.1016/j.ccep.2012.06.004

various clinical stroke risk factors identified. In patients with nonvalvular AF, the comparison of 12 published stroke risk-stratification schemes found substantial and clinically relevant differences among the published schemes, with a modest stroke predictive value for most of them.[3] The categorization of clinical risk factors for stroke into high-, moderate-, and low-risk groups has been deemphasized in the recent European guidelines,[4] given a poor predictive value of such artificial categories, and the risks have been recognized in a continuum. The widely used risk-assessment scheme is the $CHADS_2$ score, which includes the following:

- Congestive heart failure
- Hypertension
- Age (75 years or older)
- Diabetes mellitus
- History of stroke or TIA

This index is based on a points system in which 2 points are assigned for a history of TIA or stroke and 1 point for each of the other risk factors. The scoring for $CHADS_2$ is as follows:

- 0 is considered to indicate a low risk of TE
- 1 indicates moderate risk
- 2 or more indicates high risk

The limitation of this scheme is the generation of a large group (60%) of patients at intermediate TE risk.

Recently, Lip and colleagues proposed a novel stroke risk-stratification scheme reclassifying or incorporating additional risk factors as relevant with aim to consider at low risk for stroke patients with event rate truly low and to reduce the percentage of patients classified at intermediate risk.[5] This novel schema is termed CHA_2DS_2-VASc, which includes the following categories:

- Congestive heart failure
- Hypertension
- Age (75 years or older)
- Diabetes
- Stroke
- Vascular disease
- Age (65–74 years)
- Sex

CHA_2DS_2-VASc scoring considers female gender, age (65–74 years), and vascular disease (specifically, prior myocardial infarction, aortic plaque, and peripheral artery disease) as additional stroke risk factors that may influence the decision whether or not to anticoagulate. This scheme is also based on a point system in which 2 points are assigned for a history of stroke or TIA, or age (75 years or older) and 1 point each is assigned for age (65 to 74 years), a history of hypertension, diabetes, recent cardiac failure, vascular disease, and female gender.

Comparing the CHA_2DS_2-VASc score with the existing scheme in the real world, it was observed that, with this novel schema, most patients with AF (75%) were considered at high TE risk, whereas only 9% and 15% were considered at low and intermediate TE risk, respectively. This finding may affect the treatment of patients with AF with anticoagulation considering that, from this score, most of them should be treated with vitamin K antagonist (VKA). On the other hand, the percentage of TE events in the group of patients classified as low risk by the CHA_2DS_2-VASc score was truly low, whereas TE occurred in 1.4% of patients classified as low risk using the $CHADS_2$ score.[5]

In summary, as reported in the guidelines on the management of patients with AF, estimating the risk of stroke for individual patients with AF is a crucial factor in the decision to provide anticoagulation therapy. Based on the $CHADS_2$ score system, patients with a score of 2 or more have a stroke rate higher than 4% per year, whereas patients with a score of 1 or 0 have a stroke rate of 2.8% and 1.9% per year, respectively. Considering the risk-benefit ratio of oral anticoagulation therapy (OAT), patients with a stroke risk of 2% per year or less do not benefit substantially from oral anticoagulation.[2] On the contrary, in high-risk patients with AF, with stroke rates of 6% per year or greater, oral anticoagulation is strongly recommended. Routine chronic anticoagulation remains controversial in patients at an intermediate stroke risk (annual rate 3%–5%). Therefore, patients with a $CHADS_2$ score of 2 or more should be chronically anticoagulated, patients with a $CHADS_2$ score of 1 could be treated with both oral anticoagulation or aspirin, and those with a $CHADS_2$ score of 0 should take aspirin or nothing. When possible, no antithrombotic therapy should be considered for such patients, rather than aspirin, given the limited data on the benefits of aspirin in this patient group (ie, lone AF) and the potential for adverse effects, especially bleeding.[4]

In the group of patients with a $CHADS_2$ score equal to or less than 1, the recent European guidelines recommend a more detailed stroke risk assessment using the CHA_2DS_2-VASc score. However, it has been stated that the following are necessary in any case when OAT is considered: an evaluation of the pros and cons with patients, an estimation of the risk of bleeding complications, the ability to safely follow the therapy, and patient preferences. In particular, an accurate assessment of the bleeding risk should be considered before starting anticoagulation. HAS-BLED is a new, simple bleeding risk score that assigns 1 point for each of the following bleeding risk factors:

- Hypertension
- Abnormal renal function
- Abnormal liver function
- Stroke
- Bleeding history or predisposition
- Labile international normalized ratio (INR)
- Elderly
- Drug and alcohol use concomitantly

Patients with a HAS-BLED score greater than or equal to 3 are considered at high risk of bleeding and require caution in the choice of antithrombotic treatment in addition to a regular follow-up after the initiation of such therapy.[4]

ANTITHROMBOTIC THERAPY

VKA

VKA is widely used to prevent systemic embolism in patients with AF. In a meta-analysis of 6 major randomized clinical trials comparing adjusted-dose VKA with placebo or control, the average stroke rate was 4.5% per year for primary prevention and 12.0% per year for secondary prevention among patients assigned to the placebo and control groups According to this meta-analysis, adjusted-dose VKA was associated with a 64% reduction of all (ischemic and hemorrhagic) stroke.[6] This reduction was similar for both disabling and nondisabling strokes (60%). The absolute risk reduction in all strokes was 2.7% per year for primary prevention and 8.4% per year for secondary prevention. When only ischemic strokes were considered, VKA therapy was associated with a 67% RR reduction. The all-cause mortality was also substantially reduced (26%) in the group of patients treated with VKA compared with controls. However, OAT involves a risk of major hemorrhage of up to 3.4% per year[2,7,8] and the decision to administer this therapy must, therefore, be based on a thorough assessment of the risk-benefit ratio.

Underuse of VKA

Although the efficacy of VKA in preventing stroke in patients with AF has been clearly demonstrated, this therapy is still underused in clinical practice. Indeed, at least one-third of the patients with AF who are at risk for stroke have either not started the therapy or discontinued the therapy once started.

Several reasons can explain the suboptimal use of VKA in the real world, including the following:

- Risk of hemorrhage
- Restrictions in everyday life
- Frequent monitoring of the INR
- Patients' inability to comply with VKA therapy

Firstly, VKA therapy carries a risk of hemorrhage that could be underestimated in clinical practice considering the restrictive selection criteria used in randomized trials, which often enroll patients with a lower risk of bleeding. For example, in the SPINAF trial, only 7% of the 7982 patients initially screened were enrolled.[9] Moreover, the risk of hemorrhage is strictly related to patients' age. Indeed, the incidence rate of major hemorrhage has been found to increase from 1.5 per 100 patient-years for patients aged younger than 60 years to 4.2 per 100 patients-years for patients aged older than 80 years (hazard ratio [HR] 2.7).[10] In a meta-analysis of major randomized trials of VKA therapy, the mean age of patients was 69 years and only 20% of the participants were older than 75 years.[6] By contrast, in clinical practice, this latter group of patients represents more than 50% of the population that needs to be treated with VKA.

The second reason for the underuse of VKA is that this therapy is associated with restrictions in everyday life. Indeed, these drugs have significant drug, food, and alcohol interactions that limit their acceptability by patients.

Moreover, because of marked intraindividual and interindividual dose response, VKA therapy requires frequent monitoring of the INR level to adjust the therapeutic dosage. As a result of a balance between stroke and bleeding risk, an INR of 2.0 to 3.0 is considered the optimal range. Therefore, the goal of VKA therapy should be to maximize the time each patient spends within that range of INR. Connolly and colleagues[11] demonstrated that the time in the therapeutic range has a major impact on the treatment benefit of VKA therapy, and 58% to 65% of time in the therapeutic range has been estimated as the target threshold and less than which the benefit of VKA therapy may be completely offset. However, maintaining the INR in the therapeutic range is challenging as confirmed by the wide variation existing between centers in the success of maintaining the INR between 2 and 3, even within the relatively controlled setting of clinical trials. On average, the mean time spent in the therapeutic range by patients enrolled in clinical studies is of 64%. However, reports from large administrative databases indicate that, in some areas, patients were in the therapeutic range only for 29% of the time, suggesting that the time in the therapeutic range is decidedly lower in the daily practice. This finding counteracts the potential benefit of VKA therapy and increases its risks.

Finally, it is well known that a considerable percentage of patients are unable to comply with VKA therapy. In patients who are treated with VKA, the discontinuation of this therapy occurs at rates of up to 38% a year, and approximately 50% of strokes occur during inadvertent therapeutic lapses or in patients who temporarily or permanently discontinued therapy.[12] Obviously, the benefit of oral anticoagulation is more substantial in patients who are at a high risk for stroke. However, these patients are more likely to have relative or absolute contraindications to VKA treatment that prevent use of the recommended anticoagulation therapy. Indeed, it has been reported that 46% of elderly Medicare beneficiaries have contraindications to VKA, such as previous hemorrhage, blood dyscrasia, and renal or hepatic disease.[13] The management of these patients is challenging, and alternative methods of treatment to reduce embolic stroke need to been considered.

Antiplatelet Therapy

VKA therapy was substantially more efficacious than antiplatelet therapy, with an RR reduction of 39%. Aspirin reduces the risk of stroke in patients who have nonvalvular AF by only 22% in comparison with placebo or control group.[6] The absolute risk reduction was of 0.8% and 2.5% per year for primary and secondary prevention trials, respectively. Aspirin was also associated with a lower reduction of both disabling (13%) and nondisabling (29%) strokes compared with warfarin. Moreover, it is noteworthy that the 22% stroke risk reduction with aspirin in AF is broadly similar to the stroke reduction seen by antiplatelet therapy use in *high-risk patients with vascular disease*. Therefore, these results seem to be mostly related to a direct effect of aspirin on the vascular disease, usually associated in this population, rather than on its effect on the thrombogenesis. VKA was also superior to the combination of clopidogrel and aspirin for the prevention of vascular events (annual risk 3.93% vs 5.60%; RR 1.44) in patients at a high risk of stroke, especially in those already taking VKA therapy as demonstrated in the Atrial Fibrillation Clopidogrel Trial with Irbesartan for Prevention of Vascular Events (ACTIVE W) study.[14] Moreover, although major bleeding rates were similar between the two treatment arms, patients taking aspirin plus clopidogrel reported minor bleeding more frequently. In patients for whom VKA was unsuitable, the addition of clopidogrel to aspirin reduced the risk of major vascular events, especially stroke (28% relative reduction) compared with aspirin alone (6.8% vs 7.6% per year; RR 0.89; P = .01). However, major bleedings were significantly increased (2.0% vs 1.3% per year; RR 1.57; P<.001), which is broadly similar to that seen with VKA therapy.[15] Other antiplatelet agents, such as indobufen and triflusal, have been investigated in patients with nonvalvular AF, with the suggestion of some benefit, but more data are required to confirm these preliminary results.

New Oral Anticoagulant Drugs

In the last years, several new oral anticoagulants have been developed and others are on the horizon. These drugs are expected to improve the compliance of patients with respect to the VKA considering that they may not need INR monitoring and have lower interactions with food and other drugs. These drugs can be broadly grouped in 2 classes: the oral direct thrombin inhibitors (eg, dabigatran etexilate and AZD0837) and the oral factor Xa inhibitors (rivaroxaban, apixaban, edoxaban, betrixaban, YM150, among others).

Dabigatran

Dabigatran is a potent, direct, competitive inhibitor of thrombin. It has an absolute bioavailability of 6.5%, and 80% of the given dose is excreted by the kidneys. This drug needs to be administered at a fixed dose twice daily to reduce variability in the anticoagulation effect because its serum half-life is 12 to 17 hours and it does not require regular monitoring.[16] In the RE-LY study, dabigatran 110 mg twice a day was noninferior to VKA for the prevention of stroke and systemic embolism with lower rates of major bleeding, whereas dabigatran 150 mg twice a day was associated with lower rates of stroke and systemic embolism but with similar rates of major hemorrhage compared with VKA.[7] Rates of TE events were 1.69% per year in the VKA group as compared with 1.53% per year in the group that received 110 mg of dabigatran and 1.11% per year in the group that received 150 mg of dabigatran. The rate of major bleeding was 3.36% per year in the VKA group as compared with 2.71% per year in the group receiving 110 mg of dabigatran (P = .003) and 3.11% per year in the group receiving 150 mg of dabigatran (P = .31). Of note, the rates of hemorrhagic stroke were more than two-thirds higher in the warfarin group (0.38% per year) than in the group of patients treated with dabigatran 110 mg (0.12% per year) or 150 mg (0.10% per year).

The benefits of 150 mg dabigatran at reducing stroke, 110 mg dabigatran at reducing bleeding, and both doses at reducing intracranial bleeding versus warfarin were consistent regardless of the centers' quality of INR control. For all vascular events, nonhemorrhagic events, and mortality, the advantages of dabigatran were greater at the sites with poor INR control than at those with good INR control. Overall, these results show that local standards of care affect the benefits of use of new treatment alternatives.

The retrospective subanalyses of the RE-LY trial suggested that the reduction in stroke-risk achieved with dabigatran 150 mg over VKA occurred regardless of the CHA_2DS_2-VASc risk score. Indeed, dabigatran 150 mg was associated with a reductions in stroke risk compared with warfarin for any patient with a CHA_2DS_2-VASc score of 0 to 2 (RR = 0.63), 3 (RR = 0.61), 4 (RR = 0.53), and 5 to 9 (RR = 0.77) (interaction *P* value = .60). However, a significant interaction between CHA_2DS_2-VASc score and rates of major bleeding were observed in these patients. The rates of major bleeding were significantly lower for patients with a CHA_2DS_2-VASc score of 0 to 2 (RR = 0.75), 3 (RR = 0.74), and 4 (RR = 0.83) than for patients at the greatest risk (CHA_2DS_2-VASc score of 5–9, RR = 1.33).[17] Moreover, dabigatran 150 mg reduced the risk of stroke and systemic embolism compared with warfarin independently from the type of AF (permanent AF, HR = 0.7; paroxysmal AF, HR = 0.61; persistent AF, HR = 0.64; interaction *P* value = .88). The treatment with both doses of dabigatran was associated with a rate of myocardial infarction higher than warfarin. Indeed, the rate of myocardial infarction was 0.53% per year with warfarin, 0.72% per year with dabigatran 110 mg (RR = 1.35; *P* = .07), and 0.74% per year with dabigatran 150 mg (RR 1.38; *P* = .048). The only adverse effect that was significantly more common with dabigatran than with warfarin was dyspepsia occurring in about 11% and 6% (*P*<.001) of patients with dabigatran and warfarin, respectively.

Apixaban

Apixaban is a direct and competitive inhibitor of factor Xa. It has about 50% bioavailability and approximately 25% is excreted by the kidney. Connolly and colleagues[18] studied the efficacy and safety of apixaban 5 mg twice daily versus aspirin (81–324 mg/d) in the AVERROES study. This study was terminated early because of a clear benefit in favor of apixaban observed at the interim analysis of data. Indeed, during a mean follow-up of 1.1 years, the risk of stroke or systemic embolism was reduced among patients randomized to apixaban (1.6% per year) compared with those assigned to aspirin (3.7% per year; *P*<.001), whereas no differences of major bleedings have been observed between the two groups (1.4% and 1.2% per year in the apixaban and aspirin group, respectively; *P* = .57). Apixaban (5 mg twice daily) was also compared with dose-adjusted VKA in the ARISTOTLE trial that enrolled 18 201 patients with AF and at least one additional risk factor for stroke.[19] In this study, during a median follow-up of 1.8 years, apixaban was superior to VKA in preventing stroke or systemic embolism with a significant reduction of major bleeding and lower mortality. The rate of all stroke and systemic embolism was 1.27% per year in the apixaban group as compared with 1.60% per year in the VKA group. No significant differences in the rate of ischemic or uncertain type of stroke have been observed between the two groups (0.97% and 1.05% per year in the apixaban and VKA group, respectively; *P* = .42). On the contrary, the rate of hemorrhagic stroke, major bleedings, and death from any cause were lower in the apixaban group than in the VKA group (hemorrhagic stroke: 0.24% vs 0.47% per year; *P*<.001; major bleedings: 2.13% vs 3.09% per year, *P*<.001; death: 3.52% vs 3.94% per year, *P* = .047).

Rivaroxaban

Rivaroxaban is the oral factor Xa inhibitor more recently compared, at a dose of 20 mg once daily, with dose-adjusted VKA in the Rivaroxaban Once Daily Oral Direct Factor Xa Inhibition Compared with Vitamin K Antagonism for Prevention of Stroke and Embolism Trial in Atrial Fibrillation (ROCKET-AF).[8] This study enrolled 14 264 patients with AF and at least 2 risk factors for stroke. Patients with a $CHADS_2$ score of 1 were not enrolled, and only 13% of all patients had a $CHADS_2$ score of 2, whereas all other patients (87%) had a $CHADS_2$ score of greater than or equal to 3. Rivaroxaban was clearly noninferior to warfarin. Indeed, the primary end point, stroke and systemic embolism, occurred in 2.12% per year of patients treated with rivaroxaban and in 2.42% per year of patients treated with warfarin (*P* = .117). Major bleeding occurred in 3.6% of patients in the rivaroxaban-treated group versus 3.45% in the warfarin-treated group (*P* = .576). The rate of intracranial hemorrhage was significantly lower with rivaroxaban treatment compared with warfarin treatment (0.49% vs 0.74%; *P* = .019).

PERIPROCEDURAL ANTICOAGULATION

Anticoagulation Before and After Cardioversion

The TE risk after cardioversion has been reported in case-control series in a range between 1% and 5%, and it was near the low end of this spectrum when VKA was given for 3 to 4 weeks before and after conversion.[2] The TE risk is essentially caused by postcardioversion left atrial/LAA stunning that can be prolonged for several weeks after sinus rhythm restoration. Therefore, OAT is considered mandatory for the elective cardioversion of patients with AF of a 48-hour duration or longer or when the duration of AF is unknown. Dose-adjusted VKA should be given for at least 3 weeks before electrical or pharmacologic cardioversion and should be continued for at least 4 weeks after sinus rhythm restoration, maintaining an INR range between 2 and 3. Thereafter, the discontinuation of OAT or their continuation lifelong will depend on the presence of risk factors for stroke. In patients with AF greater than 48 hours and hemodynamic instability (angina, myocardial infarction, shock, or pulmonary edema), immediate cardioversion should be performed and unfractionated heparin (UFH) or low-molecular-weight heparin (LMWH) should be administered before cardioversion. After the cardioversion, heparin should be bridged with OAT and continued until the INR is at the therapeutic level. In patients with AF of less than 48 hours, the need for anticoagulation is less clear. In such patients, cardioversion can be performed expediently under the cover of UFH administered intravenously (IV) followed by subcutaneous LMWH and OAT should be started only if TE risk factors are present. An alternative to 3-week precardioversion anticoagulation is the transesophageal echocardiogram (TOE)–guided cardioversion.[20] With this strategy, if no left atrial thrombus is detected on TOE, UFH or LMWH should be started before cardioversion and continued thereafter until the target INR is achieved with OAT. On the contrary, if TOE detects a thrombus in the left atrium or LAA, VKA treatment is required for at least 3 weeks and cardioversion can be performed only after the demonstration of thrombus resolution on TOE.

Perioperative Anticoagulation of Patients Undergoing Noncardiac Surgery

Patients on OAT for AF can require surgical procedures in up to 10% of cases per year. No universally accepted recommendations exist for such patients coming from large randomized clinical trials.[21] Estimating the TE and hemorrhagic risk for individual patients with AF undergoing surgery is crucial to define the more appropriate periprocedural anticoagulation strategy. Patients with chronic AF had an approximately 2-fold greater risk of stroke in the first 30 days after surgery compared with patients without chronic AF and an absolute increase in the crude 30-day rate of stroke of approximately 1%.[22] Thus, Douketis and colleagues[23] suggested to divide surgical patients into 3 different groups according to the TE risk. Patients were considered at a high risk if they had a $CHADS_2$ score greater than or equal to 5, or recent (<3 months) stroke/TIA or rheumatic valvular heart disease. Patients with a $CHADS_2$ score of 3 or 4 were considered at moderate risk, whereas patients with a $CHADS_2$ score less than or equal to 2 and without previous stroke or TIA were considered at a low risk. On the other side, lacking strong literature data on the perioperative bleeding risk, usually this evaluation is mainly driven by the type of surgery, the presence of concomitant comorbidities, and patient age. The noncardiac surgical procedures generally associated with a higher risk of bleeding are intracranial or intraspinal surgery and major vascular (aortic aneurysm repair and peripheral artery bypass), orthopedic, plastic, cancer, and urogenital surgery (prostate and bladder resection). Moreover, an age of more than 65 years and comorbidities, such as kidney and liver dysfunction, previous bleeding, previous stroke, and hypertension, also increase the bleeding risk. In high TE risk group discontinuation of VKA has been recommended 5 days before the intervention starting, 2 days later, a bridging anticoagulation with therapeutic-dose of LMWH or UFH. In patients with a moderate TE risk, a bridging anticoagulation with LMWH at a low dose can also be used, whereas in patients at a low TE risk, a low dose of LMWH or no bridging therapy after VKA discontinuation is recommended. Patients requiring dental, cataract, or minor skin surgery should perform the procedure on warfarin, optimizing the local hemostasis.[4,21]

Generally, LMWH has several pharmacologic advantages over UFH, including a longer half-life, a more predictable clearance and bioavailability (greater than 90% after subcutaneous injection), and an antithrombotic response based on body weight. LMWH, therefore, can be administered at a fixed dose and does not need laboratory monitoring except in patients with obesity, kidney dysfunction, or pregnancy.

The resumption of antithrombotic therapy after surgical intervention is related to both the TE and bleeding risk of patients and to the type of surgery. It is reasonable to restart LMWH approximately 24 hours after the procedure if an adequate hemostasis has been obtained. However, the initiation of therapeutic-dose LMWH/UFH should be delayed for 48 to 72 hours or completely avoided after a major surgery with a high bleeding risk. VKA should be restarted approximately 12 to 24 hours after surgery at the usual maintenance dose considering that it takes 2 to 3 days to obtain a measurable anticoagulant effect and, therefore, it is unlikely to determine an increased risk of bleeding.[4,21]

Perioperative Anticoagulation of Patients Undergoing Percutaneous Coronary Intervention

Coronary artery disease affects about 20% to 30% of patients with AF, and more than 5% of patients with AF on OAT therapy undergo percutaneous coronary interventions (PCI) during their life.[24] Before PCI, patients can bridge OAT with UFH or LMWH, especially when TE risk is high.[25] However, more recent findings suggest that uninterrupted anticoagulation with VKA could replace this bridging strategy in this intervention with a favorable balance between bleeding and TE complications.[26] In anticoagulated patients, the radial approach should be preferred for PCI considering the lower risk of bleeding and other vascular complications associated with this vascular access. After PCI with stent implantation, the use of combined therapy, aspirin plus clopidogrel (4 weeks for a bare-metal stent, 6–12 months for a drug-eluting stent), is recommend. However, this strategy is less effective than VKA in the prevention of stroke in patients with AF, therefore, there is a need to combine dual antiplatelet therapy and VKA in patients with AF requiring PCI. This triple therapy seems to have an acceptable risk-benefit ratio when administered for a short time. Indeed, the prevalence of major bleeding with the association of VKA, aspirin, and clopidogrel is 2.6% to 4.6% at 30 days but increases to 7.4% to 10.3% at 12 months. From these data, in patients at a high TE risk, the use of a bare-metal stent is strongly suggested considering the shorter duration of triple therapy required. In these patients, the period of triple therapy should be limited to 4 weeks and followed by longer therapy with VKA and single antiplatelet therapy (either aspirin or copidogrel). The duration of triple therapy should also be reduced to 2 to 4 weeks in patients at a high hemorrhagic risk (HAS-BLED score $\geq$3).[4]

Perioperative Anticoagulation During Pacemaker and Implantable Cardioverter-defibrillator Implantation

The percentage of patients on OAT undergoing pacemaker implantation procedures ranges from 25% to 45%.[27] In these patients, the perioperative anticoagulation strategy is still controversial. The most common complication caused by antithrombotic therapy, following cardiac device implantation, is the development of a pocket hematoma, which can increase the risk of infections, prolong hospitalization, and expose patients to the risk of subsequent TE if anticoagulation discontinuation is needed.[28] The incidence of this complication ranges between 4% and 20% and is strictly related to the periprocedural anticoagulation strategy adopted. Recently, several studies demonstrated the safety of device implantation performed on OAT and the increased risk of bleeding when bridging OAT with UFH.[29] Therefore, 2 different anticoagulation strategies can be used in patients at high TE risk candidate to device implantation. One strategy suggests to bridge warfarin with LMWH (1 mg/kg twice a day) 48 to 72 hours before surgery. The last dose of heparin should be given 24 hours before the procedure. VKA should be resumed the same evening of the procedure and LMWH should be started 48 to 72 hours after, when hemostasis is secured. The other strategy is to perform device implantation during therapeutic INR value (2–2.5).

In patients at a moderate or low TE risk, it is reasonable to discontinue VKA 5 days before the procedure without bridging anticoagulation. Alternatively, the VKA therapy can be reduced, maintaining the INR between 1.5 and 2.0.[30]

Perioperative anticoagulation during AF ablation procedure

Catheter ablation of AF has been described as an effective curative treatment. This therapy can be associated with an increased risk of thromboembolisms, and an adequate anticoagulation strategy before, during, and after the ablation procedure plays a crucial role in preventing atrioembolic stroke.

Preablation anticoagulation strategy

In the absence of controlled trials, there is a wide practice to reflect on the guidelines for the management of patients with AF before ablation procedures.[4] In particular, the recommendations for anticoagulation at the time of cardioversion have been applied to patients who are in AF at the time of the ablation procedure and in whom AF termination is sought during an AF ablation procedure, either by catheter ablation or by cardioversion.[31] Puwanant and colleagues[32] suggested that the incidence of intracardiac thrombus was low in ablation candidates (0.6%), increasing with TE risk score. Therefore, it has been suggested that patients with a $CHADS_2$ or CHA_2DS_2-VASc score of 2 or higher should be treated with OAT in any case, maintaining an INR between 2 and 3 for at least 3 weeks before the ablation procedure.[33] On the contrary, there is little consensus regarding the need of OAT in low-risk patients, especially if they have paroxysmal AF and are in sinus rhythm at time of the ablation procedure.

Anticoagulation during the ablation procedure

AF ablation procedures can be associated with an increase risk of intraprocedural thromboembolisms. Stroke or TIA have been reported in 0.23% and 0.71% of patients, respectively.[34] These percentages can increase up to 14% if silent cerebral emboli were included.[35] Thrombus can form within the sheaths, on the catheters positioned in the left atrium, or can be promoted by the radiofrequency ablation. On the other side, major bleeding complications, such as cardiac tamponade, hemothorax, and groin complications, can occur. Therefore, the goal of intraprocedural anticoagulation is to achieve the lowest TE risk, maintaining an acceptably low bleeding complication rate.

Many centers discontinued VKA a few days before the ablation procedure and undergo bridging with UFH or LMWH.

Recently, it has been proposed to perform the ablation procedure on VKA therapy.[36–38] This strategy, combined with an open irrigation ablation catheter, has been reported to reduce the risk of periprocedural stroke without increasing the risk of pericardial effusion or other bleeding complication.[38] However, it is important to take into account the different management of bleeding and cardiac tamponade that is required with this strategy. In particular, need to be emphasized the different modalities of anticoagulation reversal requiring a higher dose of protamine and fresh frozen plasma should be used. In addition, patients on VKA are more likely to have more blood removed from the pericardial space during pericardiocentesis before stabilization and are given a larger amount of blood transfusion.

During the ablation procedure, UFH is typically given even if the procedure is performed on VKA. Based on the recent consensus document, heparin should be initiated at the time of the exchange of short vascular sheaths for transseptal sheaths and no later than immediately after transseptal puncture is safely accomplished.[33] UFH should be administered as an initial bolus dose of 100 to 140 IU/kg followed by an infusion of 15 to 18 IU/kg/h or by additional boluses. For patients with an INR range of 2.0 to 3.5, the initial bolus dose should be reduced to 80 IU/kg.[33] The target intensity of anticoagulation is not standardized among experienced investigators. Observational studies have shown that the incidence of thrombus decreased with an increase in target activated clotting time (ACT) from 250 to 300 to more than 300 seconds.[39,40] Therefore, the ACT target should be 350 to 400 seconds based on these data without differences between patients with and without a therapeutic INR.[33] UFH infusion should be discontinued in all patients after the removal of catheters from the left atrium. Protamine infusion may be administered (dose 30–50 mg) or ACT allowed to decrease less than 250 seconds before sheath removal to minimize the risk for femoral hematoma formation.

Postablation anticoagulation strategy

No universally accepted recommendations exist for OAT after the successful ablation of AF. Because of the high risk of thromboembolism in the early postprocedural period,[41] the consensus document recently published recommends that OAT, if discontinued before the ablation, should be restarted either the same evening of the ablation procedure or the next morning and maintained for at least 3 months in all patients. Based on expert opinion and small observational studies, in the initial period after the ablation, LMWH (eg, enoxaparin at a dosage of 0.5–1.0 mg/kg twice a day) is generally recommended as a bridging therapy by starting 3 to 4 hours after the ablation.[33] Less frequently, UFH is administered IV until the day after the procedure, starting about 3 hours after sheath removal. Thereafter, LMWH is administrated until the INR is greater than or equal to 2, whereas VKA should be continued for at least 3 months. Bunch and colleagues[42] recently observed that selected low-risk patients with a $CHADS_2$ score less than or equal to 1, who undergo left atrial ablation with an aggressive anticoagulation strategy with UFH and use of an open irrigated tip catheter, can be safely discharged following their procedure on aspirin alone. However, the results of this small observational single-center study need to be confirmed in larger prospective randomized trials before considered in the clinical practice.

The anticoagulation strategy after the initial 3 months is still controversial. Several reports published in the last years indicate that a low rate of stroke may occur in patients with successful ablation who discontinued OAT. In the first study on this topic, conducted by Oral and colleagues,[41] none of the 383 patients who had suspended VKA in the absence of arrhythmic recurrences suffered any TE during a 24-month follow-up, whereas 2 of the 357 patients who remained on OAT after ablation had a TE (0.56%). Moreover, 2 cerebral hemorrhages (0.56%) occurred among the patients on OAT. However, in this study, 2 important categories of high-risk patients (more than 65 years of age or with a preablation history of stroke) were underrepresented (only 49 and 10 patients, respectively) and OAT was often maintained in these groups. In a study of long-term outcomes after AF substrate ablation guided by complex fractionated atrial electrograms,

Nademanee and colleagues[43] compared the incidence of TE events and hemorrhages between 434 patients without arrhythmic recurrences who discontinued VKA and 118 patients requiring OAT following unsuccessful ablation. These patients were selected from a cohort of patients who were at least 65 years old or had 1 or more risk factors for stroke, including hypertension, diabetes, structural heart disease, prior history of stroke/TIA, congestive heart failure, or left ventricular ejection fraction less than or equal to 40%. In their population, the annual stroke rate was significantly lower in successfully treated patients who discontinued VKA than in patients with AF recurrences who remained on OAT (0.4% vs 2%). In a preliminary study conducted in the authors' center, they found that the incidence of stroke was lower among 77 patients who had discontinued OAT 3 months after successful AF ablation than among a group of patients matched for age, sex, and heart disease who had undergone electrical cardioversion (0% vs 6%).[44] Thereafter, Corrado and colleagues,[45] in a multicenter study on a selected population of 138 septuagenarians successfully treated with AF ablation and followed up for 16 $\pm$ 12 months after OAT discontinuation, observed that none suffered TE. Finally, Themistoclakis and colleagues,[46] in a larger multicenter study, enrolled 3355 patients, of whom 2692 discontinued OAT 3 to 6 months after successful ablation off antiarrhythmic drugs in the absence of severe left atrial dysfunction or severe pulmonary vein stenosis. $CHADS_2$ scores of 1 and greater than or equal to 2 were recorded in 723 and 347 patients who discontinued VKA, respectively. In this study, after about 2 years of follow-up, the percentage of TE events in patients who suspended VKA following successful AF ablation was not significantly different from that observed in patients who continued VKA after the procedure (0.07% vs 0.45%, respectively; P = .06). Moreover, the incidence of major hemorrhages was significantly lower among patients who suspended VKA than among those who continued (0.04% vs 2.0%, respectively; P<.0001). In this study, in 92% of patients, OAT was replaced with aspirin and strict monitoring for arrhythmic recurrences was performed before the decision to discontinue OAT. This monitoring included the interrogation of implanted devices (when available), daily pulse check in all patients, serial Holter recordings in 86% of patients, or transtelephonic monitoring in 90% of patients.

All of these studies, however, had the limitation of being observational, nonrandomized, and enrolling an insufficient population of patients at a high TE risk. Therefore, even if in selected patients with a $CHADS_2$ score greater than or equal to 2, normal left atrial function and without evidence of recurrent AF seems to be possible to discontinue VKA, there is a common opinion that larger prospective randomized trials are needed to confirm the safety of this strategy. Lacking any large randomized clinical trial data in postablation patients, it has been suggested to apply the same recommendations used for patients with AF not successfully treated with ablation. Therefore, patients with a $CHADS_2$ or CHA_2DS_2-VASc score of 1 may be treated with aspirin or VKA, whereas for patients with a $CHADS_2$ or CHA_2DS_2-VASc score of 2 or more, it has been suggested to continue long-term warfarin treatment with a targeted INR of 2 to 3.[4,31,33,47] The reasons for continuing anticoagulation after ablation mainly stem from studies on drug therapy and chiefly concern the risk of a long-term recurrence rate and, in particular, the risk of asymptomatic recurrences.[48] However, as previously reported, patients with a TE risk of 2% per year or less do not benefit substantially from OAT and, according to the international guidelines, should not be treated with this therapy.[2] It is important to note that all of the studies conducted to date on patients who have undergone successful AF ablation and discontinued OAT reported a decidedly lower incidence of TE events than that required by the guidelines. Moreover, there are no data that show that a benefit exists in continuing OAT in patients without recurrences of AF after the ablation.

REFERENCES

1. Wolf PA, Abbott RD, Kannel WB. Atrial fibrillation as an independent risk factor for stroke: the Framingham Study. Stroke 1991;22(8):983–8.
2. Fuster V, Rydén LE, Cannom DS, et al. ACC/AHA/ESC 2006 guidelines for the management of patients with atrial fibrillation: a report of the American College of Cardiology/American Heart Association Task Force on Practice Guidelines and the European Society of Cardiology Committee for Practice. Circulation 2006;114(7):e257–354.
3. The stroke risk in AF Working Group. Independent predictors of stroke in patients with atrial fibrillation: a systematic review. Neurology 2007;69(6):546–54.
4. Camm AJ, Kirchhof P, Lip GY, et al. Guidelines for the management of atrial fibrillation: the Task Force for the Management of Atrial Fibrillation of the European Society of Cardiology (ESC). Eur Heart J 2010; 31(19):2369–429.
5. Lip GY, Nieuwlaat R, Pisters R, et al. Refining clinical risk stratification for predicting stroke and thromboembolism in atrial fibrillation using a novel risk

factor-based approach: the euro heart survey on atrial fibrillation. Chest 2010;137(2):263–72.
6. Hart RG, Pearce LA, Aguilar MI. Meta-analysis: antithrombotic therapy to prevent stroke in patients who have nonvalvular atrial fibrillation. Ann Intern Med 2007;146:857–67.
7. Connolly S, Ezekowitz M, Yusuf S, et al. Dabigatran versus warfarin in patients with atrial fibrillation. N Engl J Med 2009;361(12):1139–51.
8. Patel MR, Mahaffey KW, Garg J, et al. Rivaroxaban versus warfarin in nonvalvular atrial fibrillation. N Engl J Med 2011;365(10):883–91.
9. Emmerich J, Le Heuzey JY, Bath P, et al. Indication for antithrombotic therapy for atrial fibrillation: reconciling the guidelines with clinical practice. Eur Heart J Suppl 2005;7(Suppl C):C28–33.
10. Torn M, Bollen WL, van der Meer FJ, et al. Risks of oral anticoagulant therapy with increasing age. Arch Intern Med 2005;165(13):1527–32.
11. Connolly SJ, Pogue J, Eikelboom J, et al. Benefit of oral anticoagulant over antiplatelet therapy in atrial fibrillation depends on the quality of international normalized ratio control achieved by centers and countries as measured by time in therapeutic range. Circulation 2008;118(20):2029–37.
12. Al-Saady NM, Obel O, Camm J. Left atrial appendage: structure, function, and role in thromboembolism. Heart 1999;82(5):547–54.
13. Rockson SG, Albers GW. Comparing the guidelines: anticoagulation therapy to optimize stroke prevention in patients with atrial fibrillation. J Am Coll Cardiol 2004;43(6):929–35.
14. Connolly S, Pogue J, Hart R, et al. Clopidogrel plus aspirin versus oral anticoagulation for atrial fibrillation in the Atrial Fibrillation Clopidogrel Trial with Irbesartan for Prevention of Vascular Events (ACTIVE W): a randomised controlled trial. Lancet 2006;367(9526): 1903–12.
15. Connolly SJ, Pogue J, Hart RG, et al. Effect of clopidogrel added to aspirin in patients with atrial fibrillation. N Engl J Med 2009;360(20): 2066–78.
16. Stangier J. Clinical pharmacokinetics and pharmacodynamics of the oral direct thrombin inhibitor dabigatran etexilate. Clin Pharmacokinet 2008;47(5): 285–95.
17. Oldgren J, Alings M, Darius H, et al. Risks for stroke, bleeding, and death in patients with atrial fibrillation receiving dabigatran or warfarin in relation to the CHADS2 score: a subgroup analysis of the RE-LY trial. Ann Intern Med 2011;155(10):660–7.
18. Connolly SJ, Eikelboom J, Joyner C, et al. Apixaban in patients with atrial fibrillation. N Engl J Med 2011; 364(9):806–17.
19. Granger CB, Alexander JH, McMurray JJ, et al. Apixaban versus warfarin in patients with atrial fibrillation. N Engl J Med 2011;365(11):981–92.
20. Lip GYH, Frison L, Halperin JL, et al. Comparative validation of a novel risk score for predicting bleeding risk in anticoagulated patients with atrial fibrillation: the HAS-BLED (Hypertension, Abnormal Renal/Liver Function, Stroke, Bleeding History or Predisposition, Labile INR, Elderly, Drug. J Am Coll Cardiol 2011;57(2):173–80.
21. Douketis JD, Berger PB, Dunn AS, et al. The perioperative management of antithrombotic therapy: American College of Chest Physicians evidence-based clinical practice guidelines (8th edition). Chest 2008;133(Suppl 6):299S–339S.
22. Kaatz S, Douketis JD, Zhou H, et al. Risk of stroke after surgery in patients with and without chronic atrial fibrillation. J Thromb Haemost 2010; 8(5):884–90.
23. Douketis JD. Perioperative management of patients who are receiving warfarin therapy: an evidence-based and practical approach. Blood 2011; 117(19):5044–9.
24. Lip GY, Huber K, Andreotti F, et al. Antithrombotic management of atrial fibrillation patients presenting with acute coronary syndrome and/or undergoing coronary stenting: executive summary–a consensus document of the European Society of Cardiology Working Group on Thrombosis. Eur Heart J 2010; 31(11):1311–8.
25. Lip GY, Huber K, Andreotti F, et al. Management of antithrombotic therapy in atrial fibrillation patients presenting with acute coronary syndrome and/or undergoing percutaneous coronary intervention/ stenting. Thromb Haemost 2010;103(1):13–28.
26. Karjalainen PP, Vikman S, Niemelä M, et al. Safety of percutaneous coronary intervention during uninterrupted oral anticoagulant treatment. Eur Heart J 2008;29(8):1001–10.
27. McComb JM, Gribbin GM. Chronic atrial fibrillation in patients with paroxysmal atrial fibrillation, atrioventricular node ablation and pacemakers: determinants and treatment. Europace 1999;1(1):30–4.
28. Wiegand UK, LeJeune D, Boguschewski F, et al. Pocket hematoma after pacemaker or implantable cardioverter defibrillator surgery: influence of patient morbidity, operation strategy, and perioperative antiplatelet/anticoagulation therapy. Chest 2004;126(4): 1177–86.
29. Thal S, Moukabary T, Boyella R, et al. The relationship between warfarin, aspirin, and clopidogrel continuation in the peri-procedural period and the incidence of hematoma formation after device implantation. Pacing Clin Electrophysiol 2010; 33(4):385–8.
30. Jamula E, Douketis JD, Schulman S. Perioperative anticoagulation in patients having implantation of a cardiac pacemaker or defibrillator: a systematic review and practical management guide. J Thromb Haemost 2008;6(10):1615–21.

31. Calkins H, Brugada J, Packer DL, et al. HRS/EHRA/ECAS expert consensus statement on catheter and surgical ablation of atrial fibrillation: recommendations for personnel, policy, procedures and follow-up. A report of the Heart Rhythm Society (HRS) Task Force on catheter and surgical ablation of. Heart rhythm 2007;4(6):816–61.
32. Puwanant S, Varr BC, Shrestha K, et al. Role of the CHADS2 score in the evaluation of thromboembolic risk in patients with atrial fibrillation undergoing transesophageal echocardiography before pulmonary vein isolation. J Am Coll Cardiol 2009;54(22):2032–9.
33. Connolly SJ, Callans D, Hocini M, et al. Periprocedural and long-term anticoagulation. In: Natale A, Raviele A, editors. Atrial fibrillation ablation. 2011 update. The state of the art based on the Venice Chart international consensus document. Chichester (United Kingdom): Wiley-Blackwell; 2011. p. 77–84.
34. Cappato R, Calkins H, Chen SA, et al. Updated worldwide survey on the methods, efficacy, and safety of catheter ablation for human atrial fibrillation. Circ Arrhythm Electrophysiol 2010;3(1):32–8.
35. Gaita F, Caponi D, Pianelli M, et al. Radiofrequency catheter ablation of atrial fibrillation: a cause of silent thromboembolism? Magnetic resonance imaging assessment of cerebral thromboembolism in patients undergoing ablation of atrial fibrillation. Circulation 2010;122(17):1667–73.
36. Wazni OM, Beheiry S, Fahmy T, et al. Atrial fibrillation ablation in patients with therapeutic international normalized ratio: comparison of strategies of anticoagulation management in the periprocedural period. Circulation 2007;116(22):2531–4.
37. Kwak JJ, Pak HN, Jang JK, et al. Safety and convenience of continuous warfarin strategy during the periprocedural period in patients who underwent catheter ablation of atrial fibrillation. J Cardiovasc Electrophysiol 2010;21(6):620–5.
38. Di Biase L, Burkhardt JD, Mohanty P, et al. Periprocedural stroke and management of major bleeding complications in patients undergoing catheter ablation of atrial fibrillation: the impact of periprocedural therapeutic international normalized ratio. Circulation 2010;121(23):2550–6.
39. Ren JF, Marchlinski FE, Callans DJ, et al. Increased intensity of anticoagulation may reduce risk of thrombus during atrial fibrillation ablation procedures in patients with spontaneous echo contrast. J Cardiovasc Electrophysiol 2005;16(5):474–7.
40. Wazni OM, Rossillo A, Marrouche NF, et al. Embolic events and char formation during pulmonary vein isolation in patients with atrial fibrillation: impact of different anticoagulation regimens and importance of intracardiac echo imaging. J Cardiovasc Electrophysiol 2005;16(6):576–81.
41. Oral H, Chugh A, Ozaydin M, et al. Risk of thromboembolic events after percutaneous left atrial radiofrequency ablation of atrial fibrillation. Circulation 2006;114(8):759–65.
42. Bunch TJ, Crandall BG, Weiss JP, et al. Warfarin is not needed in low-risk patients following atrial fibrillation ablation procedures. J Cardiovasc Electrophysiol 2009;20(9):988–93.
43. Nademanee K, Schwab MC, Kosar EM, et al. Clinical outcomes of catheter substrate ablation for high-risk patients with atrial fibrillation. J Am Coll Cardiol 2008;51(8):843–9.
44. Rossillo A, Bonso A, Themistoclakis S, et al. Role of anticoagulation therapy after pulmonary vein antrum isolation for atrial fibrillation treatment. J Cardiovasc Med 2008;9(1):51–5.
45. Corrado A, Patel D, Riedlbauchova L, et al. Efficacy, safety, and outcome of atrial fibrillation ablation in septuagenarians. J Cardiovasc Electrophysiol 2008;19(8):807–11.
46. Themistoclakis S, Corrado A, Marchlinski FE, et al. The risk of thromboembolism and need for oral anticoagulation after successful atrial fibrillation ablation. J Am Coll Cardiol 2010;55(8):735–43.
47. Natale A, Raviele A, Arentz T, et al. Venice Chart international consensus document on atrial fibrillation ablation. J Cardiovasc Electrophysiol 2007;18(5):560–80.
48. Kuch KH, Shah D, Camm AJ, et al. Patient management pre- and postablation. In: Natale A, Raviele A, editors. Atrial fibrillation ablation. Malden (MA): Blackwell Futura; 2007. p. 34–40.

AF Ablation
Do You Need a Mapping System for Ablation?

Kojiro Tanimoto, MD[a], Paul J. Wang, MD, FHRS[b], Amin Al-Ahmad, MD, FHRS, CCDS[c,*]

KEYWORDS

- Atrial fibrillation • Electroanatomical mapping • 3D cardiac mapping • Catheter ablation
- Radiofrequency ablation

KEY POINTS

- The advantages of 3-dimensional (3D) mapping systems for atrial fibrillation (AF) ablation procedures include decreased exposure to ionizing radiation, the ability to define anatomic and electrical substrate, the ability to record the location of ablation lesions, and facilitation in mapping organized atrial arrhythmias that may occur during ablation.
- Effective and safe AF ablation can be achieved with the use of a 3D mapping system as well as without.
- Although 3D mapping systems are not needed for successful ablation, the advantages of using them are important to consider. The decision to use a mapping system rests with the experience and technique of the clinician weighing the advantages and understanding the limitations.

INTRODUCTION

Radiofrequency (RF) catheter ablation has been established as the important treatment of choice for drug-refractory symptomatic paroxysmal atrial fibrillation (AF).[1] In recent years, indications for AF ablation were extended to include persistent AF. The pulmonary veins (PVs) play a critical role in the initiation and maintenance of AF. PV electrical isolation is the optimal end point for paroxysmal AF. Substrate modification in the left atrium (LA) is often required for persistent AF.

Mapping systems allow us to localize catheters in 3-dimensional (3D) space without fluoroscopy and create a 3D map of LA and PVs.[2,3] In addition, preacquired or simultaneously acquired imaging, such as computed tomography (CT), magnetic resonance imaging (MRI), rotational angiography, or intracardiac echocardiography, can be superimposed on the acquired 3D map, which will provide the detailed visualization of LA and PV.[4,5]

Currently, CARTO (Biosense Webster Inc, Diamond Bar, California) and Ensite NavX (St Jude Medical, Minnetonka, Minnesota) systems are the most commonly used for 3D mapping systems throughout the world to provide accurate visualization of the atrial anatomy and identification of the atrial substrate for catheter ablation. This article describes the advantages and limitations of the 3D mapping system in AF ablation.

ELECTROANATOMIC MAPPING SYSTEMS

The CARTO System

The CARTO mapping system uses ultralow-intensity magnetic fields emitted from a locator pad beneath

Disclosures: KT, none; PW, Fellowship support from St Jude Medical and Biosense Webster; AA, Honoraria, St Jude Medical.

[a] Cardiology Division, Keio University School of Medicine, Shinjuku, Tokyo, Japan; [b] Cardiac Arrhythmia Service, Division of Cardiovascular Medicine, Stanford University, Stanford, CA, USA; [c] Stanford Arrhythmia Service, Division of Cardiovascular Medicine, Stanford University, Stanford, CA, USA

* Corresponding author. Cardiac Electrophysiology Laboratory, Cardiac Arrhythmia Service, Stanford University School of Medicine, H2146, 300 Pasteur Drive, Stanford, CA 94305.

E-mail address: aalahmad@stanford.edu

Card Electrophysiol Clin 4 (2012) 375–381
http://dx.doi.org/10.1016/j.ccep.2012.06.008

the catheter laboratory table.[6] The magnetic field strength is detected by a location sensor embedded proximally to the tip of a mapping catheter. The strength of each coil's magnetic field decays as a function of distance from the coil; by integrating each coil's field strength and converting this measurement into a distance, the location sensor can be triangulated in space. The catheter is moved into the chamber of interest, and mapping points are taken at the sites with contact. This information is used to generate an integrated 3D chamber reconstruction with anatomic and electrical information, such as activation sequence (activation map) or local electrogram amplitude (voltage map). The resolution of the system is less than 1 mm.

The CARTO system has the capability to import 3D CT or MRI images to facilitate the identification of specific anatomic landmarks (PV ostia), this is called CARTO-MERGE (**Fig. 1**).[4] This feature helps to guide mapping and ablation using the detailed LA anatomy acquired from CT/MRI. The landmark points, such as PV ostia and left appendage ridge, are mapped and registered to the corresponding points on the CT/MRI image to integrate the electroanatomic map and the CT/MRI image. After the integration into the CT/MRI image, the mapping catheter can be moved in the detailed anatomic chamber without fluoroscopy. The clinician can use the system to define the catheter position visualized from any angle he or she desires because the map can be viewed and rotated on the screen. In addition, the endoscopic view can be visualized and helps identify the ridge between the PV and LA appendage (**Fig. 2**). Extracardiac structures, such as the esophagus, can be visualized. It is useful to avoid esophageal injury in LA posterior ablation.

The CARTO3 platform, a hybrid magnetic and current-based mapping system, is used.[7] In addition to the magnetic field to locate a proprietary catheter with a magnetic sensor, a small current is sent through the connected catheter. The strength of the current is detected and measured by the 6 patches on the patient's body surface to locate a catheter position. As a proprietary catheter with a magnetic sensor moves around the chamber, multiple locations with both magnetic and current information are created and stored by the system. A current-based field is calibrated by the magnetic field. Using the calibrated current-based field, the mapping catheters without the magnetic sensor can be located and visualized on the electroanatomic map without spatial distortion. This advanced catheter location technology provides information on the spatial relationship of the multielectrode circular mapping catheter (Lasso catheter) and anatomic landmarks without fluoroscopy. It is useful to check the spatial relationship of the Lasso catheter and ablation lesions. This practice enables the clinician to decrease the use of fluoroscopy. CARTO3 also has a fast anatomic mapping feature that allows a 3D anatomic structure to be created rapidly by using position information from a proprietary catheter with a magnetic sensor with the sampling rate of 60 per second. In addition, a specialized Lasso catheter can also be used to collect anatomic information.

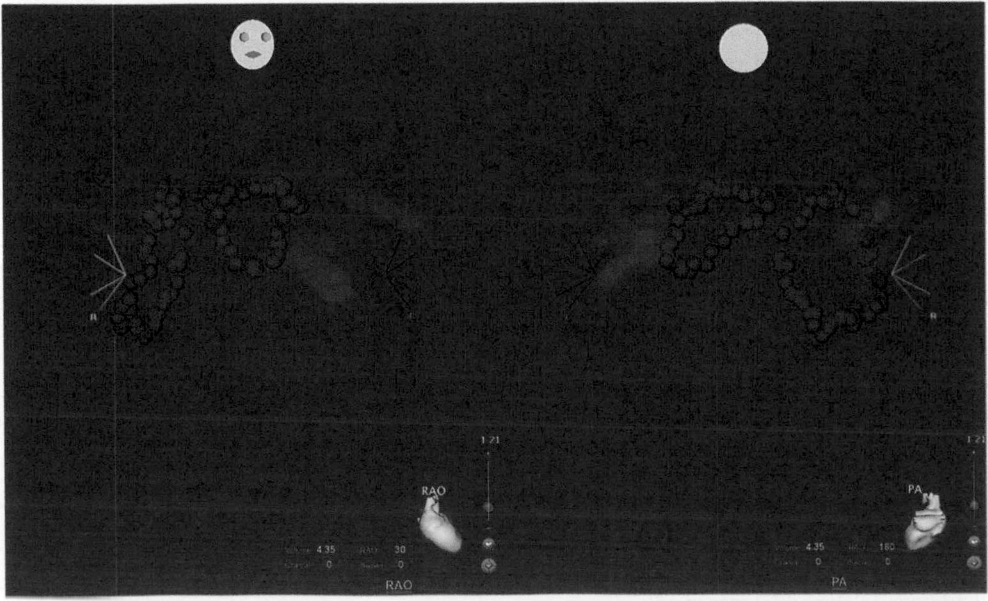

Fig. 1. CARTO-MERGE image of registration and integration of the 3D map with a previously acquired CT scan. The red circles denote the location of ablation lesions.

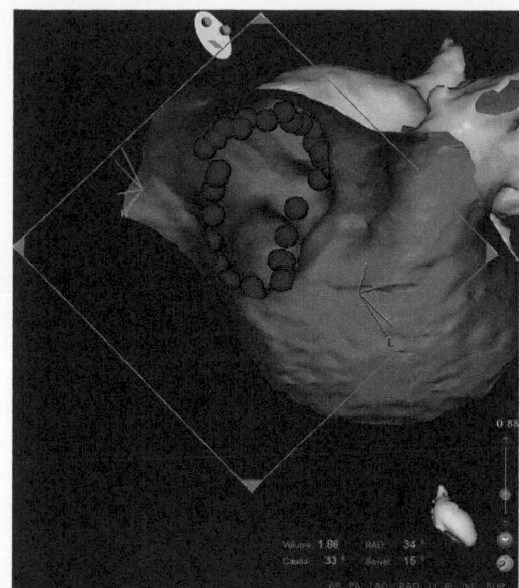

Fig. 2. Cutout view from inside the left atrium highlighting the anatomy of the left PV and the LA appendage. The red circles denote the location of ablation lesions.

The CARTO sound image integration module integrates intracardiac ultrasound (ICE) images into an electroanatomic map.[8] A 3D anatomic structure is derived from the ICE image acquired from the ICE catheter with a magnetic sensor. A 3D anatomic map of LA can be constructed by images from the ICE catheter positioned in the right atrium (RA) before the transseptal puncture. This strategy provides detailed anatomic mapping without deformity caused by catheter contact, and adjacent structures (esophagus and valves) can be imaged. The ICE images can be integrated into images from CT/MRI (**Fig. 3**). Because of the stiff ICE catheter, careful manipulation is required.

The EnSite System

The EnSite NavX system uses the voltage gradient that exists across tissue when a current is applied through the surface electrodes.[5] Electrodes from standard electrophysiology catheters sense the electrical signals transmitted between 3 pairs of surface electrode patches. This system collects electrical data from the catheters and uses this information to track or navigate their movement and to construct 3D models of the chamber. Any multielectrode catheter can be used to create a geometric model of the cardiac chamber, which involves creating a cloud of points to represent the geometry of the cardiac chamber. At the completion of the point cloud, the final anatomy is displayed as a best-fit surface projected to the point cloud. An electroanatomic map is generated by acquiring and displaying the activation and voltage data on the 3D chamber (**Fig. 4**). Similar to the CARTO system, the EnSite NavX system also has a capability to import and integrate 3D CT or MRI images to facilitate anatomically based ablation procedures.[9] Complex fractionated electrograms can be targeted in persistent AF using the software to depict the mean electrogram cycle length map (**Fig. 5**).[10]

ADVANTAGES AND LIMITATIONS OF 3D ELECTROANATOMIC MAPPING SYSTEMS

Reduction of Radiation Exposure

AF ablation procedures may be time consuming and may require significant exposure to radiation, which can cause acute skin injury and increase in lifetime risk of fatal malignancy for patients and electrophysiologists. To decrease the risk of radiation complications, the fluoroscopy time should be minimized. Prior studies have associated the use of 3D electroanatomic mapping systems with a substantial reduction in the fluoroscopic time but no significant improvement in ablation outcomes.[11,12] Recently, zero fluoroscopy for AF ablations has also been reported with the use of electroanatomic mapping systems.[13]

Anatomic Identification and Images Integration

The complex anatomy of the LA can make it challenging to move ablation catheters with fluoroscopy alone. In addition to complexity, anatomic variants of PVs are sometimes noticed.[14] Considerable variation of left atrial appendage and LA roof morphologies are also reported.[15] Both the EnSite NavX and CARTO systems allow for the integration of either CT or MRI images of the LA into the catheter display image of the mapping system.[4,9] Anatomic variability can be identified after merging the CT anatomy into the reconstructed shell. The mapping systems can also provide a clear LA image from both outside (cardiac shell) and inside (endoscopic view), and the RF application can be deployed accurately. In addition to cardiac structures, extracardiac structures, like the esophagus, can also be visualized in the electroanatomic map. These methods can be important for potentially avoiding complications.

Another useful advantage of the 3D mapping systems is the ability to mark RF lesions. Although, certainly, the red-dot ablation lesion on the 3D map should not be taken as a reliably transmural lesion, it is still useful to see the lesion cloud where ablations have been delivered and where ablation lesions have yet to be delivered or have been missed. In

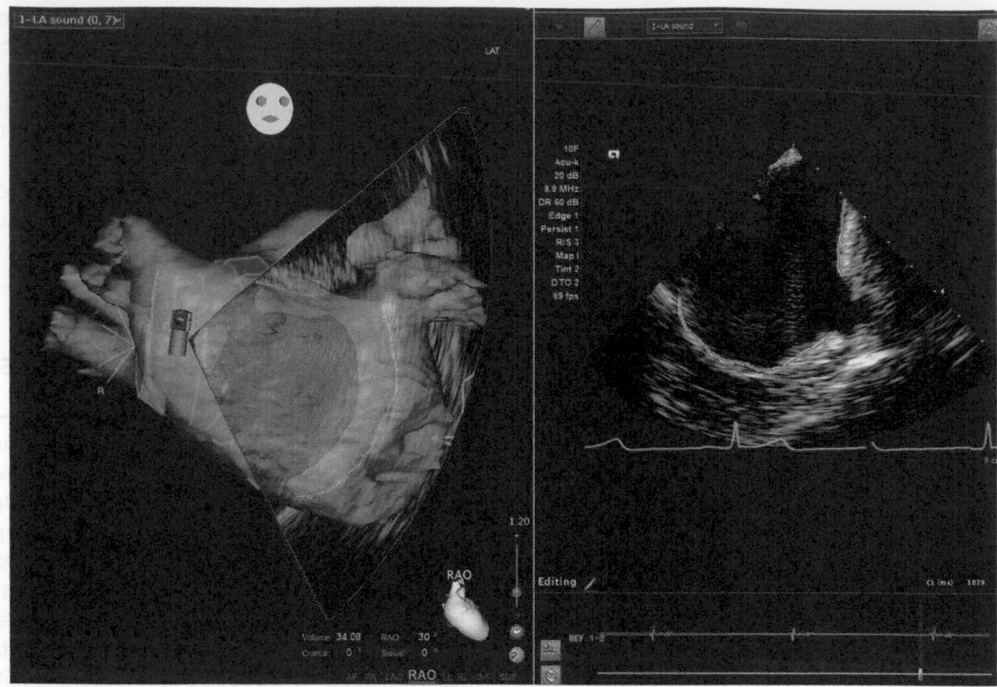

Fig. 3. Integration of ICE images with the 3D map and the previously acquired CT scan. The green line denotes the endocardial boarder that is incorporated in the CARTO-Sound mapping system.

addition to the fact that the lesion should not be taken as a transmural lesion, the location of the lesion should not always be considered accurate because of inaccuracies with the registration and differences of cardiac cycle and respiration when the lesion was acquired as compared with lesions in proximity to it. It is also worth noting that the CARTO system will assign the lesion to the catheter tip, whereas the lesion location with the EnSite NavX system is user defined.

It is important to note that both the reduction in fluoroscopy and the identification of anatomic landmarks and image integration may also have limitations. An inaccurate integration of an external 3D data set, such as CT, may cause significant errors and potentially complications. In general, surface registration is more accurate than landmark registration and both may suffer accuracy issues. For example, prior studies have demonstrated a change in the PV angle with respiration and this may lead to inaccuracies that should be taken into account during the procedure.[16] In addition, patient movement in the case of the CARTO system and movement of the reference catheter (if used) in the

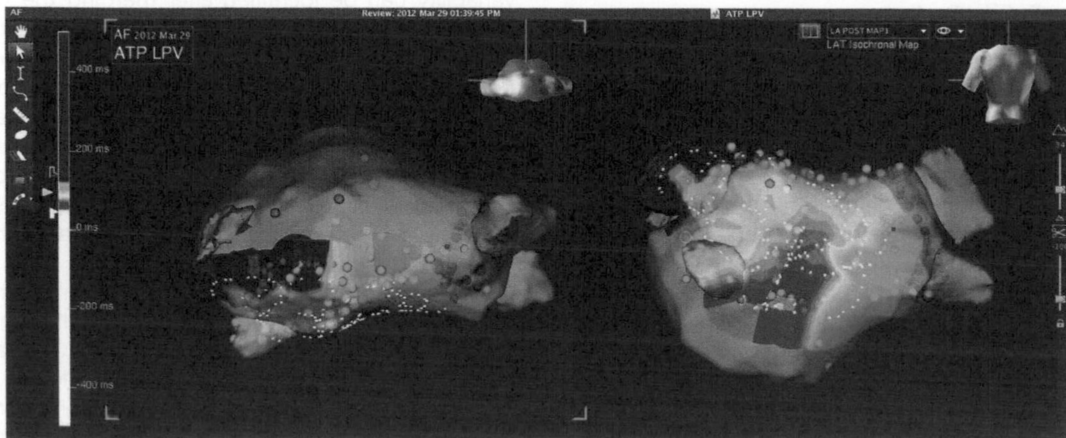

Fig. 4. EnSite NavX activation map showing the area of earliest activation in the LA.

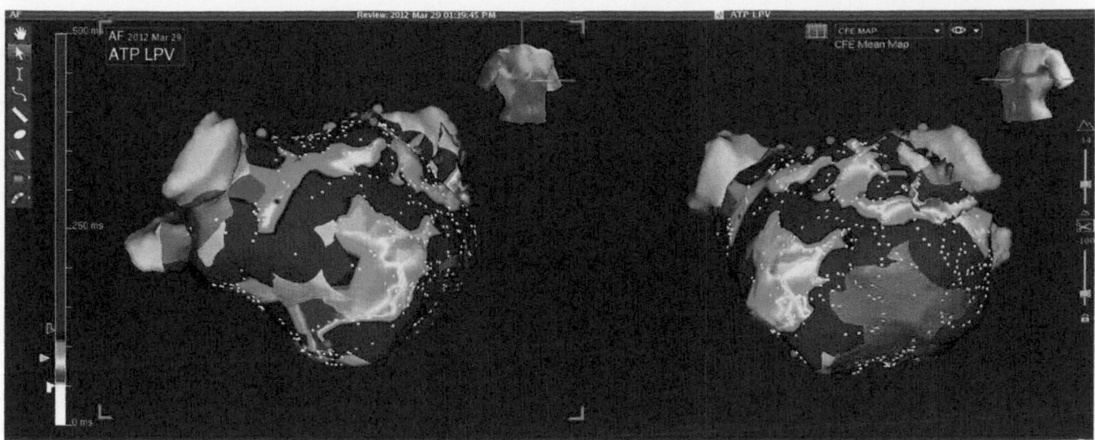

Fig. 5. EnSite NavX map depicting areas of complex fractionated electrograms.

EnSite NavX system may also lead to shifts in the 3D map that can limit the accuracy.

Atrial Substrate Modification

Substrate modification is important during the ablation procedure for persistent AF. Nademanee and colleagues[17] demonstrated that areas with complex fractionated atrial electrograms (CFE) represent arrhythmogenic substrates and ideal targets for ablation to terminate AF. During a 1-year follow-up, 73% of the patients with persistent AF and 79% of the patients with paroxysmal AF were free of any arrhythmia after a single procedure. Both of the 3D electroanatomic mapping systems also provide an automatic detection algorithm for CFE mapping. Lin and colleagues[10] showed proof of the consistency of the automatic detection algorithms using the EnSite NavX system. The assessment of the CFEs requires a recording duration of 5 seconds or more at each site to obtain a consistent fractionation. In addition to PV isolation and LA linear ablation, ablation targeted for CFEs has a better long-term efficacy.[18] Although CFE may play an important role in the maintenance of AF and the 3D mapping system is a useful tool for substrate mapping during AF, the strategy of using CFE with 3D mapping systems has not yielded a higher success rate than the use of a multielectrode catheter without the mapping system.[19]

In addition to CFE mapping, voltage mapping of the LA may help identify areas of decreased voltage that may represent atrial fibrosis and have been associated with a decreased success rate of AF ablation.[20] Voltage mapping can also be achieved without the aid of 3D mapping systems, but 3D mapping systems allow for a better 3D understanding of scar location with anatomic relationships.

Ablation of AF Ablation-Related Atrial Tachycardias

Postablation atrial tachycardia and flutter have been reported in patients undergoing catheter ablation of AF. Focal atrial tachycardias with reentrant circuit located at the PV ostia occurred after segmental PV isolation.[21] Many of the atrial tachycardias after circumferential PV isolation have a reentrant mechanism and they considered that gaps might be related to prior ablation lines.[22] However, it may not be easy to identify such gaps. Although entrainment is a conventional technique for localizing the circuit of reentrant tachycardia, it may terminate the tachycardia during the pacing maneuvers or cause the organized tachycardia to deteriorate into AF. Moreover, there are extensive low-voltage zones and scars in these patients with AF, which may cause difficulty in capturing atrial tissue during entrainment pacing. The 3D electroanatomic mapping systems provide an effective alternative to mapping and localizing postablation atrial tachycardias.[23] Using the 3D mapping system with traditional pacing maneuvers can lead to a detailed understanding of the complexity of some of the atrial arrhythmias that can occur after AF ablation. Challenges and limitations of the 3D mapping systems in these cases involve the accurate identification of early versus late signals, definition of the onset of the local electrogram in areas where it can be fractionated, and low voltage with slow conduction. In addition, the recognition that the tachycardia may have shifted or changed is crucial to perform a remap rather than risk significant inaccuracies with the map.

DOES THE USE OF 3D MAPPING SYSTEMS LEAD TO IMPROVED OUTCOMES?

Although the use of 3D mapping systems may have many advantages, RF ablation for AF can be performed rapidly, successfully, and with an acceptable complication rate without using these systems. For example, the antral isolation approach can be guided with ICE, a circular mapping catheter, and fluoroscopy.[24,25] Outcomes with this approach have been demonstrated to be favorable.[26] Prior studies that have examined this issue have not been able to conclude that the use of 3D mapping leads to improved success or decreased risk.[7,11,12] These studies do, however, show a significant decrease in the fluoroscopy time during the procedure.[7,11,12] It is worthwhile to note that CT scans are often used with 3D mapping systems and also represent radiation exposure to patients. In addition, the use of mapping systems does increase the cost of the procedure.

SUMMARY

The 3D mapping systems do add value to AF ablation procedures. Advantages include decreased exposure to ionizing radiation, the ability to define anatomic and electrical substrates, and the ability to record the location of ablation lesions and to facilitate in mapping organized atrial arrhythmias that may occur during ablation. Understanding the advantages and limitations of the 3D mapping systems has become a necessity for practicing electrophysiologists. Many techniques and approaches to the ablation of AF use 3D mapping systems, whereas others do not. Effective and safe AF ablation can be achieved with the use of a 3D mapping system as well as without. Certainly, 3D mapping systems are not needed for successful ablation but the advantages of using them are important to consider. The decision to use a mapping system rests with the experience and technique of the clinician weighing the advantages and understanding the limitations.

REFERENCES

1. Calkins H, Kuck KH, Cappato R, et al. 2012 HRS/EHRA/ECAS expert consensus statement on catheter and surgical ablation of atrial fibrillation: recommendations for patient selection, procedural techniques, patient management and follow-up, definitions, endpoints, and research trial design: a report of the Heart Rhythm Society (HRS) Task Force on Catheter and Surgical Ablation of Atrial Fibrillation. Developed in partnership with the European Heart Rhythm Association (EHRA), a registered branch of the European Society of Cardiology (ESC) and the European Cardiac Arrhythmia Society (ECAS); and in collaboration with the American College of Cardiology (ACC), American Heart Association (AHA), the Asia Pacific Heart Rhythm Society (APHRS), and the Society of Thoracic Surgeons (STS). Endorsed by the governing bodies of the American College of Cardiology Foundation, the American Heart Association, the European Cardiac Arrhythmia Society, the European Heart Rhythm Association, the Society of Thoracic Surgeons, the Asia Pacific Heart Rhythm Society, and the Heart Rhythm Society. Heart Rhythm 2012;9(4):632–696.e21.
2. Pappone C, Oreto G, Lamberti F, et al. Catheter ablation of paroxysmal atrial fibrillation using a 3D mapping system. Circulation 1999;100(11):1203–8.
3. Ouyang F, Bansch D, Ernst S, et al. Complete isolation of left atrium surrounding the pulmonary veins: new insights from the double-Lasso technique in paroxysmal atrial fibrillation. Circulation 2004; 110(15):2090–6.
4. Kistler PM, Earley MJ, Harris S, et al. Validation of three-dimensional cardiac image integration: use of integrated CT image into electroanatomic mapping system to perform catheter ablation of atrial fibrillation. J Cardiovasc Electrophysiol 2006; 17(4):341–8.
5. Estner HL, Deisenhofer I, Luik A, et al. Electrical isolation of pulmonary veins in patients with atrial fibrillation: reduction of fluoroscopy exposure and procedure duration by the use of a non-fluoroscopic navigation system (NavX). Europace 2006;8(8):583–7.
6. Gepstein L, Hayam G, Ben-Haim SA. A novel method for nonfluoroscopic catheter-based electroanatomical mapping of the heart. In vitro and in vivo accuracy results. Circulation 1997;95(6):1611–22.
7. Stabile G, Scaglione M, del Greco M, et al. Reduced fluoroscopy exposure during ablation of atrial fibrillation using a novel electroanatomical navigation system: a multicentre experience. Europace 2012; 14(1):60–5.
8. Okumura Y, Henz BD, Johnson SB, et al. Three-dimensional ultrasound for image-guided mapping and intervention: methods, quantitative validation, and clinical feasibility of a novel multimodality image mapping system. Circ Arrhythm Electrophysiol 2008;1(2):110–9.
9. Brooks AG, Wilson L, Kuklik P, et al. Image integration using NavX Fusion: initial experience and validation. Heart Rhythm 2008;5(4):526–35.
10. Lin YJ, Tai CT, Kao T, et al. Consistency of complex fractionated atrial electrograms during atrial fibrillation. Heart Rhythm 2008;5(3):406–12.
11. Sporton SC, Earley MJ, Nathan AW, et al. Electroanatomic versus fluoroscopic mapping for catheter ablation procedures: a prospective randomized study. J Cardiovasc Electrophysiol 2004;15(3):310–5.
12. Rotter M, Takahashi Y, Sanders P, et al. Reduction of fluoroscopy exposure and procedure duration

during ablation of atrial fibrillation using a novel anatomical navigation system. Eur Heart J 2005; 26(14):1415–21.

13. Reddy VY, Morales G, Ahmed H, et al. Catheter ablation of atrial fibrillation without the use of fluoroscopy. Heart Rhythm 2010;7(11):1644–53.
14. Kato R, Lickfett L, Meininger G, et al. Pulmonary vein anatomy in patients undergoing catheter ablation of atrial fibrillation: lessons learned by use of magnetic resonance imaging. Circulation 2003;107(15):2004–10.
15. Wongcharoen W, Tsao HM, Wu MH, et al. Morphologic characteristics of the left atrial appendage, roof, and septum: implications for the ablation of atrial fibrillation. J Cardiovasc Electrophysiol 2006;17(9):951–6.
16. Noseworthy PA, Malchano ZJ, Ahmed J, et al. The impact of respiration on left atrial and pulmonary venous anatomy: implications for image-guided intervention. Heart Rhythm 2005;2(11):1173–8.
17. Nademanee K, McKenzie J, Kosar E, et al. A new approach for catheter ablation of atrial fibrillation: mapping of the electrophysiologic substrate. J Am Coll Cardiol 2004;43(11):2044–53.
18. Haissaguerre M, Hocini M, Sanders P, et al. Catheter ablation of long-lasting persistent atrial fibrillation: clinical outcome and mechanisms of subsequent arrhythmias. J Cardiovasc Electrophysiol 2005; 16(11):1138–47.
19. Di Biase L, Elayi CS, Fahmy TS, et al. Atrial fibrillation ablation strategies for paroxysmal patients: randomized comparison between different techniques. Circ Arrhythm Electrophysiol 2009;2(2):113–9.
20. Verma A, Wazni OM, Marrouche NF, et al. Pre-existent left atrial scarring in patients undergoing pulmonary vein antrum isolation: an independent predictor of procedural failure. J Am Coll Cardiol 2005;45(2): 285–92.
21. Gerstenfeld EP, Callans DJ, Sauer W, et al. Reentrant and nonreentrant focal left atrial tachycardias occur after pulmonary vein isolation. Heart Rhythm 2005;2(11):1195–202.
22. Chae S, Oral H, Good E, et al. Atrial tachycardia after circumferential pulmonary vein ablation of atrial fibrillation: mechanistic insights, results of catheter ablation, and risk factors for recurrence. J Am Coll Cardiol 2007;50(18):1781–7.
23. Chang SL, Lin YJ, Tai CT, et al. Induced atrial tachycardia after circumferential pulmonary vein isolation of paroxysmal atrial fibrillation: electrophysiological characteristics and impact of catheter ablation on the follow-up results. J Cardiovasc Electrophysiol 2009;20(4):388–94.
24. Marrouche NF, Martin DO, Wazni O, et al. Phased-array intracardiac echocardiography monitoring during pulmonary vein isolation in patients with atrial fibrillation: impact on outcome and complications. Circulation 2003;107(21):2710–6.
25. Verma A, Marrouche NF, Natale A. Pulmonary vein antrum isolation: intracardiac echocardiography-guided technique. J Cardiovasc Electrophysiol 2004;15(11):1335–40.
26. Kanj M, Wazni O, Natale A. Pulmonary vein antrum isolation. Heart Rhythm 2007;4(Suppl 3):S73–9.

Percutaneous Closure of the Left Atrial Appendage

Rodney P. Horton, MD[a,b,*], Shephal K. Doshi, MD[c], Javier E. Sánchez, MD[d], Luigi Di Biase, MD, PhD[a,b,e,*], Andrea Natale, MD[a]

KEYWORDS

• Percutaneous LAA closure device • Left atrial appendage • Stroke prevention

KEY POINTS

- The left atrial appendage (LAA) is an anatomically and physiologically complex structure that plays a key role in formation of left atrial thrombus in patients with atrial fibrillation.
- Surgical removal of the LAA is invasive, technically challenging and associated with changes in volume status caused by loss of atrial natriuretic peptide.
- Several percutaneous methods of eliminating flow into or out of the LAA have been developed, including the WATCHMAN LAA closure system, the AMPLATZER cardiac plug, the LARIAT LAA closure system, and the WaveCrest LAA occluder.
- Although many of the percutaneous devices are in the early stages of testing, they each represent promise as well as unique challenges in safe and complete closure of the LAA.

INTRODUCTION

The left atrial appendage (LAA) is a curved, pouch-like structure connected to the left atrium (LA) anterior to the left superior pulmonary vein. Most of the structure extends anterior to the LA and superior to the left ventricle. It usually resides superior to the left main coronary artery or the proximal circumflex coronary artery and inferior to the left phrenic nerve (**Fig. 1**). Its embryologic origin is the primordial LA, although its inner surface is derived from the primordial pulmonary vein. The developed LA is almost entirely derived from the primordial pulmonary vein.[2] Structurally, the LAA differs from the LA considerably. Whereas the entire endocardial surface of the LA is smooth, only the proximal tubular portion of the LAA is smooth.[3] Beyond this region, the LAA becomes highly pectinate and varies widely with regard to overall shape, length, and degree of lobulation. This complex endocardial texture combined with blood stasis during atrial fibrillation (AF) is believed to be the source of thrombus formation.[4] At the cellular level, LAA cells appear similar to LA cells but distinct from pulmonary venous cells.[5] However, chronic AF seems to cause smoothing and thickening of the endocardium of the appendage, particularly in the portions overlying the left ventricle.[6]

The primary morbidity associated with AF is the development of a stroke. During AF, the LAA allows for intracavitary thrombus formation, which can subsequently embolize. In the 1940s, the LAA was believed to be responsible for 50% of strokes associated with AF.[7] More recent studies suggest a more prominent role of the LAA in the formation of thrombi, which may be responsible for more than 90% of strokes in nonvalvular AF cases.[8,9]

For decades, the gold standard for lowering stroke risk in patients with AF has been oral

[a] Texas Cardiac Arrhythmia Institute at St David's Medical Center, Austin, TX, USA; [b] Department of Biomedical Engineering, University of Texas, Austin, TX, USA; [c] Pacific Heart Institute/St Johns Hospital, Santa Monica, CA, USA; [d] Seton Heart Institute, Austin, TX, USA; [e] Department of Cardiology, University of Foggia, Foggia, Italy
* Corresponding author. Texas Cardiac Arrhythmia Institute at St David's Medical Center, Austin, TX.
E-mail addresses: rodney.horton@gmail.com; dibbia@gmail.com

Card Electrophysiol Clin 4 (2012) 383–394
http://dx.doi.org/10.1016/j.ccep.2012.06.001

cardiacEP.theclinics.com

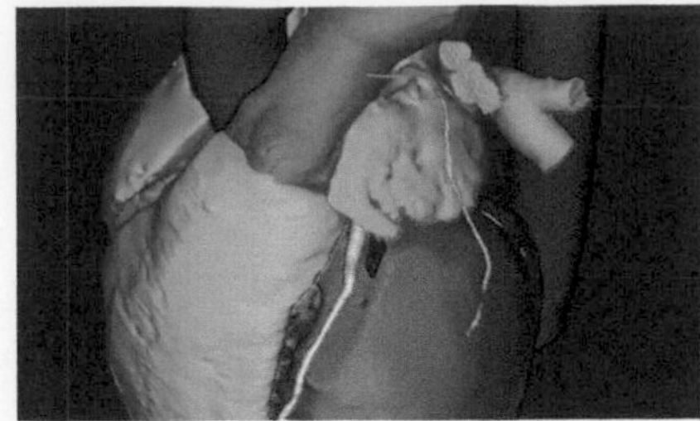
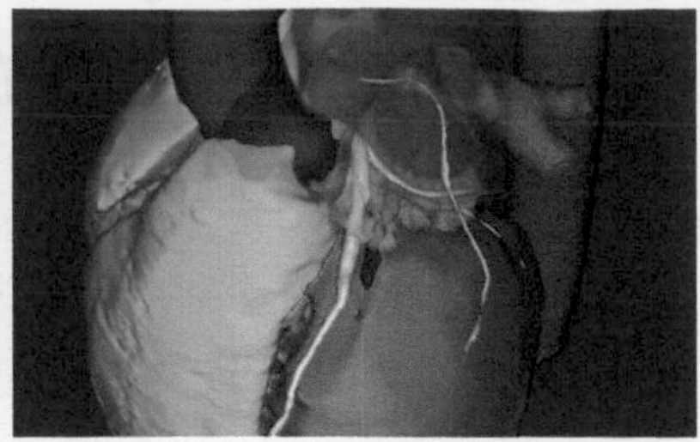

Fig. 1. (*Left*) The orientation of the LAA with the surrounding structures. The phrenic nerve (*yellow*), located by segmenting the pericardiocophrenic artery,[1] courses superiorly to the LAA (*green*). (*Right*) The orientation of the circumflex coronary artery (*white*) and CS (*blue*), which courses between the LAA and the mitral annulus.

anticoagulation (typically with warfarin). Although this strategy is effective, it is still poorly tolerated by many patients. Bleeding risks, frequent dose titration and phlebotomy, drug interactions with other medications, and foods have led to the pursuit of alternatives to this treatment strategy.[10] In 1948, amputation of the LAA was first proposed as a means of lowering subsequent stroke risk during heart surgery.[7] Over the subsequent 60 years, closure or removal of the LAA has become a focus of therapy for both surgeons and cardiologists alike to prevent embolic stroke in the setting of AF.

LAA removal (obliteration) has been performed as a concomitant procedure to other open chest surgical procedures for 2 decades.[11–13] Although this seems effective in eliminating thrombus formation for a dysfunctional LAA, it is technically difficult and not possible in patients whose LAA ostium is broad. Also, volume retention has been reported in the first few months after this procedure.[14] Volume retention is believed to be caused by the loss of LAA-associated atrial natriuretic peptide (ANP) production. Surgical ligation (closure at the base with suture or staples) has become more popular in recent years because it is less anatomically challenging and leaves a functioning organ for ANP release.[15,16] Although expedient, the incidence of incomplete closure with surgical ligation can be high (36%–40%).[17,18] The risk of subsequent embolism from an incompletely closed LAA is concerning and seems to be higher than in intact LAAs.[12] Occlusion of the LAA by percutaneous methods has been an area of active investigation for more than a decade. This article describes and contrasts currently studied closure systems undergoing investigation in the United States and Europe.

WATCHMAN LAA CLOSURE SYSTEM

The WATCHMAN device (Atritech, Plymouth, MN) consists of the self-expanding nitinol metal frame with a porous 160-μm polyester membrane covering the proximal face. The membrane serves to filter blood, thereby preventing LAA thrombus EMBOLIZATION and promoting endothelial growth over the device. Small barbs are positioned radially around the midportion of the device to prevent migration after deployment. Before release, the device is mounted on a detachable deployment catheter, which is housed in a 12-F delivery catheter. The delivery catheter is required to prevent premature opening of the device. The WATCHMAN device and delivery catheter are inserted into the heart within a 14-F access sheath. The device is manufactured in sizes ranging between 21 and 33 mm (3-mm increments) in diameter and in long and short device lengths. The size measurement represents the width of the device at the widest point (shoulder) on deployment from the delivery catheter (**Fig. 2**). Although the device size relates to the uncompressed cross-sectional diameter at the widest point, each of the device sizes fit in a 12-F delivery catheter. The LAA dimensions seen during

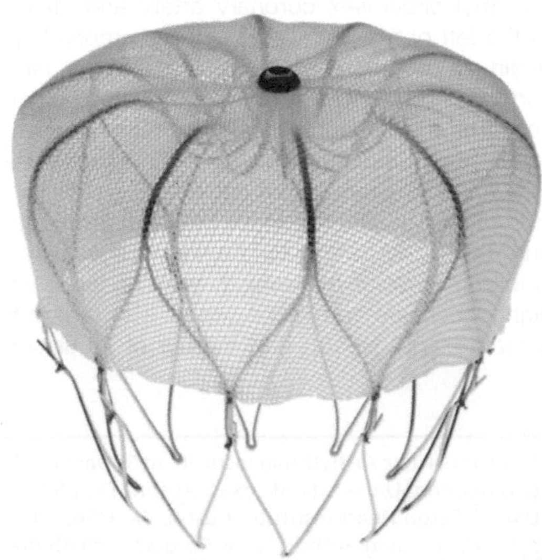

Fig. 2. The WATCHMAN device in an uncompressed form. (*Courtesy of* Atritech; with permission.)

transesophageal echocardiography (TEE) are used to determine the appropriate device size.

Patients usually arrive in the procedure room having withdrawn from warfarin therapy (international normalized ratio [INR] <1.7) and in a fasting state. Aspirin or clopidogrel may be continued for this procedure. As with other medical device implants, strict sterile technique is followed and prophylactic antibiotics are administered intravenously. Central venous access is obtained from the femoral vein; LA imaging is used using TEE or intracardiac echocardiography. With this imaging, all physical characteristics of the LAA are observed, with particular focus on the ostial dimensions of the LAA in 2 obliquities, the length of the main structure from ostium to distal tip, the number and orientation of the appendage lobes, and orientation of the LAA to the left pulmonary veins. Based on these observations, the device size and access sheath shape are determined. The device size is selected by the largest ostial diameter of the LAA with a desired 10% to 20% approximate (company instructions for use) device compression. For example, a measured LAA ostial diameter of 20 mm usually requires a 24-mm WATCHMAN device for adequate coverage with 20% device compression. While using echocardiographic guidance to visualize the fossa ovalis, transseptal catheterization is performed in the interatrial septum using a standard transseptal sheath and needle. Although transseptal perforation anywhere along the fossa ovalis allows for LAA cannulation, a more inferior and posterior puncture usually offers a more direct route to the appendage. Heparin anticoagulation is administered either before or immediately after transseptal puncture with an activated clotting time (ACT) range of 200 to 300 seconds pursued. On advancement of the sheath into the LA, a long exchange wire is advanced through the sheath and into the left superior pulmonary vein. The sheath is then removed while maintaining the wire in the LA. Under fluoroscopy, the 14-F access sheath is advanced across the interatrial septum and the wire and dilator are removed.

Accessing the LAA with the sheath can be operator dependent. The 2 recommended strategies involve a pigtail catheter approach or a direct sheath approach. For the pigtail catheter approach, a pigtail catheter is inserted into the access sheath and then advanced into the LAA. Once engaged, the sheath can be advanced over the pigtail catheter. The pigtail is then replaced by the WATCHMAN device housed in the delivery catheter. The access sheath is positioned in the distal portion of the LAA. The access sheath position is maintained and the device/containment sheath combination is advanced to the end of the access sheath. Because the device shortens on deployment, marker bands on the access sheath offer guidance as to the position on the proximal surface of the deployed device on opening (**Fig. 3**). After fluoroscopic confirmation of position, the access and containment sheaths are withdrawn en bloc and the distal position of the WATCHMAN device is maintained. This strategy allows the device to spring into the open (deployed) position. Contrast fluoroscopy and echocardiographic and mechanical (tug) tests are performed to confirm proper position of the device, show adequate device compression, confirm an acceptable LAA seal with color Doppler, and confirm stability of the final position. Once these criteria are confirmed, the device is released from the delivery catheter by counterclockwise rotation of the deployment knob. Final echocardiographic measurements are recorded and the access sheath and delivery catheter are withdrawn into the right atrium (**Fig. 4**).

After the procedure, the patient is placed on warfarin therapy with a target therapeutic INR range of 2.0 to 3.0. After 45 days, an outpatient TEE is performed to assess device closure. Once complete endothelization over the device is confirmed, warfarin may be discontinued and aspirin therapy initiated.

THE AMPLATZER CARDIAC PLUG

The AMPLATZER Cardiac Plug (St Jude Medical, St Paul, MN) is a self-expanding device originally designed for atrial septal defect closure. This basic design was later modified to function as an endocardial plug to seal the LAA. Like the WATCHMAN device, this product is made of nitinol. However, the design has 2 primary components: a lobe and a disk. The lobe is a soft, deformable mesh

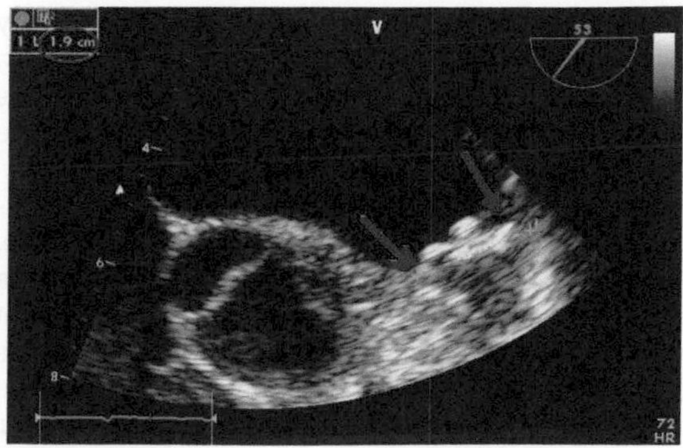

Fig. 3. A TEE image of a 24-mm WATCHMAN device deployed in an LAA. Note the measurement of the widest point on the device, reflecting the degree of compression (area contained between the *red arrow*).

A

Device Size *(uncompressed diameter)*	Compressed **Short** Device Length*
21 mm	20.2 mm
24 mm	22.9 mm
27 mm	26.5 mm
30 mm	29.4 mm
33 mm	31.5 mm

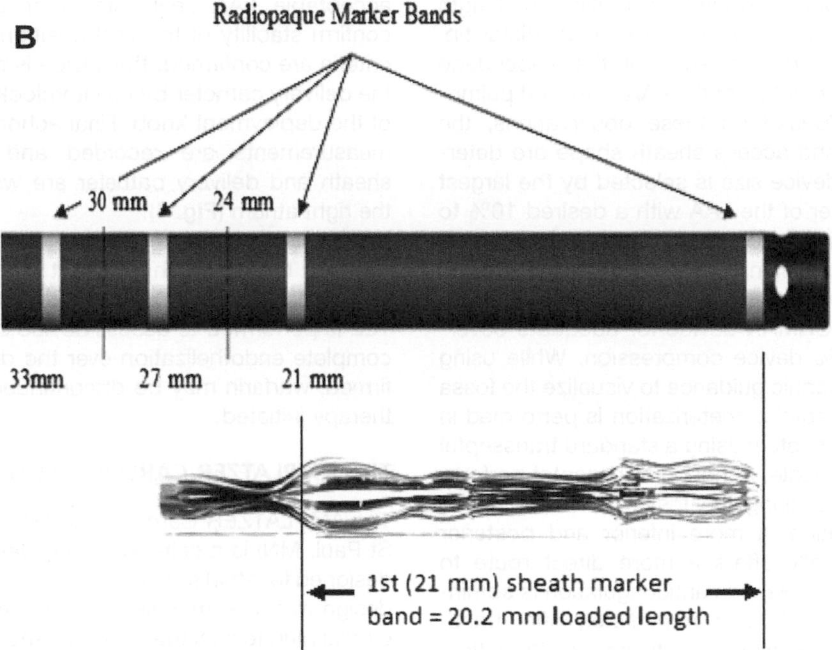

Fig. 4. (*A*) Table of compressed device length (before deployment). (*B*) Magnified view of a compressed device and distal end of the access sheath. (*Courtesy of* Atritech; with permission.)

with nitinol anchors that insert into the LAA cavity on deployment. The lobe is connected to a disk, which on deployment is intended to cover the ostium of the LAA, thereby sealing the structure (**Fig. 5**).

Patients are taken to the laboratory after withdrawal of anticoagulation and in a fasting state. Access to the femoral vein is performed and a standard transseptal sheath is placed in the right atrium. Using a standard Brockenbrough needle with TEE or intracardiac echocardiography visualization, the LA is accessed with a transseptal puncture. Heparin is administered either before or immediately after transseptal puncture with ACT monitoring (target 250–300 seconds). Using the transseptal sheath itself or a pigtail catheter, the LAA ostium is engaged and a contrast injection with cineangiography recording is performed. This procedure is required to determine LAA ostial dimensions for selection of appropriate AMPLATZER sheath and device size. **Table 1** shows the recommended sheath and device sizes for the LAA dimensions. The device is mounted on a 145-cm delivery cable. Once the sheath/device size is selected, a stiff exchange wire is advanced into the transseptal sheath and positioned in the left superior pulmonary vein. Using this wire for retained LA access, the standard transseptal sheath is replaced with the selected delivery sheath. Once placed in the LA, the wire and dilator are removed and the sheath is advanced into the LAA. Before insertion into the delivery sheath, the AMPLATZER

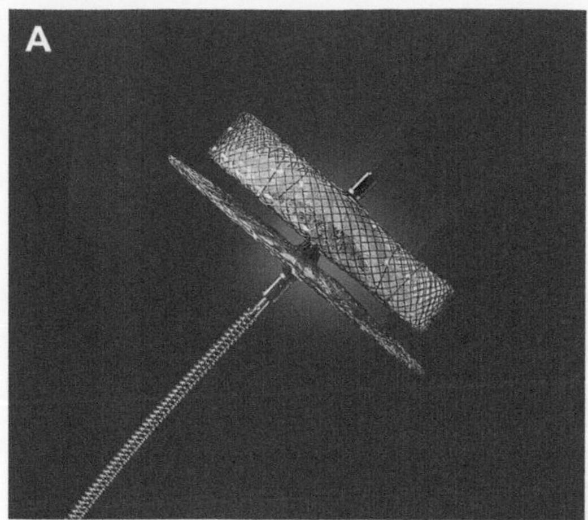

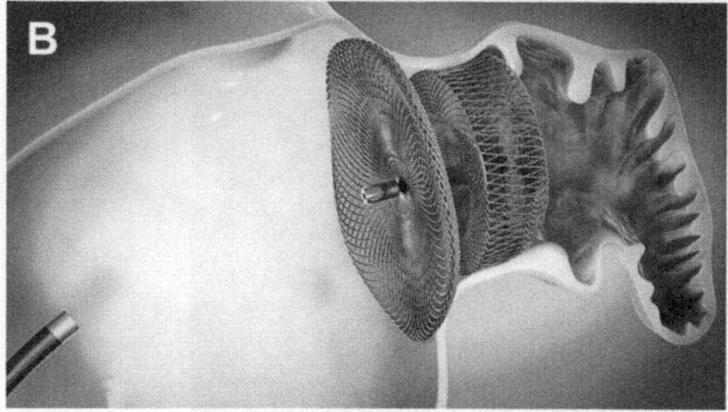

Fig. 5. The AMPLATZER device positioned in the LAA (*A, B*). (*Courtesy of* St Jude Medical, St Paul, MN; with permission.)

device is prepared for placement into a loading hub. This procedure requires front loading the distal end of the device onto a loading cable and into the loading hub (this process is necessary to avoid damage to the nitinol anchors on the lobe portion of the device). The proximal end is then connected to the delivery cable and inserted completely into the loading hub. The leading cable is then removed and the device is connected to the side port of the delivery sheath, evacuated of any introduced air, and advanced into the sheath. The sheath is carefully advanced into the LAA approximately 10 mm beyond the ostium. The device delivery cable is fixed and the sheath is slowly withdrawn to permit deployment of the distal mesh lobe. The delivery cable is advanced slightly to allow complete deployment of the lobe. Injection through the sheath allows for assessment of the lobe placement, which should be 3 to 6 mm within the LAA. While gentle tension is maintained on the delivery cable, the sheath is further retracted, allowing deployment of the proximal disk. All of the proximal disk should be in contact with the LA surrounding the entire LAA ostium in all angles. Confirmation of LAA closure should be performed with contrast injection through the sheath under fluoroscopy as well as echocardiography. Once complete closure is confirmed, the device is released with counterclockwise rotation of the delivery cable. Dual antiplatelet therapy (clopidogrel and aspirin) is usually used for 1 month after the initial procedure followed by 5 months of low-dose aspirin. Follow-up TEEs at 1 month and 6 months after implant are also recommended.[18]

THE LARIAT LAA CLOSURE SYSTEM

The LARIAT system for percutaneous ligation of the LAA (SentreHeart, Palo Alto, CA) involves 3 components: a 20-mm compliant balloon, 0.025 mm and 0.035 mm magnetically tipped guide wires, and a 12-F suture delivery device (**Fig. 6**A–C). The novel components of this design include 2 magnetically tipped guide wires, a suture delivery system, and an endocardial balloon. The

Table 1
AMPLATZER cardiac plug sizing guide

Lobe Diameter (mm)	Disk Diameter (mm)	Lobe Length (mm)	Minimum Sheath Size (F)	Minimum Sheath ID mm (in)	Recommended Sheath Length (cm)	Minimum Orifice Depth (mm)	Maximum Orifice Width (mm)	AMPLATZER Cardiac Plug Size (mm)
16	20	6.5	9	3.0 (0.118)	≤100	≤10	12.6–14.5	16
18	22	6.5	10	3.3 (0.130)	≤100	≤10	14.6–16.5	18
20	24	6.5	10	3.3 (0.130)	≤100	≤10	16.6–18.5	20
22	26	6.5	10	3.3 (0.130)	≤100	≤10	18.6–20.5	22
24	30	6.5	13	4.3 (0.170)	≤100	≤10	20.6–22.5	24
26	32	6.5	13	4.3 (0.170)	≤100	≤10	22.6–24.5	26
28	34	6.5	13	4.3 (0.170)	≤100	≤10	24.6–26.5	28
30	36	6.5	13	4.3 (0.170)	≤100	≤10	26.6–28.5	30

Abbreviation: ID, inner diameter.

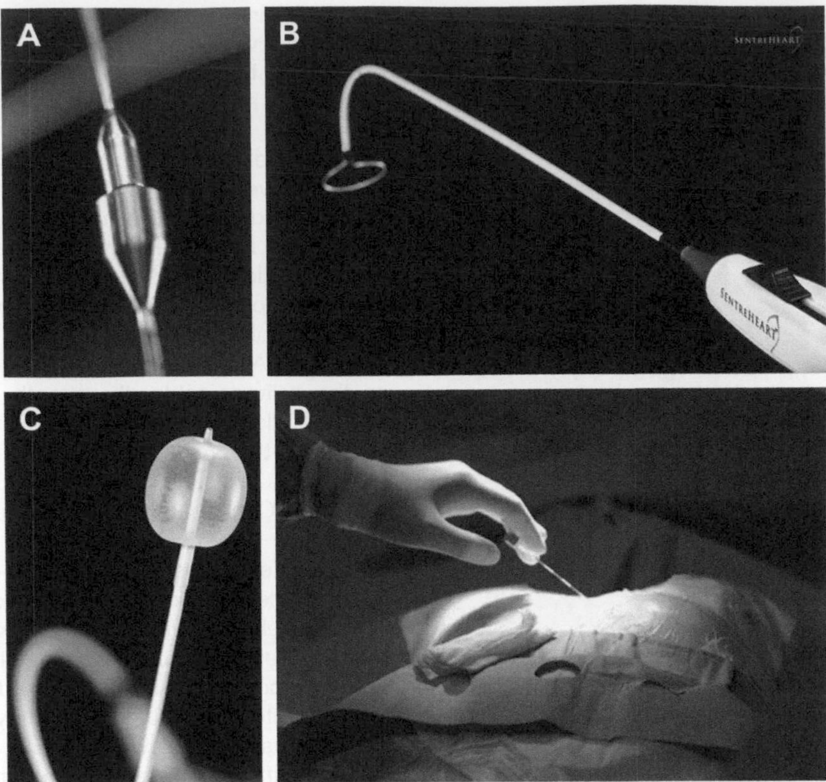

Fig. 6. (*A*) Endocardial and pericardial components of the LARIAT system magnetically bound. (*B*) The LARIAT suture delivery device placed through the pericardial access point and positioned over the LAA. (*C*) The balloon device in the LAA endocardial with the LARIAT system to facilitate epicardial suture position and avoid suture migration. (*D*) Subxiphoid access into the pericardial space. (*Courtesy of* SentreHeart, Palo Alto, CA; with permission.)

0.025 wire is designed for placement in the endocardium and lumen of the LAA. The 0.035 wire is designed for placement in the pericardial space. When the 2 wires are close to each other, they are magnetically guided to meet end to end, allowing for delivery of the suture device over the pericardial wire and advancing over the endocardial wire until the suture device is positioned at the ostium of the LAA. The suture device is composed of a size 0 Teflon-coated, braided polyester suture that is mounted on the delivery device in a pretied loop. The loop size is variable but has a maximum diameter of 40 mm.

The pericardial space is accessed first with a subxiphoid puncture angled for anterior access using a 17-gauge Tuhoy needle (see **Fig. 6**D). An anterior puncture (anterior to the right ventricle) angled to the apex of the LAA is essential for proper positioning of the suture delivery device over the LAA. On pericardial access, a long guide wire is advanced into the pericardium. Sequential dilation procedures are performed at the access point to dilate up to a 14-F sheath in the pericardial space.

Once pericardial and femoral venous access is achieved, heparin is administered and full anticoagulation maintained, with ACT measurements followed for the remainder of the procedure. The LA is accessed using a standard transseptal approach with an SL-1 transseptal sheath (St Jude Medical) and a standard Brockenbrough needle. The balloon is then prepared and the 0.025 magnetic-tipped wire is inserted into the lumen of the balloon. The balloon/wire combination is then inserted into the transseptal sheath and advanced into LAA. Using fluoroscopic and echocardiographic visualization, the 0.025 wire is advanced into the LAA and positioned at the tip (apex) of the LAA. The balloon may be advanced to the ostium of the LAA and used for contrast injections to confirm position.

The 0.035 magnetic-tipped guide wire is loaded into the suture delivery device and these components are inserted into the pericardial sheath. The 0.035 wire (pericardial) is advanced with fluoroscopic guidance until it comes beside the endocardial wire and magnetically binds with the endocardial wire that was previously placed endocardially at the tip of the LAA. This magnetic bond requires approximately 112 g of force to separate the wires. This bond allows for some measure of traction from the pericardial wire to facilitate advancement of the suture delivery device, which is advanced over the endocardial wire in a monorail fashion until the suture loop is properly positioned at the base of the LAA. Fluoroscopy and intracardiac or TEE are used to confirm the position. The endocardial balloon may be advanced into the proximal portion of the LAA to help confirm position. This technique may also be useful in preventing slippage of the suture away from the base of the LAA. As the suture is slowly tightened, the balloon is deflated and removed from the LAA along with the guide wire. The suture is then tightened fully and the LAA is excluded. Once the transseptal sheath is withdrawn from the LA, heparin may be reversed and sheaths removed. **Fig. 7** shows the step-by-step process of LARIAT suture closure of the LAA.

THE WAVECREST LAA OCCLUDER

The WaveCrest LAA occluder (Coherex Medical, Salt Lake City, UT) is an umbrella-shaped device with a nitinol frame designed to cover the LAA at the ostium (**Fig. 8**). Before deployment, the device is preloaded into a 15.4-F delivery sheath. It is deployed through a curved access sheath specifically designed for the procedure. Unlike the WATCHMAN device, the covering material is deployed first, followed by the anchoring frame. Housed on the frame are small barbs intended to secure the device and prevent migration. The covering material includes 2 components: a nonpermeable, Teflon material intended for contact blood pool and a foam cuff around the perimeter intended for direct contact with the atrial endocardium.

Similar to the WATCHMAN and AMPLATZER procedures, patients in a fasting state are brought to the laboratory and femoral vein access is performed. Using either TEE or ICE, the LA is accessed in the interatrial septum, with a preference for low and posterior puncture sites with a standard transseptal sheath and Brockenbrough needle. Heparin is given before or immediately after transseptal puncture, and full heparin anticoagulation is maintained and monitored. Using either echocardiographic method, the anatomy of the LAA ostium is analyzed for size and ostial orientation (**Fig. 9**). A contrast injection at the ostium with the sheath may also be useful in this evaluation. Based on the findings, 1 of 4 delivery sheaths is selected (each with a different distal curve to facilitate device placement). Using a stiff 0.035 exchange wire to retain access, the transseptal sheath is removed and replaced by the access sheath. The device is made in 3 sizes to accommodate LAA ostial dimensions between 14 and 30 mm. Once device size is selected, the device and delivery sheath are prepared for insertion by flushing thoroughly to remove any air. Using constant flushing from the access sheath, the

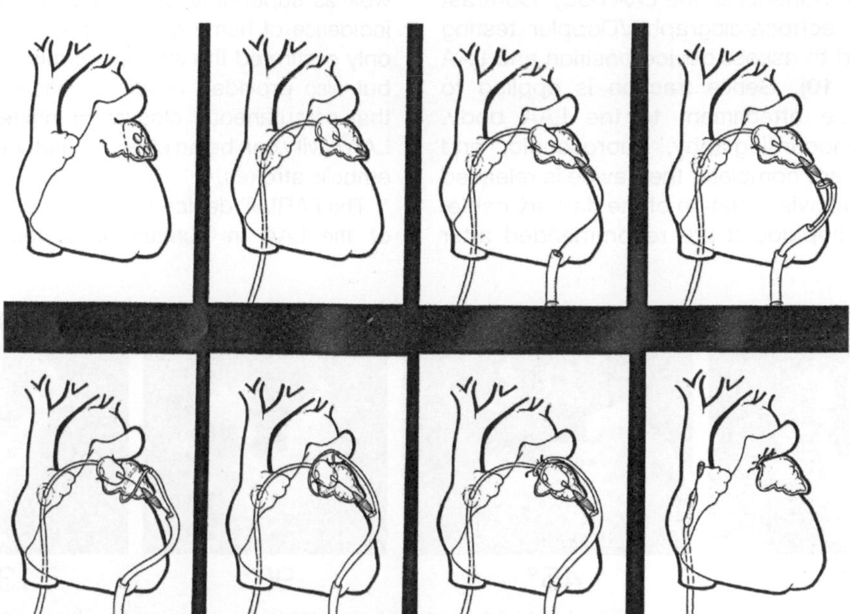

Fig. 7. The progression of LARIAT closure from access to completion. (*Courtesy of* SentreHeart, Palo Alto, CA; with permission.)

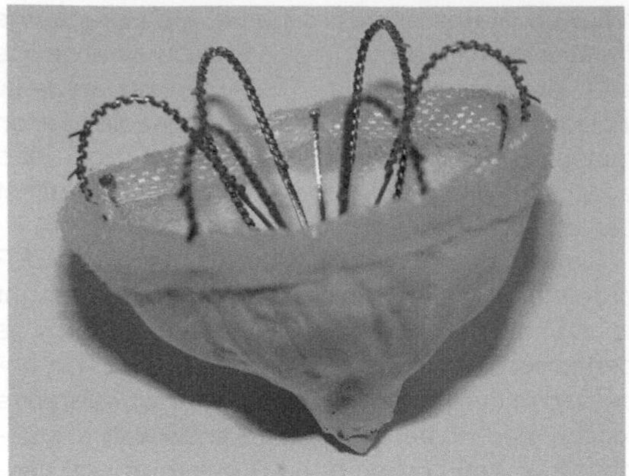

Fig. 8. A deployed WaveCrest LAA closure device. (*Courtesy of* Coherex Medical, Salt Lake City, UT; with permission.)

delivery sheath is inserted into the proximal end of the access sheath and advanced toward the distal end of the access sheath. Contrast can be injected directly through the delivery sheath to facilitate access sheath position at the LAA ostium. Deployment of the device involves 2 steps. The first is advancement of the outer covering portion of the device into the LAA. Because this portion of the device is atraumatic, it can be advanced forward out of the sheath. This situation is in contrast to deployment techniques with the WATCHMAN and AMPLATZER devices, which require sheath placement inside the LAA and withdrawal of the sheath over a fixed device to avoid trauma. The second deployment step is advancement of the anchoring component into the LAA body. Contrast injection and echocardiographic/Doppler testing are performed to assess device position and LAA closure (**Fig. 10**). Gentle traction is applied to confirm device attachment to the LAA body. Once all echocardiography, fluoroscopic, and traction tests are complete, the device is released by counterclockwise rotation of the delivery cable. Aspirin and clopidogrel are recommended after implantation. TEE is required several weeks after implantation to confirm complete closure.

DISCUSSION

The LAA is an anatomically and physiologically complex structure, which plays a key role in formation of LA thrombus in patients with AF. Numerous strategies have been pursued to address this complication, including surgical removal, surgical closure, and percutaneous closure.[12,13,16,19–28] Surgical removal is invasive, technically challenging, and associated with changes in volume status caused by loss of ANP. The 4 devices described are designed to accomplish a similar goal: percutaneous exclusion of the LAA cavity, thereby eliminating that source of thrombus formation in patients with AF.

Small studies and registries have shown the ease of implantation of the AMPLATZER device and have suggested a high likelihood of clinical effectiveness. The WATCHMAN device has been extensively studied, having completed a multicenter, multinational randomized, controlled study (PROTECT AF [WATCHMAN Left Atrial Appendage System for Embolic Protection in Patients with AF]) and there have been numerous single-center reports of safety and efficacy. The PROTECT AF trial reported noninferiority of the WATCHMAN device compared with warfarin therapy in the prevention of strokes during the study period. The analysis also reported a relative risk reduction in thrombotic stroke incidence, and mortality as well as superiority over warfarin therapy in the incidence of hemorrhagic strokes.[28] This trial not only confirmed the efficacy of this specific device but also provided proof of concept, suggesting that percutaneous closure or obliteration of the LAA cavity can be an effective method for reducing embolic strokes.

The LARIAT device showed successful closure of the LAA in humans in a feasibility trial.[29]

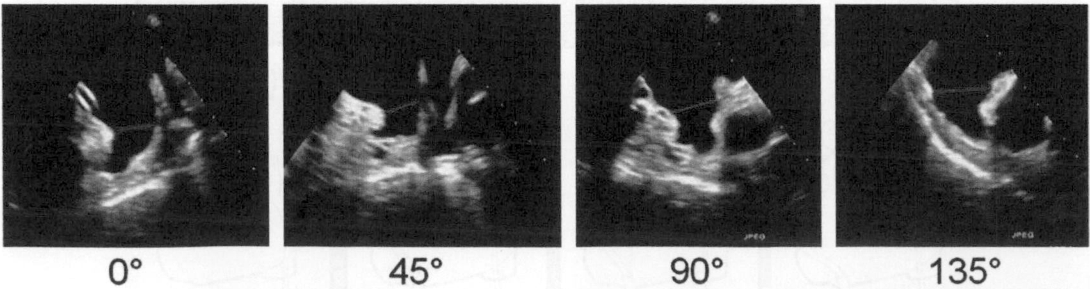

Fig. 9. The different TEE angles required for LAA analysis before WaveCrest access sheath selection and device size. The red arrows indicate the ostium of the LAA at the different TEE angles. (*Courtesy of* Coherex Medical, Salt Lake City, UT; with permission.)

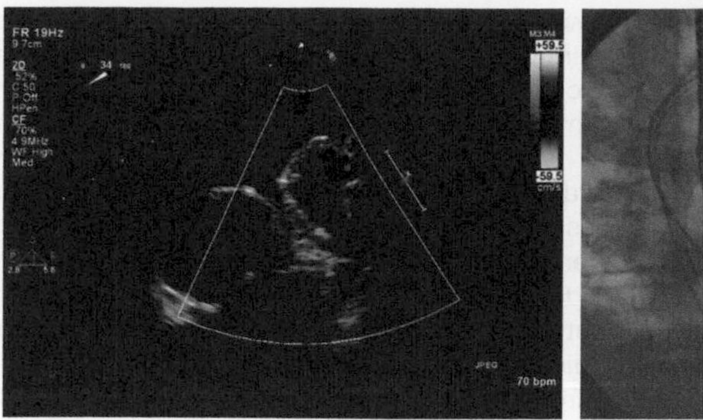

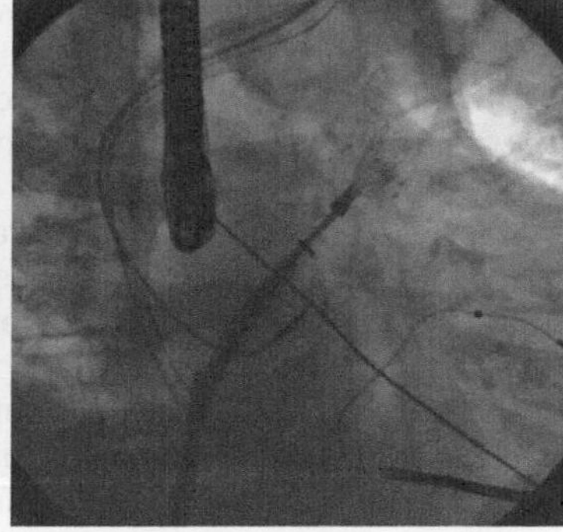

Fig. 10. (*Left*) A TEE image of the LAA after WaveCrest device closure. (*Right*) A fluoroscopic image of a deployed WaveCrest device in the LAA (right anterior obliquity).

Although long-term efficacy data have yet to be published, it has been argued that data from surgical closure of the LAA apply to this technology because it functionally accomplishes the same result. Although this claim may prove to be true, the technique is significantly different from any of the surgical closure procedures. Moreover, closure of the LAA ostium from a single loop of suture may have unexpected consequences on LAA tissue viability. Only with extensive registry data for a protracted follow-up period could such an assumption be proved valid.

LAA anatomy is highly variable and should be considered when using any of these technologies. Long, single-lobed LAA with well-defined tubular necks are the easiest structures to close using any of these devices. **Fig. 11** shows an ostial dimension measurement in 2 obliquities of an LAA using a computerized tomographic angiogram. The 2 measurements are averaged to determine the appropriate device size. The WATCHMAN device is made in several sizes, all of which fit into the same delivery sheath. Device size is based on LAA ostial dimensions. However, the larger devices have a longer compressed and deployed length. This fact is relevant when considering LAA anatomy. Primary LAA length should be long enough to accommodate the compressed (undeployed) device. LAAs with wide ostia and short bodies cannot be occluded with this device because there is inadequate space for the device before deployment. In the AMPLATZER device, LAA ostia/body length issues are less significant because this device can be deployed with as little as 10 mm of sheath placement inside the LAA cavity on deployment. In this aspect, the WaveCrest device seems to have an advantage by permitting safe deployment of the atraumatic covering portion forward out of the sheath. This option offers the possibility of sealing shorter LAAs than can be achieved with the other endocardial devices.

With the LARIAT device, anatomic issues are perhaps more significant than the other devices. LAA ostial orientation should be anteriorly directed, with minimal posterior bend. This strategy allows for placement of the suture loop around the proximal portion of the LAA neck and provides a

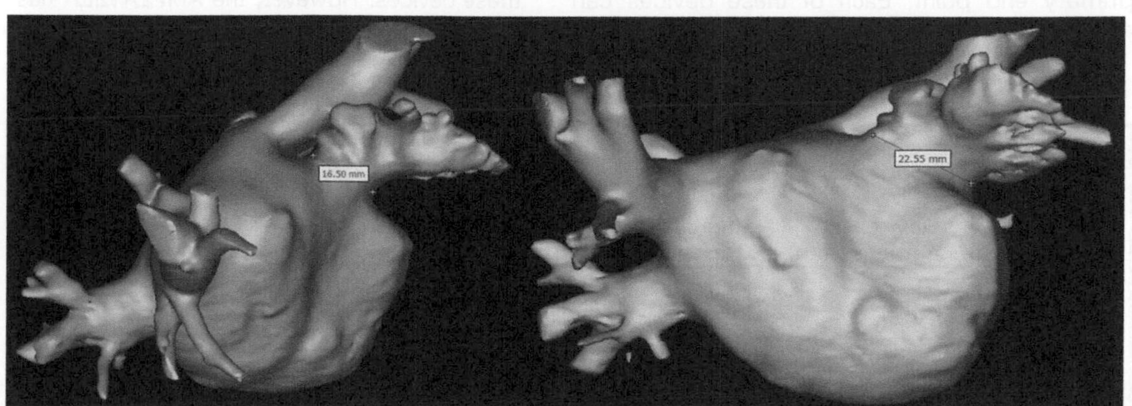

Fig. 11. Ostial dimension measurement in 2 different obliquities of an LAA.

clear path for safe removal of the delivery device after deployment. The suture loop has a maximal diameter of 40 mm. As a result, the device should not be used to close LAAs wider than 40 mm. Unlike the entirely endocardial approaches, the LARIAT procedure is also affected by thoracic anatomy. Patients with pectus excavatum present a unique problem for this approach.[29] The sternal orientation makes anterior pericardial access difficult. Moreover, the 1 reported case of suture ligation in a patient with this anatomy required thoracoscopy to remove the delivery device from the appendage because the sternal compression of that region of the heart prevented conventional removal.

The main complication reported in the PROTECT AF trial involving the WATCHMAN device was pericardial effusion.[27,28] Although some of these complications could be treated conservatively, most required pericardial drainage. Strokes were reported in the device treatment arm but at a lower rate than with warfarin therapy. One hemorrhagic stroke was reported in the device treatment arm, occurring during the protocol prescribed 45 days of warfarin therapy after placement of the device. Device migration was a rare complication, but required sternotomy for removal except for 1 incidence of percutaneous snare retrieval in a case of device migration to the descending aorta. Less is known about the AMPLATZER, although pericardial effusions and device migrations have been reported, the latter requiring surgical retrieval.[30,31] Thrombi have been identified on the WATCHMAN device within the first 12 months of deployment on TEE.[28] No embolic event has been reported from this finding because all cases have resumed warfarin therapy. Complications from the LARIAT device include acute pericarditis after device placement as well as pericardial effusions.[29]

Complete closure of the LAA is the obvious primary end point. Each of these devices can accomplish this goal. However, each has shown an incidence of incomplete closure. In the PROTECT AF trial, complete closure occurred in 87% of cases, allowing for withdrawal of warfarin at 45 days after placement. This percentage increased to 91% at 6 months.[28] The most likely reason for incomplete closure appeared to be undersizing of the device, final positioning too distal, or an unrecognized side lobe in the area of the proximal device face, allowing for flow around the device, and these factors have been reported acutely and in follow-up.[32] A recent report shows that residual leaks less than 5 mm wide measured on TEE Doppler did not increase stroke incidence in the WATCHMAN device.[33] In the AMPLATZER device, incomplete closure seems related to device positioning too proximally, allowing for blood flow between the proximal disk and the LAA ostium. With the LARIAT device, reports from the first human study showed small residual flow into the LAA in 2 of 6 patients at 60-day follow-up.[29] Although no long-term data are yet available for the WaveCrest device, early reports showed no incidence of residual flow in any of the patients who received early implant.

The described percutaneous closure devices involve a complex sequence of techniques and measurements for proper placement. Each has a unique design, method, and a different recommended LAA ostial target dimension. Moreover, some seem to be more complex to deploy than others. **Table 2** shows key differences in devices, sheath, and target LAA ostial dimension options. The AMPLATZER device requires a complicated manual loading process into the delivery sheath compared with the other devices, which are preloaded at the time of packaging. The AMPLATZER device has been reported to become released in the sheath before deployment. This complication has not been reported with the preloaded devices. LAA ostial dimension measurements play an important role in appropriate sizing of each of these devices. However, the AMPLATZER has 3 different sheath sizes, corresponding to different

Table 2
Implanting tool options

Device	Device Size Options (mm)	Sheath Curve Options	Sheath Size Options (F)	Preassembly	LAA Ostial Dimensions (mm)
WATCHMAN	21–33	2	14	No	16–30
AMPLATZER	16–30	1	9, 10, 13	Yes	12.6–28.5
WaveCrest	25–35	4	15.4	No	14–30
LARIAT	Not applicable	1	8 (endocardial), 14 (pericardial)	No	<40 at widest point

device sizes. This feature makes resizing more complicated than the other devices. Partial recapture is a term used to describe resheathing a deployed device up to the area of the anchoring barbs. This technique is required for repositioning of the WATCHMAN and AMPLATZER devices without damage to the device itself. Once the device is fully recaptured, it is considered damaged and should be replaced. This limitation does not occur with the WaveCrest device, which can be fully recaptured and deployed without damage. The LARIAT presents a series of unique complexities, including elective pericardial access, coupling of endovascular and pericardial wires, and confirmation of ostial suture placement without slippage.

The goal of each of these technologies is reduction of embolic stroke risk in the nonvalvular AF patient without the need for long-term oral anticoagulation therapy. In this regard, the device material left in contact with endocardial blood is relevant. The WATCHMAN and AMPLAZER devices use polyethylene terephthalate (Dacron) as the covering in contact with blood pool. In contrast, the WaveCrest device uses expanded polytetrafluoroethylene (Teflon) as its covering. Teflon has been extensively tested in the surgical literature as a safe and effective material used in vascular and structural cardiac repairs without the need for warfarin therapy.[31,34] Because all of these devices involve an endocardial, left atrial component during placement, heparin therapy is required during each of these procedures. The WATCHMAN device also requires resumption of warfarin after device placement for 45 days. TEE confirmation of LAA closure at that time permits withdrawal of warfarin and initiation of clopidogrel and aspirin therapy. It is recommended to remain on this antiplatelet therapy for 12 months, followed by aspirin therapy alone.[31] AMPLATZER implantation guidelines suggest that warfarin may not be required after placement of the device. However, until proved with a randomized trial, anticoagulation after the procedure is advised. The WaveCrest device requires antiplatelet therapy (aspirin and clopidogrel) after insertion, but warfarin is not required. This requirement is based on the surgical experience with this covering material.[35] However, given the possibility of incomplete closure, short-term warfarin therapy could be advisable until more clinical evidence is available. Because the LARIAT procedure leaves no endovascular foreign object, anticoagulation may not be required after this procedure; however, given the stroke risk shown in the surgical literature from incomplete surgical closure, anticoagulation with warfarin until confirmation of chronic closure is a reasonable precaution. With the exception of the WATCHMAN device, no studies have been completed that define the postprocedure anticoagulation/antiplatelet therapy for these devices.

SUMMARY

LAA mechanical function remains a complex issue with regard to stroke prevention in patients with AF. Elimination of flow into or out of the structure has been shown to be an effective means of reducing stroke risk. Several percutaneous methods of accomplishing this goal have been developed. Although many of these devices are in the early stages of testing, they each represent promise as well as unique challenges in safe and complete closure of the LAA. Although each technology provides a means of mechanical closure of the LAA, prospective study is required to determine the timing and appropriateness of anticoagulation withdrawal.

REFERENCES

1. Horton RP, Di Biase L, Reddy V, et al. Locating the right phrenic nerve by imaging the right pericardiophrenic artery with computerized tomographic angiography: implications for balloon-based procedures. Heart Rhythm 2010;7(7):937–41.
2. Moore KL. The developing human: clinically oriented embryology. 6th edition. Philadelphia: WB Saunders; 1998.
3. Ho SY, Anderson RH, Sánchez-Quintana D. Atrial structure and fibres: morphologic basis of atrial contraction. Cardiovasc Res 2002;54:325–36.
4. Shively BK, Gelgand EA, Crawford MH. Regional left atrial stasis during atrial fibrillation and flutter: determinants and relation to stroke. J Am Coll Cardiol 1996;27(7):1722–9.
5. Perez-Lugones A, McMahon JT, Ratliff NB, et al. Evidence of specialized conduction cells in human pulmonary veins of patients with atrial fibrillation. J Cardiovasc Electrophysiol 2003;14(8):803–9.
6. Shirani J, Alaeddini J. Structural remodeling of the left atrial appendage in patients with chronic nonvalvular atrial fibrillation: implications for thrombus formation, systemic embolism, and assessment by transesophageal echocardiography. Cardiovasc Pathol 2000;9(2):95–101.
7. Madden J. Resection of the left auricular appendix. J Am Med Assoc 1948;140:769–72.
8. Wolf PA, Dawber TR, Thomas HE Jr, et al. Epidemiologic assessment of chronic atrial fibrillation and risk of stroke: the Framingham study. Neurology 1978;28(10):973–7.
9. Kannel WB, Wolf PA, Benjamin EJ, et al. Prevalence, incidence, prognosis, and predisposing conditions

for atrial fibrillation: population-based estimates. Am J Cardiol 1998;82(8A):2N–9N.

10. Levine MN, Raskob G, Landefeld S, et al. Hemorrhagic complications of anticoagulant treatment. Chest 2001;119:S108–21.
11. Lindsay BD. Obliteration of the left atrial appendage: a concept worth testing. Ann Thorac Surg 1996; 61(2):515.
12. Kanderian AS, Gillinov AM, Pettersson GB, et al. Success of surgical left atrial appendage closure: assessment by transesophageal echocardiography. J Am Coll Cardiol 2008;52(11):924–9.
13. Blackshear JL, Odell JA. Appendage obliteration to reduce stroke in cardiac surgical patients with atrial fibrillation. Ann Thorac Surg 1996;61(2):755–9.
14. Nishimura K. Does atrial appendectomy aggravate secretory function of atrial natriuretic polypeptide? J Thorac Cardiovasc Surg 1991;101(3):502–8.
15. Landymore R, Kinley CE. Staple closure of the left atrial appendage. Can J Surg 1984;27(2):144–5.
16. DiSesa VJ, Tam S, Cohn LH. Ligation of the left atrial appendage using an automatic surgical stapler. Ann Thorac Surg 1988;46(6):652–3.
17. Katz ES, Tsiamtsiouris T, Applebaum RM, et al. Surgical left atrial appendage ligation is frequently incomplete: a transesophageal echocardiographic study. J Am Coll Cardiol 2000;36(2):468–71.
18. Lynch M, Shanewise JS, Chang GL, et al. Recanalization of the left atrial appendage demonstrated by transesophageal echocardiography. Ann Thorac Surg 1997;63(6):1774–5.
19. Khattab AA, Meier B. Transcatheter left atrial appendage exclusion, gold or fool's gold? Eur Heart J Suppl 2010;12(Suppl E):E35–40.
20. Odell JA, Blackshear JL, Davies E, et al. Thoracoscopic obliteration of the left atrial appendage: potential for stroke reduction? Ann Thorac Surg 1996;61(2):565–9.
21. Nakai T, Lesh MD, Gerstenfeld EP, et al. Percutaneous left atrial appendage occlusion (PLAATO) for preventing cardioembolism: first experience in canine model. Circulation 2002;105(18):2217–22.
22. Ostermayer SH, Reisman M, Kramer PH, et al. Percutaneous left atrial appendage transcatheter occlusion (PLAATO system) to prevent stroke in high-risk patients with non-rheumatic atrial fibrillation: results from the international multi-center feasibility trials. J Am Coll Cardiol 2005;46(1):9–14.
23. Healey JS, Crystal E, Lamy A, et al. Left Atrial Appendage Occlusion Study (LAAOS): results of a randomized controlled pilot study of left atrial appendage occlusion during coronary bypass surgery in patients at risk for stroke. Am Heart J 2005;150(2):288–93.
24. Sick PB, Shuler G, Hauptmann KE, et al. Initial worldwide experience with the WATCHMAN left atrial appendage system for stroke prevention in atrial fibrillation. J Am Coll Cardiol 2007;49(13): 1490–5.
25. Möbius-Winkler S, Shuler GC, Sick PB. Interventional treatments for stroke prevention in atrial fibrillation with emphasis on the WATCHMAN device. Curr Opin Neurol 2008;21:64–9.
26. Fountain RB, Holmes DR, Chandrasekaran K, et al. The PROTECT AF (WATCHMAN left atrial appendage system for embolic protection in patients with atrial fibrillation) trial. Am Heart J 2006;151(5): 956–61.
27. Holmes DR, Reddy VY, Turi ZG, et al. Percutaneous closure of the left atrial appendage versus warfarin therapy for prevention of stroke in patients with atrial fibrillation: a randomised non-inferiority trial. Lancet 2009;374:534–42.
28. Reddy VY, Holmes D, Doshi SK, et al. Safety of percutaneous left atrial appendage closure results from the Watchman Left Atrial Appendage System for Embolic Protection in Patients with AF (PROTECT AF) clinical trial and the continued access registry. Circulation 2011;123:417–24.
29. Bartus K, Bednarek J, Myc J, et al. Feasibility of closed-chest ligation of the left atrial appendage in humans. Heart Rhythm 2011;8(2):188–93.
30. Meier B, Palacios I, Windecker S, et al. Transcatheter left atrial appendage occlusion with Amplatzer devices to obviate anticoagulation in patients with atrial fibrillation. Catheter Cardiovasc Interv 2003; 60(3):417–22.
31. Park JW, Bethencourt A, Sievert H, et al. Left atrial appendage closure with Amplatzer cardiac plug in atrial fibrillation: initial European experience. Catheter Cardiovasc Interv 2011;77(5):700–6.
32. Bai R, Horton RP, Di Biase L, et al. Intraprocedural and long-term incomplete occlusion of the left atrial appendage following placement of the WATCHMAN device: a single center experience. J Cardiovasc Electrophysiol 2012;23:455–61.
33. Viles-Gonzalez JF, Kar S, Douglas P, et al. The clinical impact of incomplete left atrial appendage closure with the watchman device in patients with atrial fibrillation: a PROTECT AF substudy. J Am Coll Cardiol 2012;59:923–9.
34. Piéchaud JF. Closing down: transcatheter closure of intracardiac defects and vessel embolisations. Heart 2004;90:1505–10.
35. Jonas RA, Castaneda AR. Modified Fontan procedure: atrial baffle and systemic venous to pulmonary artery anastomotic techniques. J Card Surg 1988; 3(2):91–6.

Surgical Atrial Fibrillation Ablation

An Electrophysiologist's Perspective

Elad Anter, MD[a], David J. Callans, MD[b,*]

KEYWORDS

• Atrial fibrillation • Surgery • Electrophysiology • Heart

KEY POINTS

- The beginning of surgery to treat atrial fibrillation.
- The evolution of the Cox-Maze procedure.
- The benefit of concomitant excision of the left atrial appendage during atrial fibrillation surgery.
- New approaches to surgical atrial fibrillation ablation: from discovery of pulmonary vein triggers to epicardial radiofrequency isolation of the pulmonary veins.
- The role of autonomic modulation and ganglionated plexi ablation during surgery of atrial fibrillation.
- Atrial fibrillation: surgery versus catheter-based ablation. What approach should be taken?

THE IMPACT OF SURGICAL ABLATION ON THE DEVELOPMENT OF ELECTROPHYSIOLOGY

The experience and insight obtained during surgical ablation of all types of arrhythmias was formative for electrophysiology and catheter ablation. The early surgical ablation experience provided proof of concept as well direct operative observation of anatomy and pathophysiologic mechanisms. For the specific case of atrial fibrillation (AF), surgical ablation also anticipated many of the problems that catheter ablation would subsequently encounter (the importance of transmural lesions, proarrhythmia of incomplete linear lesions, and the possibility of atrioesophageal fistula), although in general these lessons were not promptly appreciated. Rather than competition, greater cooperation and communication between surgeons and electrophysiologists in the future would be more likely to enhance understanding of the underlying pathophysiology of AF.

The History of AF Surgery

Surgical techniques for treatment of AF began in the early 1980s. Most of these have only historical significance now because they were unable to address major detrimental sequelae of AF, including restoration of sinus rhythm and vulnerability to systemic thromboembolism. The left atrial isolation procedure, introduced by Williams and colleagues[1] in 1980, confined AF to the left atrium and left the remainder of the heart in normal sinus rhythm. This procedure allowed conduction through the atrioventricular node and thus alleviated the compromised hemodynamics associated with an irregular heart rate and a rapid ventricular response. However, the left atrium continued to fibrillate and the vulnerability to systemic thromboemboli was not altered.

In 1982, His bundle ablation was developed to control the irregular and rapid ventricular response associated with AF.[2] This procedure required the

[a] Division of Cardiology, Department of Medicine, Beth Israel Deaconess Medical Center, 185 Pilgrim Road, Baker 4, Boston, MA 02215, USA; [b] Division of Cardiology, Department of Medicine, University of Pennsylvania, 3400 Spruce Street, 9 Founders Pavilion, Philadelphia, PA 19104, USA

* Corresponding author.

E-mail address: david.callans@uphs.upenn.edu

Card Electrophysiol Clin 4 (2012) 395–402

http://dx.doi.org/10.1016/j.ccep.2012.06.002

implantation of a permanent ventricular pacemaker and restored regular ventricular rate. However, the atria continued to fibrillate and the risk for systemic thromboembolism was not addressed.

In 1985, Leitch and colleagues[3] introduced the corridor procedure for the treatment of AF. In this open heart technique, a strip of septal corridor containing the sinoatrial and atrioventricular nodes was isolated from both atria. The procedure corrected the irregular heart rate associated with AF, but both atria continued to fibrillate. Moreover, the atria were also isolated from their respective ventricles, precluding atrioventricular synchrony. Therefore, although the sinus node was allowed to control the heart rate, patients were still at risk for thromboembolism and did not benefit from atrioventricular synchrony. Furthermore, His bundle ablation could accomplish a similar physiologic result without the need for an open heart surgery.

The Maze Procedure

Development of the Maze procedure began with the recognition of the need for better appreciation of the relationship between atrial anatomy and atrial electrophysiology in both normal and pathologic states. Cox and colleagues[4–6] developed the Maze procedure in 1987.[4–6] The Cox-Maze procedure was an empiric operation involving the creation of a myriad of incisions in both the left and right atria, designed to interrupt the macroreentrant circuits thought at the time to be responsible for AF (**Fig. 1**). In effect, these incisions directed the electrical impulse from the sinoatrial node while preventing reentrant circuits from forming. It also allowed all of the atrial myocardium to be activated, preserving atrial transport function. The Maze procedure includes multiple left and right atrial incisions including en bloc isolation of the pulmonary veins and posterior left atrium along with excision of the left atrial appendage (LAA). Unlike earlier procedures, the Cox-Maze procedure addressed all 3 detrimental sequelae of AF by restoring sinus rhythm, normalizing the ventricular rate response, and decreasing the risk of thromboembolism and stroke.[7] After 2 iterations addressing procedure complications and technical difficulty, the Cox-Maze III was developed (see **Fig. 1**) and become the gold standard for the surgical treatment of AF.

Long-term results of the Cox-Maze procedure vary between different groups, but success rates have been reported in the range of 70% to 96% in patients undergoing both an isolated and combined procure.[8–10] These data suggested that the temporal pattern of AF (paroxysmal, persistent, or permanent) did not have an impact on the results of the Maze procedure.[11]

The Cox-Maze procedure also proved to be safe. Although technically complex and adding cardiopulmonary bypass and cardiac arrest time, experienced surgeons have performed the classic operation in large numbers of patients undergoing concomitant cardiac surgery without increased operative mortality or morbidity.[8,10,12–14] Major complications included reoperation for bleeding and a 5% to 10% incidence of pacemaker implantation, thought to be the result of incisions placed

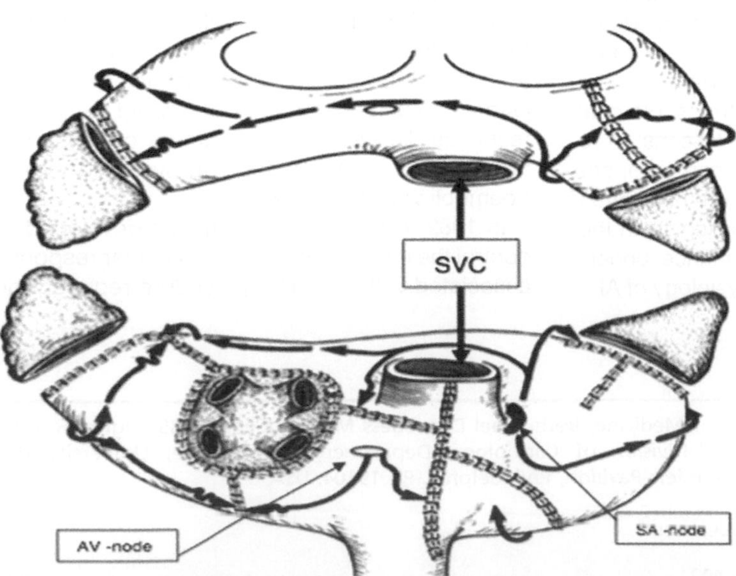

Fig. 1. The original Cox-Maze III procedure atriotomies with propagation of the sinus impulse represented by arrows. AV, atrioventricular; SA, sinoatrial; SVC, superior vena cava. (*From* Cox JL, Schuessler RB, D'Agostino HJ, et al. The surgical treatment of atrial fibrillation. III. Development of a definitive surgical procedure. J Thorac Cardiovasc Surg 1991;101:571; with permission.)

near the sinus node resulting in chronotropic incompetence.[15]

However, these outcome data need to be interpreted with caution. Major limitations include the small number of patients and the limited long-term rhythm monitoring. Long-term follow-up was studied in a diverse group of roughly 500 patients undergoing both concomitant and lone procedures; a small number of patients compared with the large-scale catheter ablation studies. Follow-up rhythm data were limited to noncontinuous atrial rhythm monitoring (ie, 24-hour Holter) or office electrocardiograms, likely associated with an uncertain number of undetected and asymptomatic AF recurrences. Thus, the success rate of surgical AF ablation by conventional rhythm monitoring is potentially overestimated.

The LAA

An important benefit of the Cox-Maze procedure is the concomitant excision of the LAA. Because most thromboembolic events are associated with mechanical dysfunction of the LAA and thrombus formation, its removal can potentially reduce or eliminate the risk for stroke associated with AF.[16,17] One early study showed significant reduction in the stroke risk to less than 1% at 1 year in nonanticoagulated patients, a rate similar to patients fully anticoagulated with warfarin for AF.[18] Furthermore, in a retrospective study, the risk for stroke was significantly reduced in patients who underwent LAA exclusion during mitral valve replacement compared with those who did not.[19] However, there are no randomized studies corroborating this conclusion, and, in a subsequent observational study, a higher subsequent stroke rate was seen in patients who had LAA exclusion during mitral valve surgery if anticoagulation was stopped.[17] This rate is likely secondary to the rate of incomplete surgical LAA exclusion reported in 36% to 55% of patients after surgery and the presence of thrombus documented in these partially excluded appendages.[20]

New Approaches to Surgical AF Ablation

Despite its success, the Cox-Maze procedure did not gain widespread acceptance owing to its complexity and technical difficulty. However, the Maze procedure provided the basic framework for contemporary nonpharmacologic treatment of AF in the form of lines of electrical block within the atrium. The key observation made later by Haissaguerre and colleagues[21] that AF could be triggered from ectopic activity originating from the pulmonary veins, and that ablation of these triggers can eliminate AF, shifted the emphasis away from the Maze-based linear lesions toward treating and isolating the pulmonary veins.

In 1999, The Cox-Maze III procedure was modified to include bilateral isolation of the pulmonary veins with a connecting posterior line to replace the original posterior box lesion set (**Fig. 2**). Moreover, to simplify the procedure, the cut-and-sew operation was replaced with newer ablation technologies, including radiofrequency (RF) energy, microwave, cryoablation, laser, and high-frequency ultrasound. These new technologies have also supported efforts to develop more limited lesion sets that can be performed less invasively, often through small incisions or ports without the

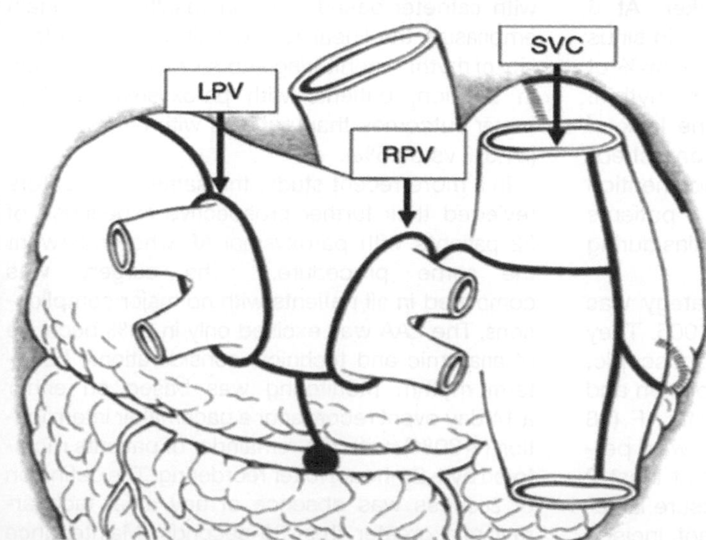

Fig. 2. Cox-Maze IV procedure lesion set. Most of the incisions of the original Cox-Maze III procedure have been replaced with bipolar radiofrequency ablation. Modification included independent isolation of the pulmonary veins with connecting lesion, and no atrial septal incision (originally used for exposure). IVC, inferior vena cava. (*From* Cox JL, Schuessler RB, D'Agostino HJ, et al. The surgical treatment of atrial fibrillation. III. Development of a definitive surgical procedure. J Thorac Cardiovasc Surg 1991;101:572; with permission.)

need for cardiopulmonary bypass. The early use of intraoperative RF ablation led to the initial appreciation of atrioesophageal fistula, later encountered with catheter-based approaches.[22]

The procedure would ideally (1) reliably create transmural lesions with conduction block, (2) have a predicted dose-response curve, and (3) be adaptive to a minimally invasive approach that can be done on the beating heart. To date, each of the ablation technologies have different advantages and disadvantages and none have fulfilled all of these criteria. The principal shortcoming of many of these energy sources is their inability to create reliable transmural lesions on the beating heart. This failing has been thought to be caused by the heat-sink effect of the circulating intracardiac blood. In this regard, bipolar RF energy is an attractive energy source, because the heat sink is potentially overcome by clamping the tissue between the 2 closely approximated electrodes so that the circulating blood is excluded and has little effect on ablation lesion formation.

In 2007, Moten and colleagues[23] reported the initial experience with a minimally invasive Cryo-Maze procedure in patients with lone AF. In a single-center, retrospective study, 41 patients with lone AF (26.8% with paroxysmal AF) were studied. The operation was performed via a 4-cm right inframammary incision using femorofemoral cardiopulmonary bypass. The cryoablation strategy included isolation of the pulmonary veins, mitral isthmus line, right atrial cavotricuspid isthmus line, and a line from the superior to the inferior vena cava. The LAA was oversewn. Electrophysiologic measures of block across these lines were not confirmed during surgery. The procedure was not associated with major complications; however, 4 patients (10%) required implantation of a permanent pacemaker. At 6 months of follow-up, 87.2% (34/39) were in sinus rhythm. Follow-up at 1 year included only 56% of patients, of whom 87% were in sinus rhythm. Additional major limitations included the lack of continuous rhythm monitoring (based on scheduled office electrocardiograms) and no mention of antiarrhythmic drug use. Moreover, 3 patients developed new organized atrial arrhythmias during the follow-up period.

An innovative minimally invasive strategy was reported by Wolf and colleagues[24] in 2005. They performed bilateral video-assisted thoracoscopic, off-pump, epicardial pulmonary vein isolation and excision of the LAA on 27 patients with AF (18 paroxysmal). Pulmonary vein isolation was performed using a bipolar RF device and at least 2 overlapping lesions were created to ensure isolation. In this procedure, the heart is not incised and no additional lines are made. The procedure was performed successfully, without major complications, in all patients. Although the follow-up data were limited to 3 months, 91% of patients were free of AF with the concomitant use of antiarrhythmic drugs, the procedure was noted to be feasible and safe, and it offered a minimally invasive, beating-heart approach for surgical treatment of AF.

In 2007, Edgerton and colleagues.[25] reported the efficacy of a minimally invasive surgical approach to treat AF that combined off-pump, bilateral antral pulmonary vein isolation with targeted partial autonomic denervation. Seventy-four patients (46 paroxysmal, 14 persistent, 14 long-standing persistent) underwent minimally invasive, video-assisted thoracoscopic antral pulmonary isolation using bipolar RF energy. The pulmonary veins were mapped at baseline and entrance block was confirmed following ablation. The ablation was repeated at slightly different orientations until entrance block was achieved. In addition, ganglionated plexi were located by high-frequency stimulation and ablated until repeated stimulation turned negative (less than 50% increase in R to R interval). In addition, the ligament of Marshall was ligated, and the LAA was excised. Rhythm was monitored by office electrograms at 1, 3, and 6 months. At 6 months, the burden of AF was assessed by 14-day to 21-day autotriggered event monitor. There were 4 major complications, including 1 death related to tearing of the base of the LAA. Efficacy was related to the intensity of rhythm follow-up: 92.9% of patients were free of AF at 6 months based on office electrograms, whereas 74.2% who had event monitoring had no detectable AF (AF > 15 seconds). These outcome data are more in line with catheter-based ablation results, and again emphasize the linear relationship between intensity of rhythm monitoring and AF recurrence rates. In addition, patients with paroxysmal AF had better outcomes than patients with persistent AF (81.5% vs 56.5%).

In a more recent study, the same investigators reviewed their further prospective experience of 52 patients with paroxysmal AF who underwent the same procedure.[26] The surgery was completed in all patients with no major complications. The LAA was excised only in 88% because of anatomic and technical considerations. Long-term rhythm monitoring was based on either a 14-day event recorder or a pacemaker interrogation (~80%), with the remainder of patients monitored by a 24-hour Holter reordering. The definition of success was absence of any atrial tachyarrhythmia greater than 30 seconds. Maintenance of sinus rhythm was 86.6% at 6 months and 80.8% at 1 year. In addition, 81.4% of these patients were off antiarrhythmic medications at 6 months and 89.2% at 12 months. Two patients in this series developed atrial flutters, were considered failures, and underwent a subsequent catheter-based ablation of a right atrial flutter.

In this regard, both complete and incomplete surgical lesions created during surgical ablation procedures can be proarrhythmic by promoting a macroreentrant circuit.[27–29] The extent to which epicardial pulmonary vein isolation performed using a minimally invasive thoracoscopic surgery can predispose patients to other arrhythmias was studied by Kron and colleagues.[30] In this series, 50 patients with AF (paroxysmal 74%, persistent 26%) underwent a minimally invasive, thoracoscopy-assisted antral isolation of the pulmonary veins and ablation of ganglionated plexi using bipolar RF energy. Isolation of the pulmonary veins was shown by the presence of entrance and exit block. Of the 50 patients, 20 had recurrent atrial tachyarrhythmia. Of the 20 patients, 13 chose to undergo an electrophysiologic study. The most common arrhythmia was AF (8/13), followed by atrial flutter (4/13). Of the 44 pulmonary veins examined, 50% were reconnected. The most common veins to reconnect were the right inferior vein (73%) followed by the left superior vein (64%). Four atrial flutters were seen in 3 patients. Two had cavotricuspid isthmus-dependent flutter. One patient with typical flutter also had an atypical flutter mapped to the posterior right atrium, and 1 patient had a left-sided atrial flutter. These data are consistent with modern catheter-based pulmonary vein isolation: despite achieving entrance and exit block during the index procedure, pulmonary vein reconnection is common in patients with recurrent AF. Pulmonary vein reconnection probably represents recovery of tissue that was incompletely destroyed during the initial procedure .Focal areas of reconnections are similar with both endocardial and epicardial approaches.

The first prospective and randomized trial comparing catheter ablation and surgical ablation was published in 2011.[31] Inclusion criteria included patients with symptomatic paroxysmal or persistent AF who were refractory to, or intolerant of, at least 1 antiarrhythmic drug. Major exclusion criteria were long-standing AF (>12 months), left atrial size greater than 65 mm, and left ventricular ejection fraction less than 45%. The catheter ablation procedure consisted of pulmonary vein isolation with demonstration of entrance block. Additional lines were performed at the discretion of the operator. Surgical ablation was performed with video-assisted thoracoscopy and included isolation of the pulmonary veins with demonstration of both entrance and exit block. In addition, the ganglionic plexi were ablated as described. The primary end point was freedom from any left atrial arrhythmia lasting more than 30 seconds during a 12-month follow-up. Rhythm monitoring consisted of office electrograms at 3, 6, and 12 months, with a 7-day Holter performed at 6-month and 12-month periods. A 3-month blanking period was allowed, following which antiarrhythmic drug therapy was discontinued. Sixty-three patients were randomized to catheter ablation, whereas 61 patients were randomized to surgical ablation. Freedom from left atrial arrhythmia for more than 30 seconds off antiarrhythmic drugs at 1 year was 36.5% for catheter ablation and 65.6% for surgical ablation. Patients randomized to surgical ablation experienced significantly more major adverse effects, including pneumothorax, major bleeding, and need for permanent pacemaker. Although this was the first prospective and randomized study, several important limitations are worthy of consideration. First, the success of catheter ablation in this experience is inferior to contemporary reports using the same intensity of postprocedural monitoring. This may, at least in part, be because ablation was performed with a standard, nonirrigated, 4-mm ablation catheter in approximately half the patients randomized to a catheter-based procedure. Second, persistent AF was twice as common in patients randomized to catheter ablation (42.1% vs 21.2%). Nonetheless, this experience suggests the conventional wisdom that surgical ablation techniques are more powerful than catheter-based techniques, but are delivered with greater risk of morbidity.

A 2-decade single-center experience with the Cox-Maze procedure in patients with lone AF was recently published.[32] In this retrospective study, 212 patients (48% paroxysmal) underwent a stand-alone Cox-Maze procedure. In the first decade, 112 patients underwent the Cox-Maze III procedure using the cut-and-sew technique. The remainder of patients afterward underwent the Cox-Maze IV procedure using either a bipolar RF or cryoablation energy with isolation of the pulmonary veins. All patients underwent open heart surgery with cardiopulmonary bypass. The LAA was excised in all patients. Median follow-up period was 3 years. Rhythm monitoring was conducted by office visits and increasingly with 24-hour Holter monitoring every 6 to 12 months. The study showed excellent long-term success rates with 93% freedom from AF and 82% freedom from AF off antiarrhythmic medications at a mean follow-up of 3.6 years. The less invasive Cox-Maze IV had significantly shorter cross-clamp time but still achieved high success rates with 90% freedom from AF and 84% freedom from AF off antiarrhythmic drugs at 2 years. Only 1 late stroke occurred over a total of 763 patient years of follow-up, with 80% of patients being off anticoagulation therapy. However, CHADS2 (congestive heart failure, hypertension, age, diabetes, prior stroke) scores for the study patients were not provided.

IS SURGERY MORE EFFECTIVE THAN CATHETER ABLATION?

The limited data comparing catheter-based ablation with surgical ablation were presented earlier and are confounded by several important factors: (1) the small number of studies and patients, (2) predominance of retrospective study design, (3) patient diversity, (3) technical operative diversity, and (4) limited rhythm monitoring.

Long-term, long-duration rhythm monitoring is crucial for measuring the performance of any intervention to treat AF. From catheter ablation of paroxysmal AF, we have learned that, although the 1-year success rate, defined as freedom from symptomatic AF, is as high as 85%, true freedom from AF is more in the range of 70%. In addition, this success rate after a single catheter ablation procedure decreases with the duration of follow-up: 40% at 1 year, 36% at 2 years, and 29% after 5 years.[33]

Available data show that isolation of the pulmonary veins can be successfully achieved either endocardially or epicardially, and the durability of such isolation, although not fully studied, seems to be the same, at least in the case of minimally invasive surgical approaches. Surgical ablation offers 2 additional advantages: excision of the LAA and ablation of the ganglionated plexi. Although data regarding surgical excision of the LAA are controversial, it is still an important treatment, especially for patients unable to take anticoagulation. It seems that LAA exclusion using current technology does not afford appreciable benefit. The importance of ganglionic plexus ablation is discussed later. Catheter ablation offers distinct advantages as well: (1) it can be provided with a lower risk of procedural morbidity; (2) it is repeatable; and (3) it is more likely to be guided by electrophysiologic study, so it is capable of diagnosing other (non-AF) arrhythmias that are specific to individual patients.

In summary, available data do not allow comparison between catheter and surgical treatments for AF. The mainstay of both technologies is isolation of the pulmonary veins. Large and well-designed studies are needed to answer this question, but this is unlikely to happen given the nature of the disease, patient referral bias, and significant difference in the invasiveness of the 2 approaches. However, as more is learned about the pathophysiology of AF, mysteries surrounding different aspects of the procedure are likely to be uncovered.

A new strategy, hybrid ablation, has recently emerged for treatment of persistent and long-standing AF. This strategy has the potential to combine the strengths of each approach and reduce the risk for complications. Surgeons may be able to isolate the pulmonary veins, divide the ligament of Marshall, ablate the ganglionated plexi, exclude the LAA, and safely isolate the superior vena cava when indicated. In contrast, electrophysiologists have an easier approach to the right atrium and cavotricuspid isthmus, and are able to perform an electrophysiology study and identify triggers and other arrhythmias in addition to confirmation of block across the lines. Randomized controlled studies comparing standard catheter and surgical approaches with a hybrid approach are underway.

THE ROLE OF GANGLIONATED PLEXI

The past 5 years have seen advances in the knowledge of neural mechanisms of atrial arrhythmogenesis. There is ample evidence from animal studies that neurohumoral influence plays an important role in the initiation of AF. Direct autonomic nerve recordings show that simultaneous sympathovagal discharges and intrinsic cardiac nerve activities are common triggers of paroxysmal AF.[34] This may also be true for persistent AF, because a high incidence of sympathovagal activation at baseline has been associated with a high vulnerability to pacing-induced sustained AF.[35] Modulation of autonomic nervous activity may constitute an important therapeutic strategy for the management of AF. Continuous, low-level stimulation of the left cervical vagus nerve effectively suppresses AF by reducing the nerve activity of the stellate ganglion.[36] During epicardial AF surgery, localization of the ganglionated plexi is achievable both visually and by high-frequency stimulation, and the absence of a vagal response to high-frequency stimulation after ablation is considered proof of destruction of the ganglionated plexus. Ablation of ganglionated plexi has been added to many minimally invasive surgery protocols. However, its value in the epicardial treatment of AF has not been fully established. In a recent study that included 20 patients undergoing concomitant Maze procedure, adjunctive ganglion ablation was associated with higher rates

Box 1
Reasonable indications for surgical AF ablation

Concomitant heart surgery
Failed catheter-based procedures
Moderate or severe mitral regurgitation
Hypertrophic cardiomyopathy
Long persistent AF
Contraindication for anticoagulation
Severe obesity

of success: freedom from AF at 1 year was 90% in patients undergoing adjunctive ganglion plexus ablation compared with 50% in patients who underwent Maze procedure alone (P = .01). However, this study suffers from common limitations of other AF surgery studies: most importantly, small sample size, patient and procedure diversity, and method of rhythm monitoring. The possible clinical value of ganglion ablation is also available from catheter ablation data showing that a vagal response during ablation, likely representing injury of the ganglionated plexi, is associated with a lower recurrence of AF.[37] However, the overall data regarding the importance of ganglionated plexi ablation in the therapy for AF require further investigation.

FURTHER THOUGHTS

Based on the Heart Rhythm/European Heart Rhythm Association (EHRA)/European Cardiac Arrhythmia Society expert consensus statement on catheter and surgical ablation of AF, standalone AF surgery should be considered for patients with symptomatic AF patients who have failed 1 or more attempts at catheter ablation, or are not candidates for catheter ablation who prefer a surgical approach.[38]

In addition, **Box 1** lists several populations of patients who are likely to be better served by surgical ablation, including patients with AF undergoing concomitant heart surgery; patients who have failed catheter-based procedures; patients with moderate or severe mitral regurgitation without indication for surgery, in whom catheter ablation is less successful[39]; patients with hypertrophic cardiomyopathy; patients with long persistent AF; and patients with contraindications for anticoagulation.

REFERENCES

1. Williams JM, Ungerleider RM, Lofland GK, et al. Left atrial isolation: new technique for the treatment of supraventricular arrhythmias. J Thorac Cardiovasc Surg 1980;80:373–80.
2. Scheinman MM, Morady F, Hess DS, et al. Catheter-induced ablation of the atrioventricular junction to control refractory supraventricular arrhythmias. JAMA 1982;248:851–5.
3. Leitch JW, Klein G, Yee R, et al. Sinus node-atrioventricular node isolation: Long-term results with the "corridor" operation for atrial fibrillation. J Am Coll Cardiol 1991;17:970–5.
4. Cox JL. The surgical treatment of atrial fibrillation. IV. Surgical technique. J Thorac Cardiovasc Surg 1991; 101:584–92.
5. Cox JL, Canavan TE, Schuessler RB, et al. The surgical treatment of atrial fibrillation. II. Intraoperative electrophysiologic mapping and description of the electrophysiologic basis of atrial flutter and atrial fibrillation. J Thorac Cardiovasc Surg 1991;101: 406–26.
6. Cox JL, Schuessler RB, D'Agostino HJ Jr, et al. The surgical treatment of atrial fibrillation. III. Development of a definitive surgical procedure. J Thorac Cardiovasc Surg 1991;101:569–83.
7. Cox JL, Ad N, Palazzo T. Impact of the maze procedure on the stroke rate in patients with atrial fibrillation. J Thorac Cardiovasc Surg 1999;118:833–40.
8. Prasad SM, Maniar HS, Camillo CJ, et al. The Cox maze III procedure for atrial fibrillation: long-term efficacy in patients undergoing lone versus concomitant procedures. J Thorac Cardiovasc Surg 2003; 126:1822–8.
9. Gillinov AM. Ablation of atrial fibrillation with mitral valve surgery. Curr Opin Cardiol 2005;20:107–14.
10. Schaff HV, Dearani JA, Daly RC, et al. Cox-Maze procedure for atrial fibrillation: Mayo Clinic experience. Semin Thorac Cardiovasc Surg 2000;12:30–7.
11. Gillinov AM, Sirak J, Blackstone EH, et al. The Cox maze procedure in mitral valve disease: predictors of recurrent atrial fibrillation. J Thorac Cardiovasc Surg 2005;130:1653–60.
12. Cox JL. Intraoperative options for treating atrial fibrillation associated with mitral valve disease. J Thorac Cardiovasc Surg 2001;122:212–5.
13. Ad N, Cox JL. Combined mitral valve surgery and the maze III procedure. Semin Thorac Cardiovasc Surg 2002;14:206–9.
14. McCarthy PM, Gillinov AM, Castle L, et al. The Cox-Maze procedure: the Cleveland Clinic experience. Semin Thorac Cardiovasc Surg 2000;12:25–9.
15. Cox JL, Jaquiss RD, Schuessler RB, et al. Modification of the maze procedure for atrial flutter and atrial fibrillation. II. Surgical technique of the maze III procedure. J Thorac Cardiovasc Surg 1995;110: 485–95.
16. Belcher JR, Somerville W. Systemic embolism and left auricular thrombosis in relation to mitral valvotomy. Br Med J 1955;2:1000–3.

17. Almahameed ST, Khan M, Zuzek RW, et al. Left atrial appendage exclusion and the risk of thromboembolic events following mitral valve surgery. J Cardiovasc Electrophysiol 2007;18:364–6.
18. Cox JL, Schuessler RB, Lappas DG, et al. An 8 1/2-year clinical experience with surgery for atrial fibrillation. Ann Surg 1996;224:267–73 [discussion: 273–5].
19. Garcia-Fernandez MA, Perez-David E, Quiles J, et al. Role of left atrial appendage obliteration in stroke reduction in patients with mitral valve prosthesis: a transesophageal echocardiographic study. J Am Coll Cardiol 2003;42:1253–8.
20. Katz ES, Tsiamtsiouris T, Applebaum RM, et al. Surgical left atrial appendage ligation is frequently incomplete: a transesophageal echocardiographic study. J Am Coll Cardiol 2000;36:468–71.
21. Haissaguerre M, Jais P, Shah DC, et al. Spontaneous initiation of atrial fibrillation by ectopic beats originating in the pulmonary veins. N Engl J Med 1998;339:659–66.
22. Doll N, Borger MA, Fabricius A, et al. Esophageal perforation during left atrial radiofrequency ablation: is the risk too high? J Thorac Cardiovasc Surg 2003;125:836–42.
23. Moten SC, Rodriguez E, Cook RC, et al. New ablation techniques for atrial fibrillation and the minimally invasive Cryo-Maze procedure in patients with lone atrial fibrillation. Heart Lung Circ 2007;16(Suppl 3):S88–93.
24. Wolf RK, Schneeberger EW, Osterday R, et al. Video-assisted bilateral pulmonary vein isolation and left atrial appendage exclusion for atrial fibrillation. J Thorac Cardiovasc Surg 2005;130:797–802.
25. Edgerton JR, Edgerton ZJ, Weaver T, et al. Minimally invasive pulmonary vein isolation and partial autonomic denervation for surgical treatment of atrial fibrillation. Ann Thorac Surg 2008;86:35–8 [discussion: 39].
26. Edgerton JR, Brinkman WT, Weaver T, et al. Pulmonary vein isolation and autonomic denervation for the management of paroxysmal atrial fibrillation by a minimally invasive surgical approach. J Thorac Cardiovasc Surg 2010;140:823–8.
27. McElderry HT, McGiffin DC, Plumb VJ, et al. Proarrhythmic aspects of atrial fibrillation surgery: mechanisms of postoperative macroreentrant tachycardias. Circulation 2008;117:155–62.
28. Akar JG, Al-Chekakie MO, Hai A, et al. Surface electrocardiographic patterns and electrophysiologic characteristics of atrial flutter following modified radiofrequency maze procedures. J Cardiovasc Electrophysiol 2007;18:349–55.
29. Magnano AR, Argenziano M, Dizon JM, et al. Mechanisms of atrial tachyarrhythmias following surgical atrial fibrillation ablation. J Cardiovasc Electrophysiol 2006;17:366–73.
30. Kron J, Kasirajan V, Wood MA, et al. Management of recurrent atrial arrhythmias after minimally invasive surgical pulmonary vein isolation and ganglionic plexi ablation for atrial fibrillation. Heart Rhythm 2010;7:445–51.
31. Boersma LV, Castella M, van Boven W, et al. Atrial fibrillation catheter ablation versus surgical ablation treatment (fast): a 2-center randomized clinical trial. Circulation 2012;125(1):23–30.
32. Weimar T, Schena S, Bailey MS, et al. The Cox-Maze procedure for lone atrial fibrillation: a single center experience over two decades. Circ Arrhythm Electrophysiol 2012;5(1):8–14.
33. Weerasooriya R, Khairy P, Litalien J, et al. Catheter ablation for atrial fibrillation: are results maintained at 5 years of follow-up? J Am Coll Cardiol 2011;57:160–6.
34. Tan AY, Zhou S, Ogawa M, et al. Neural mechanisms of paroxysmal atrial fibrillation and paroxysmal atrial tachycardia in ambulatory canines. Circulation 2008;118:916–25.
35. Shen MJ, Choi EK, Tan AY, et al. Patterns of baseline autonomic nerve activity and the development of pacing-induced sustained atrial fibrillation. Heart Rhythm 2011;8:583–9.
36. Shen MJ, Shinohara T, Park HW, et al. Continuous low-level vagus nerve stimulation reduces stellate ganglion nerve activity and paroxysmal atrial tachyarrhythmias in ambulatory canines. Circulation 2011;123:2204–12.
37. Pappone C, Santinelli V, Manguso F, et al. Pulmonary vein denervation enhances long-term benefit after circumferential ablation for paroxysmal atrial fibrillation. Circulation 2004;109:327–34.
38. Calkins H, Brugada J, Packer DL, et al. HRS/EHRA/ECAS expert consensus statement on catheter and surgical ablation of atrial fibrillation: recommendations for personnel, policy, procedures and follow-up. A report of the Heart Rhythm Society (HRS) task force on catheter and surgical ablation of atrial fibrillation developed in partnership with the European Heart Rhythm Association (EHRA) and the European Cardiac Arrhythmia Society (ECAS); in collaboration with the American College of Cardiology (ACC), American Heart Association (AHA), and the Society of Thoracic Surgeons (STS). Endorsed and approved by the governing bodies of the American College of Cardiology, the American Heart Association, the European Cardiac Arrhythmia Society, the European Heart Rhythm Association, the Society of Thoracic Surgeons, and the Heart Rhythm Society. Europace 2007;9:335–79.
39. Gertz ZM, Raina A, Mountantonakis SE, et al. The impact of mitral regurgitation on patients undergoing catheter ablation of atrial fibrillation. Europace 2011;13:1127–32.

Ablate and Pace: Is There Still a Role?

Alexandru B. Chicos, MD*, Bradley P. Knight, MD

KEYWORDS

• Ablation • Atrioventricular junction • Atrioventricular node • Ablate and pace

KEY POINTS

- Atrioventricular junction (AVJ) ablation still has a role in the management of selected patients with atrial fibrillation (AF) who are refractory to medical therapy, to improve symptoms, prevent ventricular dysfunction, and to optimize cardiac resynchronization therapy (CRT).
- "Ablate and pace" can be a very safe and effective strategy for controlling rapid ventricular rates and their negative consequences.
- Individually tailored decision making and careful planning are essential, as are genuine attempts to maximize medical therapy and careful consideration of alternatives, before proceeding to an irreversible intervention.
- If the left ventricular ejection fraction (LVEF) is 35% or less, symptoms of heart failure persist, or deterioration in LVEF occurs after AVJ ablation and right ventricular pacing, upgrading to CRT should be strongly considered.
- Observational studies suggest that ablating the AVJ in patients with heart failure and CRT improves their outcomes, and should be considered in patients who have suboptimal CRT (biventricular-paced beats <85%–95% of total beats); randomized trials are needed.

INTRODUCTION

The management of patients with atrial fibrillation (AF) has been broadly categorized into rhythm-control and rate-control strategies. The merits of either strategy have been studied and debated, and continue to be under investigation. A significant number of patients, however, fail or do not tolerate the pharmacologic management used to implement these strategies. In a subset of these patients, ablation of the atrioventricular junction (AVJ) and implantation of a permanent pacemaker ("ablate and pace" approach) may be a reasonable option.

WHO MIGHT BENEFIT FROM AVJ ABLATION?

Some patients with AF (or other atrial tachyarrhythmias: atrial flutter, atrial tachycardia) have ventricular rates that are difficult to control, despite the best attempts to slow atrioventricular (AV) conduction using medications (**Box 1**). It is important in this situation to rule out transient and correctable causes of rapid ventricular rates, such as hyperthyroidism, infection or other acute illness, and medication noncompliance. There is no clearly defined ventricular rate that is detrimental. A randomized trial[1] found that a more lenient rate control (resting heart rate <110 beats/min) may be equivalent to a stricter one (resting heart rate <80 beats/min, exercise heart rate <110 beats/min). The adequacy of rate control should be informed by this but also by clinical judgment tailored to the individual patient. Poorly controlled, fast, and irregular ventricular rates may result in symptoms (such as palpitations, dizziness, syncope, congestive heart failure, and myocardial ischemia), worsening of underlying cardiomyopathy, or even a tachycardia-mediated cardiomyopathy. It is not clear

Financial disclosures: A.B. Chicos: None. B.P. Knight: Consultant and Speaker for Boston Scientific, Speaker for Biosense Webster, Medtronic, St. Jude, and Biotronik.
Division of Cardiology, Department of Internal Medicine, Northwestern University Feinberg School of Medicine, Chicago, IL, USA
* Corresponding author. Northwestern University, 251 East Huron Street, Einberg 8-503, Chicago, IL 60611.
E-mail addresses: alex.chicos@gmail.com; achicos@nmff.org

Card Electrophysiol Clin 4 (2012) 403–412
http://dx.doi.org/10.1016/j.ccep.2012.05.003
1877-9182/12/$ – see front matter

Box 1
Indications for AVJ ablation

1. Achieve adequate rate control during AF[a]
   a. Symptoms related to rhythm and/or rate (palpitations, defibrillator shocks)
   b. Symptoms of heart failure
   c. Prevent or treat tachycardia-mediated cardiomyopathy[b]
   d. Failed or cannot tolerate medical therapy
2. Optimize CRT delivery in patients with AF

[a] Rule out hyperthyroidism, infection, acute illness, noncompliance, or other causes of rapid ventricular rates.
[b] Consider waiting and attempting conservative treatment for 1 to 3 months.

as to what is the cutoff for fast ventricular rates that may cause a tachycardia-mediated cardiomyopathy, and it is likely that this depends on the underlying cardiac substrate. In these patients, rhythm control with either antiarrhythmic medications or ablation should be considered. AF, and most atrial flutters and atrial tachycardias, are potentially curable by ablation. However, in some patients ablation may not be the best option, because of comorbid conditions, patient preference, or other factors, or because it may fail. Ablating the AVJ and pacing can provide adequate rate control and regularization of rhythm, and thus alleviate symptoms and potentially allow reversal of the tachycardia-mediated systolic dysfunction. In patients experiencing symptoms related to heart failure, it is important to consider that AVJ ablation does not restore the atrial pump function and its potential contribution to ventricular filling; however, the potential role of the atrial pump function may vary from patient to patient, and may be obviated in many by the restoration of physiologic heart rates. It is also important to consider the possible detrimental effects of right ventricular (RV) pacing causing ventricular dyssynchrony, as well the option of minimizing this by implanting a cardiac resynchronization therapy (CRT) device.

In other patients, the use and dose of medications can be limited by various side effects that limit their tolerability, including hypotension; or the drugs can interact significantly with other medications (such as the interaction between verapamil and some of the immunosuppressive agents used after transplantation). For these patients, AVJ ablation and pacing provides an alternative for rate and symptom control, and allows them to eliminate from their regimens the medications used strictly for rate control.

Another situation whereby AVJ ablation can be beneficial is in optimizing CRT in patients with AF. This situation is discussed in more detail later in the section "Role of AVJ ablation after CRT."

TIMING OF AVJ ABLATION RELATIVE TO PACEMAKER IMPLANTATION AND THE TREATMENT PLAN

While AVJ ablation and pacing may be a good option for some patients, the decision to proceed with AVJ ablation should be carefully considered, given the irreversible nature of the intervention and the fact that it frequently results in pacemaker dependence. An appropriate trial of alternative treatments should be considered, and it is prudent to try these for some period of time, depending on the rate and tolerance of the ventricular rate, as well as the rest of the clinical context of the individual patient.

It is frequently difficult to distinguish between cause and consequence when patients present with AF with rapid ventricular rates and left ventricular systolic dysfunction, given that each of these conditions can cause or worsen the other, establishing a vicious pathophysiologic circle. Individualized clinical judgment and appropriate medical therapy can frequently provide answers and avoid unnecessary and/or irreversible interventions.

In terms of timing of AVJ ablation relative to the pacemaker implantation, it is preferable to have a reliable pacing lead in place first, so it is common to perform the AVJ ablation several days to weeks after the pacemaker implantation. However, it is acceptable and common practice to perform the AVJ ablation and placement of the permanent pacemaker within the same session. Implant timing is discussed in more detail in the section "Device implantation: timing, technique, type of device."

HISTORY AND TECHNIQUE

Early AVJ ablations were performed during surgical, open-chest procedures,[2,3] and its application for controlling "life-threatening or disabling atrial arrhythmias" was first described in the surgical literature.[4] Closed-chest transcatheter techniques were then developed, initially using fulguration with high-voltage DC shocks[5–7] and subsequently radiofrequency (RF) energy,[8] which continues to be the preferred method.

The anatomic target is generally the superior angle of the triangle of Koch, the area where the compact AV node resides. Because the most common AVJ ablation technique targets the compact AV node, the term atrioventricular nodal (AVN) ablation is also frequently used. Targeting the more proximal level of the AVJ is preferred, as it leaves intact the more distal AV node and the His bundle, and is more likely to result in preservation of a stable junctional escape rhythm, thus avoiding complete pacemaker dependence. AVJ ablation can also target the His bundle, but this has the disadvantage of being much more likely to leave the patient pacemaker dependent. The His bundle dives into the fibrous trigone as it crosses the tricuspid annulus. Occasionally it may be difficult to ablate the AVJ from the right side, requiring a left-sided approach that targets the His bundle after it exits the fibrous sheath. The anterior and posterior atrial inputs into the AV node can also be targeted at the regions of the fast and slow AV nodal pathways, respectively.

The usual approach is to position a deflectable 4-mm ablation catheter on the superior and septal tricuspid annulus on the ventricular aspect, where the largest His bundle electrogram can be recorded. The catheter is then gradually withdrawn while maintaining gentle clockwise torque to preserve septal contact until a large atrial electrogram with A/V ratio greater than 1 (in sinus rhythm) and a small or barely visible His electrogram are recorded in the distal pair of electrodes. If the rhythm is AF, atrial electrograms may be small, and the catheter may be pulled until the His signal disappears under the fibrillatory atrial electrograms (**Fig. 1**). The His signal can be identified among the fibrillatory atrial electrograms by its temporal relationship to the QRS. Rarely, cardioversion may be useful to allow clear visualization of the His electrogram, but only after preparations are made with anticoagulation and transesophageal echocardiogram to rule out intracardiac thrombi, as needed. Fluoroscopically, the successful catheter tip position is generally in an area approximately 2 cm below and to the left of the His bundle area in the right anterior oblique view. RF energy is delivered while monitoring for AV block. An accelerated junctional rhythm is commonly observed during ablation at successful ablation sites (**Fig. 2**). If block is not achieved within 10 to 15 seconds, or if right bundle branch block is created, the catheter is repositioned in search of the compact AV node, slightly more posteriorly and inferiorly, in the area between the apex of the Triangle of Koch and the superior lip of the coronary sinus os.

When AV block cannot be achieved after multiple attempts from the right side (5–10), the His bundle can be targeted from the left ventricular septum just below the aortic valve.[9] This location is in the area of the membranous septum, where the catheter tip records the largest His bundle electrogram and small atrial electrograms.[10] One report describes a supravalvular approach from the noncoronary aortic cusp.[11] Intravenous heparin should be given during the left-sided procedure, which creates an increased risk of pacemaker pocket hematoma if the pocket was recently created. An

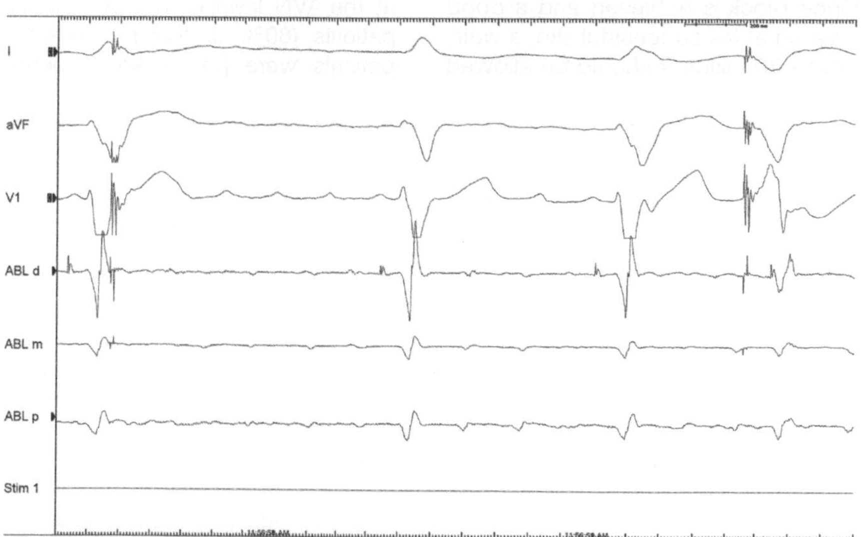

Fig. 1. Example of a successful ablation site during AVJ ablation. Shown are recordings from surface leads 1, aVF, and V1, and the intracardiac recordings from the distal (d), middle (m), and proximal (p) bipoles of the ablation catheter. The baseline rhythm is atrial fibrillation. As can be seen, the pacemaker is programmed to deliver asynchronous ventricular pacing so that pacing is not inhibited during the delivery of RF energy and is thus available after heart block is achieved. Note the large amplitude atrial and His-bundle electrograms on the recordings from the distal ablation electrode.

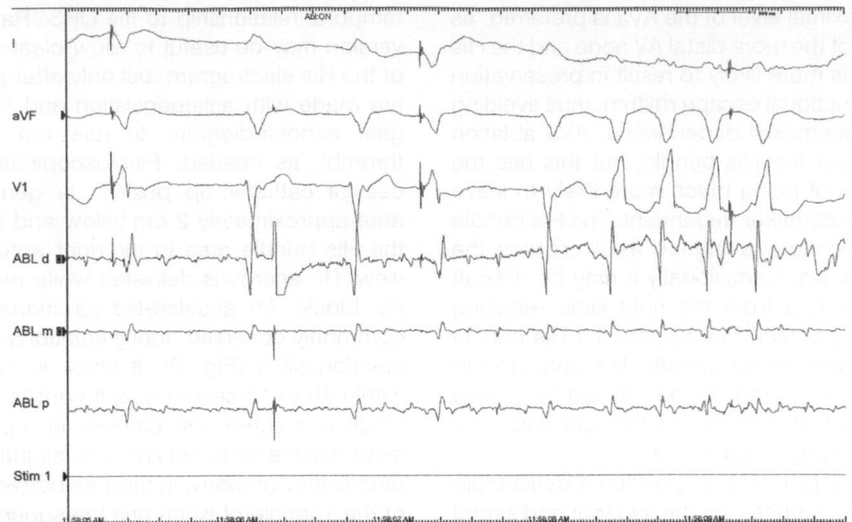

Fig. 2. An accelerated rhythm during RF ablation within seconds after the onset of energy delivery. Abbreviations and format are the same as in **Fig. 1**.

alternative approach for right-sided ablation is via the subclavian or axillary vein at the time of pacemaker implantation through a separate access sheath. The atrial pacing lead can then be advanced via the same sheath after catheter withdrawal.[12]

Typical energy delivery settings for 4-mm catheters are 50 W, with temperature targets of 60° to 70°C, for 30 to 120 seconds. In the occasional case when these approaches are not successful, an 8-mm or an irrigated-tip catheter can be considered. Once block is achieved and a good lesion was delivered at the successful site, a waiting period of 20 to 30 minutes should be allowed before withdrawing the catheters, to make sure that AV conduction does not recur (**Fig. 3**). If ablation fails despite multiple right-sided and left-sided attempts, it may be reasonable to proceed with pacemaker implantation anyway, and plan a repeat attempt later, allowing local edema to subside.

OUTCOMES OF AVJ ABLATION

Complete block can be achieved in nearly all patients, with a low recurrence rate (**Table 1**). Block at the AVN level is, however, achieved in fewer patients (80% to 90%).[15] In one study, most patients were pacemaker dependent after the

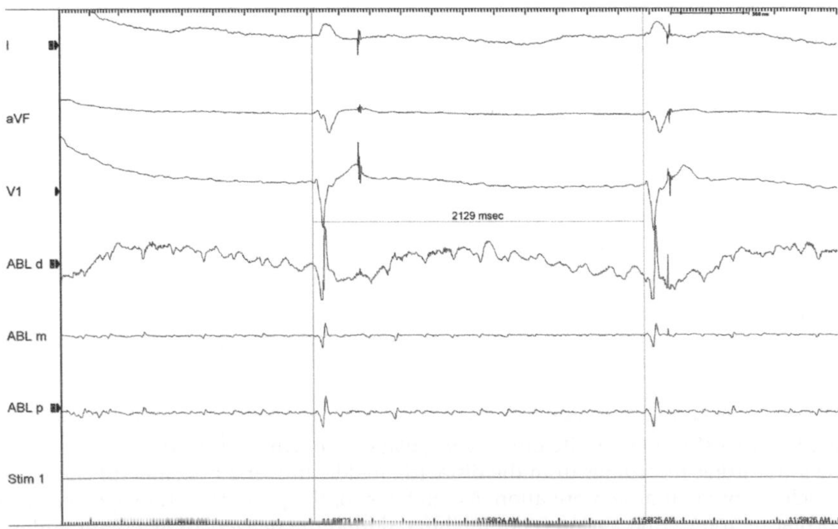

Fig. 3. Complete heart block with a junctional escape rhythm at 28 beats/min is achieved after the first ablation lesion. Abbreviations and format are the same as in **Fig. 1**.

Table 1
"Ablate and pace" outcomes

Success rate of AVJ ablation (including redo procedures)	98%–100%[13–15]
Need for left-sided ablation	~7%[16]
Recurrence rate after acute procedural success	~3%[16]
Death within 30 d of procedure	0.27%[16]
Lead failure	0.23%[16]
Presence of stable escape rhythm	35%–98%[15,17–21]

procedure,[15] as defined by absence of an escape rhythm greater than 40 beats/min. A more recent published series[18] of 96 patients looked at the presence of escape rhythms higher than 30 beats/min and found that 79% of patients had an escape rhythm immediately after ablation. However, by 1 year of follow-up nearly one-third of patients (28%) had a labile escape rhythm, defined as absence of an escape rhythm at any 1 of the 5 postablation follow-up time points. Other published series report the presence of escape rhythms in 35% to 98% of patients,[17,19–21] and it seems reasonable that an escape rhythm should be aimed for and achievable in at least 70% to 80% of patients. The use of unipolar His electrograms has been proposed to help map the proximal His bundle (QS electrograms) versus the more distal His bundle (RS electrograms), but this approach did not result in any significant improvement in the escape rhythm after ablation, although it did reduce the number of lesions required to achieve block, perhaps by better mapping the His bundle before it becomes protected by the fibrous sheath.[22]

The evidence documenting the clinical results of AVJ ablation has significant limitations, and is based on numerous small, heterogeneous, and mostly nonrandomized retrospective studies. There is no large, randomized controlled trial comparing AVJ ablation with other strategies. A recent meta-analysis and systematic review of the literature on AVJ ablation for AF addressed the efficacy and effectiveness of the procedure compared with pharmacotherapy, as well as its safety.[16] The investigators identified 5 randomized controlled trials and prospective cohorts with contemporaneous controls comparing AVN ablation and RV-only pacing versus pharmacotherapy, totaling 314 patients, of whom 161 underwent AVN ablation and 153 received pharmacotherapy, followed for a mean of 10 months. There were small but insignificant differences in mortality, changes in exercise tolerance testing, and ejection fraction (EF), although statistically significant improvements were found in quality of life measures and specific symptoms, such as palpitations, exertional dyspnea, or "easy fatigue." There were 5 deaths in each group, and all deaths in the AVN ablation group occurred more than 1 month after the AVN ablation. Thus, overall mortality was similar after AVN ablation when compared with pharmacotherapy. In the 2 studies that included patients with an abnormal EF (weighted mean EF 44% ± 4%), there was a small increase in EF, which was statistically significant (+4%, 95% confidence interval [CI] 3.1–4.9). In one retrospective analysis[15] that included 350 patients followed for 36 ± 26 months, there was also no statistically significant mortality difference between AVN ablation and pharmacotherapy. Some observational studies reporting exercise duration (5 studies, 191 patients) suggest a slight improvement (1.19 minutes, 95% CI 0.81–1.60) following AVN ablation, but there were different protocols used for exercise. Five observational studies reporting changes in EF in patients with an EF less than 45% included 196 patients and showed a significant increase in EF following AVN ablation (+7.44%, 95% CI 5.4–9.5). There was significant change in EF in 5 other observational studies in 272 patients with an EF greater than 45%.

In terms of procedural safety, the incidence of sudden cardiac death was 2.1% (range 0%–11.3%) in 3756 patients from 37 studies, followed for a weighted mean of 26.5 months. This result compares favorably with the general reported incidence of sudden cardiac death in patients with AF receiving pharmacotherapy (3.1%–3.8% in the RACE and AFFIRM trials[23,24]). The need for a left-sided approach after a failed right-sided ablation was reported in 6.9% of cases, and the incidence of recurrence of AV conduction requiring redo procedures was 2.9%. The reported incidence of malignant arrhythmias (sustained ventricular tachycardia or ventricular fibrillation within 30 days of the procedure) was 0.57%. Other reported procedure-related morbidities included lead failure (0.23%), stroke (0.19%), and hematoma (0.7%), and death within 30 days of AVN ablation occurred in 0.27%. There were a total of 12 deaths, of which 5 were reported in one study where the postprocedure pacing rate was lower than 70 beats/min. Most studies reported a mandated postablation pacing rate of at least 70 or 80 beats/min for at least 7 days. Other complications, including infection, pleural effusion, pericarditis, pseudoaneurysm, RV perforation, and pneumothorax, occurred in 1.1% of cases.

The investigators of this systematic review conclude that "AVN ablation (with RV-only pacing) is a safe intervention that improves symptoms and quality of life in patients with drug-refractory AF" and that, "compared with pharmacotherapy alone, AVN ablation may be of particular benefit to patients with baseline reduced systolic function in regards to echocardiographic improvement, although the clinical impact" is uncertain.

ALTERNATIVE TO AVJ ABLATION: AVN MODIFICATION

In an attempt to control ventricular rates during AF while avoiding the need for a permanent pacemaker, AVJ modification has been suggested.[25] Although there are fewer advantages to AV nodal modification compared with complete AV node ablation now that CRT is available to minimize the adverse consequences of postablation pacing, there is evidence that it is more cost effective than AVJ ablation and implantation of a pacemaker.[26] This procedure consists of modifying the compact AV node or the atrial inputs to the node that have the shortest refractory periods and thus can conduct at the fastest rates, without causing complete AV block. The anatomic target is the area considered the residence of the slow AV nodal pathway and/or posterior atrionodal input, between the coronary sinus ostium and the tricuspid annulus. Ablation energy is delivered and ventricular rate control is assessed during and after each lesion, often while the patient is being infused with isoproterenol. It has been suggested that RF modification of the AVJ can be expected to be more effective, safe, and expeditious in patients with a bimodal distribution pattern of their RR intervals during chronic AF, perhaps as a reflection of dual-pathway AV node physiology and significant role of the slow pathway in AV conduction in this subset of patients.[27,28] In practical terms, when adequate rate control was attempted the risk of complete AV block or need for a pacemaker was 8% to 21%.[25,27] Therefore, the procedure should only be performed in a patient who is either prepared for, or already has, a pacemaker.

DEVICE IMPLANTATION: TIMING, TECHNIQUE, TYPE OF DEVICE

The permanent pacemaker is probably best implanted before the AVJ ablation. Given the very high success rate (98%–100%[13–15]) in achieving complete AV block and the low recurrence rate (~3%) after acute procedural success, delaying the pacemaker implantation is not justified. Additional reassurance regarding ventricular lead stability is gained by implanting the pacing system several days to weeks before AVJ ablation. However, given the low rate of ventricular lead dislodgement or perforation, the implant is frequently done in the same session, just before the ablation. Ablating the AVJ with a temporary pacing wire in place and implanting the pacemaker immediately afterward can also be done; this approach avoids the risk of pocket hematoma if heparin administration becomes necessary for left-sided ablation. An adequate pacing threshold and electrode stability during ablation and during patient transfer and transportation should be ensured.

When the patient is expected to stay in AF, a single RV lead can be implanted. For patients with paroxysmal AF, a dual-chamber system is standard so as to avoid AV dyssynchrony. Ablation is performed with careful catheter maneuvering to avoid dislodging the recently implanted leads. The permanent or temporary pacemaker used for backup during ablation should be set in VVI mode at 30 to 40 beats/min, to allow identification of AV block when it is achieved. The pacemaker can be programmed in VOO mode if inhibition of pacing is noted during ablation.

In patients with depressed left ventricular ejection fraction (LVEF) who may qualify for an implantable cardioverter-defibrillator (ICD) under the current guidelines, a judgment needs to be made as to whether their EF is likely to recover after AVJ ablation and rate control, depending on the likelihood that the cardiomyopathy is totally or partially tachycardia mediated. A biventricular pacemaker may be a good initial option, although it may later require upgrade to an ICD if the LVEF does not improve. These probabilities and the additional risk related to an upgrade procedure need to be integrated into the individualized decision analysis and discussed with the patient.

SUDDEN DEATH FOLLOWING AVJ ABLATION

There has been a persistent concern related to the incidence of sudden death early after AVJ ablation. Cases of early postprocedure sudden death were reported in 5.1% of patients undergoing direct-current (DC) fulguration of the AV node.[29] In this series of 136 patients, there were 9 incidents of ventricular fibrillation or polymorphic ventricular tachycardia (2 were nonfatal). An analysis of the arrhythmic episodes and the QT intervals led to the hypothesis that prolonged QTc interval and bradycardia-dependent QT prolongation played an important role, leading to onset of torsades de pointes. The investigators noted, however, that "the patients who died were gravely ill and had other potential contributing or causative factors: two were being considered for cardiac transplantation, three were hypotensive on entry to the laboratory, two required intravenous inotropic support, and one required intra-aortic balloon counterpulsation."

Based on these findings, the investigators suggested that "the postablation pacing rate should be adequate to suppress ventricular ectopic activity, shorten the QT interval, and maximize cardiac output. The rate of the pacemaker may need to be set at a faster rate than usual, possibly at more than 80 beats/min." This practice has continued to the present day, and most texts recommend pacing faster than 80 to 90 beats/min for at least 1 week to 1 month, then decreasing the rate gradually during follow-up. Possibly validating this view, it is worth noting that in the recent systematic review of the literature,[16] 5 of 12 procedure-related deaths occurred in patients with postablation pacing rates of less than 70 beats/min. It has been suggested that it may also be reasonable to monitor patients, at least those deemed at high risk, for the first 48 hours. A comparison between DC and RF ablation showed no sudden deaths in the RF group compared with 5.1% in the DC group (similar to prior reported rate).[30] It was assumed that DC ablation was producing more extensive damage not only to the AV node but also to the surrounding myocardium, which might play a role in its higher risk of sudden death. However, in 3 patients who died suddenly in the prior series and had a pathologic examination performed, no myocardial damage was reported, at least in the high septum.[29] Subsequent reports also suggested a role for bradycardia and/or pacing-dependent repolarization abnormalities in patients who were previously tachycardic.[31–33] Another possible mechanism for early sudden death is pacemaker failure in the absence of an escape rhythm.

As already discussed, the incidence of sudden cardiac death of 2.1% compares favorably with the general reported incidence of sudden cardiac death in patients with AF receiving pharmacotherapy.[16] Many patients undergoing AVJ ablation have significant comorbidities, including left ventricular systolic dysfunction and congestive heart failure, which place the patients at increased risk for sudden death, thus making it difficult to assess the exact role played by the AVJ ablation. It is unclear which patients are at high risk, but it appears that structural heart disease, left ventricular systolic dysfunction (before the standard use of ICDs for primary prophylaxis in these patients), and coronary artery disease may be risk factors.[16,34,35]

ROLE OF CRT AFTER AVJ ABLATION

The potential detrimental effects of chronic RV pacing are a concern in patients managed with the "ablate and pace" strategy. Several studies have suggested that a high percentage of RV pacing may result in higher incidence of hospitalizations or death due to heart failure.[36,37] Acute or chronic apical RV pacing causes ventricular dyssynchrony and may result in left ventricular dysfunction,[38,39] which can be particularly detrimental in patients who have preexisting systolic dysfunction. Various studies showed inconsistent effects of the RV "ablate and pace" strategy on the LVEF, which can either decrease, increase, or stay unchanged. However, a recent systematic review of the literature[16] suggests that, overall, LVEF may increase, particularly in patients with baseline EF of less than 45%, as already presented. The LVEF outcome is likely to be the result of the interplay and relative contributions of resolution of tachycardia-mediated cardiomyopathy component, the effects of RV-pacing–induced dyssynchrony, and the underlying structural heart disease. Several studies have compared biventricular with RV pacing after AVJ ablation.[13,40–43] The PAVE trial[41] randomized 184 patients undergoing AVJ ablation for AF to either RV pacing or CRT. There were statistically significant improvements noted in the 6-minute walk and LVEF at 6 months. The Ablate and Pace in Atrial Fibrillation (APAF) trial[13] randomized 186 patients after AVJ ablation and CRT device implantation to either optimized echo-guided CRT or RV apical pacing, and followed them for a median of 20 months. Total mortality was not significantly different between the 2 groups, but the primary composite end point of death from heart failure, hospitalization due to heart failure, or worsening heart failure was significantly better in the "optimized CRT" group (11% vs 26%), driven by the soft end points. The advantage of optimized CRT was consistent in subgroups with EF up to 35% and higher than 35%, native QRS 120 ms and greater or less than 120 ms, New York Heart Association (NYHA) Class III or higher and lower than Class III. The studies available at this point suggest that CRT may be better than RV pacing after AVJ ablation for permanent AF, at least in reducing symptoms of heart failure, but future large trials are needed to investigate the effect on mortality and in patients with preserved systolic function. The most recent (2008) applicable guidelines[44] recommend CRT devices for the following indications:

- Class IIa
  - For patients with LVEF up to 35% with NYHA Class III or ambulatory Class IV symptoms who are receiving optimal recommended medical therapy and

who have frequent dependence on ventricular pacing, CRT is reasonable (level of evidence: C)

- Class IIb
  - For patients with LVEF up to 35% with NYHA Class I or II symptoms who are receiving optimal recommended medical therapy and who are undergoing implantation of a permanent pacemaker and/or ICD with anticipated frequent ventricular pacing, CRT may be considered (level of evidence: C)

In addition, if symptoms of heart failure persist or deterioration in LVEF occurs after AVJ ablation and RV pacing, upgrading to CRT becomes a stronger recommendation, and should be strongly considered.

ROLE OF AVJ ABLATION AFTER CRT

AF is the most common reason for interruption of CRT.[45] If ventricular rates are not maintained below the pacing rates, the rate of resynchronized beats drops, frequently to a rate lower than what is thought to be optimal (>95%). Even occasional conducted beats result in dyssynchronous activation of the ventricles and may cancel the potential benefit of resynchronized beats. In patients with AF, the percentage of biventricular (BIV)-paced beats is an overestimate, as many beats are counted as BIV-paced but are actually pseudofused.[46] AF has been associated with a higher percentage of nonresponders to CRT and all-cause mortality.[47] In the same systematic review of the literature, the presence of AF was also associated with less improvement in quality-of-life score, 6-minute walk distance, and left ventricular end-systolic volume, but not LVEF. Among patients with AF, AVN ablation appeared favorable, with a lower risk of clinical nonresponse and a reduced risk of death.[47] A recent large series found that AF with uncontrolled ventricular rates occurs in a third of patients with CRT devices, and is associated with suboptimal CRT (<95% BIV-paced beats), heart-failure hospitalizations, and death.[48] Data from a registry of 1285 patients[49] suggested that patients with AF and CRT who underwent AVJ ablation had improved symptomatic relief and mortality when compared with patients treated only with pharmacotherapy. Patients with AF in this registry derived the same benefit from CRT as patients in sinus rhythm, as long as they were BIV-paced more than 85% of the beats.

Thus, observational studies suggest that ablating the AVJ in patients with heart failure and CRT improves their outcomes, presumably by improving the percentage of resynchronized beats, although it is not clear how much of the clinical improvement is due to eliminating some of the rapid and/or irregular ventricular rates. Large randomized trials are not available, but it is reasonable to consider AVJ ablation in patients with AF and symptoms of refractory heart failure despite maximal medical therapy, and who have suboptimal CRT (percentage of BIV-paced beats <85%–95%).[50]

SUMMARY

Ablation of the AVJ has been performed for more than 3 decades. Despite the development of newer drugs and procedures to improve rhythm control, there is still a place for AVJ ablation in the management of selected patients with AF who are refractory to medical therapy, to improve quality of life, prevent ventricular dysfunction, and to optimize CRT. While enthusiasm for its use should be tempered by the potential for pacemaker dependence, AVJ ablation can provide dramatic symptomatic relief in appropriately selected patients and potentially improve ventricular function. It is likely that there is a large number of unrecognized patients with ventricular dysfunction that is at least partially tachycardia-mediated cardiomyopathy, or who are not deriving the full benefits of CRT because of AF with inadequate rate control, who might benefit from an "ablate and pace" strategy. Large randomized trials are needed to further clarify the role of this therapy. Individually tailored decision making is essential, as are genuine attempts to maximize medical therapy and careful consideration of alternatives such as pulmonary vein isolation.

REFERENCES

1. Van Gelder IC, Groenveld HF, Crijns HJ, et al. Lenient versus strict rate control in patients with atrial fibrillation. N Engl J Med 2010;362:1363.
2. Harrison L, Gallagher JJ, Kasell J, et al. Cryosurgical ablation of the A-V node-His bundle: a new method for producing A-V block. Circulation 1977;55:463.
3. Klein GJ, Sealy WC, Pritchett EL, et al. Cryosurgical ablation of the atrioventricular node-His bundle: long-term follow-up and properties of the junctional pacemaker. Circulation 1980;61:8.
4. Sealy WC, Gallagher JJ, Kasell J. His bundle interruption for control of inappropriate ventricular responses to atrial arrhythmias. Ann Thorac Surg 1981;32:429.
5. Gallagher JJ, Svenson RH, Kasell JH, et al. Catheter technique for closed-chest ablation of the atrioventricular conduction system. N Engl J Med 1982;306:194.
6. Gonzalez R, Scheinman M, Margaretten W, et al. Closed-chest electrode-catheter technique for His

bundle ablation in dogs. Am J Physiol 1981;241: H283.

7. Scheinman MM, Morady F, Hess DS, et al. Catheter-induced ablation of the atrioventricular junction to control refractory supraventricular arrhythmias. JAMA 1982;248:851.
8. Huang SK, Bharati S, Graham AR, et al. Closed chest catheter desiccation of the atrioventricular junction using radiofrequency energy—a new method of catheter ablation. J Am Coll Cardiol 1987;9:349.
9. Zivin A, Knight BP, Souza J, et al. Predictors of cross-over to a left ventricular approach for atrioventricular junction ablation. Am J Cardiol 1997;80:1611.
10. Sousa J, el-Atassi R, Rosenheck S, et al. Radiofrequency catheter ablation of the atrioventricular junction from the left ventricle. Circulation 1991;84:567.
11. Cuello C, Huang SK, Wagshal AB, et al. Radiofrequency catheter ablation of the atrioventricular junction by a supravalvular noncoronary aortic cusp approach. Pacing Clin Electrophysiol 1994;17:1182.
12. Issa ZF. An approach to ablate and pace: AV junction ablation and pacemaker implantation performed concurrently from the same venous access site. Pacing Clin Electrophysiol 2007;30:1116.
13. Brignole M, Botto G, Mont L, et al. Cardiac resynchronization therapy in patients undergoing atrioventricular junction ablation for permanent atrial fibrillation: a randomized trial. Eur Heart J 2011;32:2420.
14. Kay GN, Ellenbogen KA, Giudici M, et al. The Ablate and Pace Trial: a prospective study of catheter ablation of the AV conduction system and permanent pacemaker implantation for treatment of atrial fibrillation. APT Investigators. J Interv Card Electrophysiol 1998;2:121.
15. Ozcan C, Jahangir A, Friedman PA, et al. Long-term survival after ablation of the atrioventricular node and implantation of a permanent pacemaker in patients with atrial fibrillation. N Engl J Med 2001; 344:1043.
16. Chatterjee NA, Upadhyay GA, Ellenbogen KA, et al. Atrioventricular nodal ablation in atrial fibrillation: a meta-analysis and systematic review. Circ Arrhythm Electrophysiol 2011;5:68.
17. Alison JF, Yeung-Lai-Wah JA, Schulzer M, et al. Characterization of junctional rhythm after atrioventricular node ablation. Circulation 1995;91:84.
18. Arora R, Spatz E, Vijayaraman P, et al. Just how stable are escape rhythms after atrioventricular junction ablation? Pacing Clin Electrophysiol 2010;33:939.
19. Curtis AB, Kutalek SP, Prior M, et al. Prevalence and characteristics of escape rhythms after radiofrequency ablation of the atrioventricular junction: results from the registry for AV junction ablation and pacing in atrial fibrillation. Ablate and Pace Trial Investigators. Am Heart J 2000;139:122.
20. Piot O, Sebag C, Lavergne T, et al. Initial and long-term evaluation of escape rhythm after radiofrequency ablation of the AV junction in 50 patients. Pacing Clin Electrophysiol 1988;19:1996.
21. Strohmer B, Hwang C, Peter CT, et al. Selective atrionodal input ablation for induction of proximal complete heart block with stable junctional escape rhythm in patients with uncontrolled atrial fibrillation. J Interv Card Electrophysiol 2003;8:49.
22. Ito S, Tada H, Naito S, et al. Randomized comparison of bipolar vs unipolar plus bipolar recordings during atrioventricular junction ablation: importance and efficacy of unipolar recording. Circ J 2007;71:874.
23. Hagens VE, Rienstra M, Van Veldhuisen DJ, et al. Determinants of sudden cardiac death in patients with persistent atrial fibrillation in the rate control versus electrical cardioversion (RACE) study. Am J Cardiol 2006;98:929.
24. Steinberg JS, Sadaniantz A, Kron J, et al. Analysis of cause-specific mortality in the Atrial Fibrillation Follow-up Investigation of Rhythm Management (AFFIRM) study. Circulation 2004;109:1973.
25. Williamson BD, Man KC, Daoud E, et al. Radiofrequency catheter modification of atrioventricular conduction to control the ventricular rate during atrial fibrillation. N Engl J Med 1994;331:910.
26. Knight BP, Weiss R, Bahu M, et al. Cost comparison of radiofrequency modification and ablation of the atrioventricular junction in patients with chronic atrial fibrillation. Circulation 1997;96:1532.
27. Rokas S, Gaitanidou S, Chatzidou S, et al. Atrioventricular node modification in patients with chronic atrial fibrillation: role of morphology of RR interval variation. Circulation 2001;103:2942.
28. Tebbenjohanns J, Schumacher B, Korte T, et al. Bimodal RR interval distribution in chronic atrial fibrillation: impact of dual atrioventricular nodal physiology on long-term rate control after catheter ablation of the posterior atrionodal input. J Cardiovasc Electrophysiol 2000;11:497.
29. Evans GT Jr, Scheinman MM, Bardy G, et al. Predictors of in-hospital mortality after DC catheter ablation of atrioventricular junction. Results of a prospective, international, multicenter study. Circulation 1991;84: 1924.
30. Olgin JE, Scheinman MM. Comparison of high energy direct current and radiofrequency catheter ablation of the atrioventricular junction. J Am Coll Cardiol 1993;21:557.
31. Brandt RR, Shen WK. Bradycardia-induced polymorphic ventricular tachycardia after atrioventricular junction ablation for sinus tachycardia-induced cardiomyopathy. J Cardiovasc Electrophysiol 1995; 6:630.
32. Geelen P, Brugada J, Andries E, et al. Ventricular fibrillation and sudden death after radiofrequency catheter ablation of the atrioventricular junction. Pacing Clin Electrophysiol 1997;20:343.

33. Peters RH, Wever EF, Hauer RN, et al. Bradycardia dependent QT prolongation and ventricular fibrillation following catheter ablation of the atrioventricular junction with radiofrequency energy. Pacing Clin Electrophysiol 1994;17:108.
34. Gasparini M, Mantica M, Brignole M, et al. Long-term follow-up after atrioventricular nodal ablation and pacing: low incidence of sudden cardiac death. Pacing Clin Electrophysiol 2000;23:1925.
35. Ozcan C, Jahangir A, Friedman PA, et al. Sudden death after radiofrequency ablation of the atrioventricular node in patients with atrial fibrillation. J Am Coll Cardiol 2002;40:105.
36. Sweeney MO, Hellkamp AS, Ellenbogen KA, et al. Adverse effect of ventricular pacing on heart failure and atrial fibrillation among patients with normal baseline QRS duration in a clinical trial of pacemaker therapy for sinus node dysfunction. Circulation 2003;107:2932.
37. Wilkoff BL, Cook JR, Epstein AE, et al. Dual-chamber pacing or ventricular backup pacing in patients with an implantable defibrillator: the Dual Chamber and VVI Implantable Defibrillator (DAVID) Trial. JAMA 2002;288:3115.
38. Lupi G, Sassone B, Badano L, et al. Effects of right ventricular pacing on intra-left ventricular electromechanical activation in patients with native narrow QRS. Am J Cardiol 2006;98:219.
39. Tops LF, Schalij MJ, Holman ER, et al. Right ventricular pacing can induce ventricular dyssynchrony in patients with atrial fibrillation after atrioventricular node ablation. J Am Coll Cardiol 2006;48:1642.
40. Brignole M, Gammage M, Puggioni E, et al. Comparative assessment of right, left, and biventricular pacing in patients with permanent atrial fibrillation. Eur Heart J 2005;26:712.
41. Doshi RN, Daoud EG, Fellows C, et al. Left ventricular-based cardiac stimulation post AV nodal ablation evaluation (the PAVE study). J Cardiovasc Electrophysiol 2005;16:1160.
42. Leclercq C, Walker S, Linde C, et al. Comparative effects of permanent biventricular and right-univentricular pacing in heart failure patients with chronic atrial fibrillation. Eur Heart J 2002;23:1780.
43. Orlov MV, Gardin JM, Slawsky M, et al. Biventricular pacing improves cardiac function and prevents further left atrial remodeling in patients with symptomatic atrial fibrillation after atrioventricular node ablation. Am Heart J 2010;159:264.
44. Epstein AE, DiMarco JP, Ellenbogen KA, et al. ACC/AHA/HRS 2008 Guidelines for Device-Based Therapy of Cardiac Rhythm Abnormalities: a report of the American College of Cardiology/American Heart Association Task Force on Practice Guidelines (Writing Committee to Revise the ACC/AHA/NASPE 2002 Guideline Update for Implantation of Cardiac Pacemakers and Antiarrhythmia Devices) developed in collaboration with the American Association for Thoracic Surgery and Society of Thoracic Surgeons. J Am Coll Cardiol 2008;51:e1.
45. Knight BP, Desai A, Coman J, et al. Long-term retention of cardiac resynchronization therapy. J Am Coll Cardiol 2004;44:72.
46. Kamath GS, Cotiga D, Koneru JN, et al. The utility of 12-lead Holter monitoring in patients with permanent atrial fibrillation for the identification of nonresponders after cardiac resynchronization therapy. J Am Coll Cardiol 2009;53:1050.
47. Wilton SB, Leung AA, Ghali WA, et al. Outcomes of cardiac resynchronization therapy in patients with versus those without atrial fibrillation: a systematic review and meta-analysis. Heart Rhythm 2011;8:1088.
48. Boriani G, Gasparini M, Landolina M, et al. Incidence and clinical relevance of uncontrolled ventricular rate during atrial fibrillation in heart failure patients treated with cardiac resynchronization therapy. Eur J Heart Fail 2011;13:868.
49. Gasparini M, Auricchio A, Metra M, et al. Long-term survival in patients undergoing cardiac resynchronization therapy: the importance of performing atrio-ventricular junction ablation in patients with permanent atrial fibrillation. Eur Heart J 2008;29:1644.
50. Kaszala K, Ellenbogen KA. Role of cardiac resynchronization therapy and atrioventricular junction ablation in patients with permanent atrial fibrillation. Eur Heart J 2011;32:2344.

Totally Thoracoscopic Surgical Ablation or Catheter Ablation of Atrial Fibrillation

A Systematic Review and Preliminary Meta-Analysis

James R. Edgerton, MD, FHRS[a,b,*], Lindsey M. Philpot, MPH[c], Brandi Falley, MS[c], Sunni A. Barnes, PhD[c]

KEYWORDS

• Atrial fibrillation • Lone surgical ablation • Systematic review • Freedom from atrial fibrillation • Normal sinus rhythm • Pulmonary vein isolation • Dallas Lesion Set • Cox Maze

KEY POINTS

- When atrial fibrillation (AF) patients are selected for an ablative procedure, it is unclear whether they should have a catheter approach or a surgical approach.
- Across all categories of AF, surgical ablation has a better success rate than does catheter ablation (CA).
- For paroxysmal AF (PAF), the results of CA approach those of surgical ablation and have less morbidity. Therefore, patients with PAF planning to have an ablative procedure should be initially treated with CA.
- For patients with persistent AF, the data are insufficient to recommend one approach over the other. The ablative approach to these patients should be individualized and based on their comorbid conditions, with poorer-risk patients having surgical ablation.
- For long-standing persistent (LSP) AF, the results of surgery are clearly superior to those of CA. Therefore, patients with LSP AF planning to have an ablative procedure should be initially treated with minimal-access surgical ablation.

INTRODUCTION

Atrial fibrillation (AF) is defined as supraventricular tachyarrhythmia characterized by the uncoordinated activation and deterioration of mechanical function of the atria.[1] As the most common cardiac arrhythmia encountered in clinical practice, the estimated prevalence of AF is 0.4% to 1% in the general population.[2] Management of AF may include pharmacologically achieved rate control, mechanistic prevention of thromboembolism, and the correction of the rhythm abnormality through surgical or catheter-based approaches.[1]

Commercial disclosure: Dr Edgerton is a paid consultant for AtriCure, Inc.

[a] The Heart Hospital, Baylor Regional Medical Center at Plano, 4716 Allied Boulevard, Pavilion Two, Suite 310, Plano, TX 75093, USA; [b] Cardiopulmonary Research Science and Technology Institute, 7777 Forest Lane, Suite C-742, Dallas, TX 75230, USA; [c] Institute for Health Care Research and Improvement, Baylor Health Care System, 8080 North Central Expressway, Suite 500, Dallas, TX 75206, USA

* Corresponding author. The Heart Hospital, Baylor Regional Medical Center at Plano, 4716 Allied Boulevard, Pavilion Two, Suite 310, Plano, TX 75093.

E-mail address: edgertonjr@aol.com

Card Electrophysiol Clin 4 (2012) 413–423
http://dx.doi.org/10.1016/j.ccep.2012.05.001

Ablation of AF began with the introduction of the Maze procedure by Cox and colleagues.[3] Although attended by a high success rate,[4] the operation required sternotomy access and arrest of the heart on cardiopulmonary bypass. The associated morbidities and complex nature of the procedure resulted in a relatively low adoption rate.[4,5] Although the Cox Maze III is still widely performed for AF concomitant to another cardiac surgical procedure, it is rarely performed as a stand-alone procedure for AF.[6] For the treatment of stand-alone AF, surgery has largely been supplanted by ever-improving catheter-based techniques. However, catheter ablation (CA) is known to cause endocardial trauma, therapeutic thrombus, and high reablation rates because of limited efficacy.[7] More recently, the development of enabling technology has allowed surgical ablation to be performed on the beating heart with minimal-access techniques. This approach eliminates much of the morbidity associated with the original cut-and-sew Cox Maze III procedure. These minimally invasive surgical techniques hold the promise of higher potential curative benefits than those of CA for stand-alone AF but have been only minimally discussed in the academic literature. Therefore, this article describes the available publications from 2009 to 2011 of surgical intervention for stand-alone AF and provides an early depiction of summative results via preliminary meta-analysis. Results are then compared with published meta-analyses of CA success rates, and treatment recommendations are drawn.

METHODS

Search Strategy

A comprehensive literature search was performed using the United States National Library of Medicine and the National Institutes of Health PubMed engine. The search criteria included all English-language observational studies of human subjects published from January 1, 2009 to September 10, 2011, using the following MeSH terms: ("surgical procedures, operative"[MeSH Terms] OR ("surgical"[All Fields] AND "procedures"[All Fields] AND "operative"[All Fields]) OR "operative surgical procedures"[All Fields] OR "surgical"[All Fields]) AND ablation[All Fields] AND ("atrial fibrillation"[MeSH Terms] OR ("atrial"[All Fields] AND "fibrillation"[All Fields]) OR "atrial fibrillation"[All Fields]).

All studies were identified by 2 independent reviewers (L.P. and B.F.) to meet the inclusion criteria of longitudinal evaluation of freedom from AF, atrial tachycardia (AT), or atrial flutter (Aflutter) following stand-alone ablative surgery with at least 3 months of follow-up data. Also included were studies that had a combination of patients receiving concomitant ablative surgery and stand-alone ablative surgery, but for which the results of the stand-alone-ablative group could be assuredly differentiated. Studies were excluded if information was published as an abstract, review, or case report; if the focus of the publication was description of a surgical technique; or if the primary outcome of interest was different from freedom from AF or return to normal sinus rhythm (NSR). All remaining articles were subject to detailed review by 3 individuals (L.P., B.F., J.R.E.).

Data Analysis

The following data elements were taken from each of the articles: total size of the study population, subset who received stand-alone ablative surgery (if applicable), mean age of study population, length of follow-up time in months, surgical technique used, primary outcome of interest, outcome assessment method, percentage of patients who had previously undergone CA, mean left atrial size, and ejection fraction (EF), if available. The research team's surgical expert (J.R.E.) classified surgical techniques (lesion set) into groups. Type of AF was assigned according to the terminology recommended in the 'Heart Rhythm Society (HRS)/European Heart Rhythm Association (EHRA)/European Cardiac Arrhythmia Society (ECAS) Expert Consensus Statement on Catheter and Surgical Ablation of Atrial Fibrillation,' in which paroxysmal AF is referred to as recurrent AF that terminates spontaneously within 7 days, persistent AF as AF sustained longer than 7 days or lasting less than 7 days but requiring either pharmacologic or electrical cardioversion, and long-standing persistent (LSP) AF as continuous AF of duration longer than 1 year.

The primary outcome was postoperative freedom from AF, AT, and Aflutter. All analyses were performed by stratifying included studies based on the described primary outcome: freedom from AF or return to NSR according to the definitions provided within each article. Estimates and pooled outcomes with 95% confidence intervals (CI) were calculated using fixed-effects models. Statistical heterogeneity between studies was tested with the Cochrane test. The I^2 statistic was also examined, and I^2 values greater than 50% were considered to signify heterogeneity between studies. Publication bias was assessed via funnel plots. In a funnel plot, larger studies are expected to be near the average and small studies to be spread on both sides of the average. Variation from this assumption can indicate publication bias, and this is seen in a funnel plot that shows an asymmetric shape. Statistical analyses were performed with R (version 2.13.1).

RESULTS

A total of 1364 published articles were initially identified by MeSH key words and the identified time period (**Fig. 1**). Exclusion of publications printed in languages other than English, as well as of nonhuman populations, decreased the total to 1185 articles. Publication on catheter intervention eliminated an additional 837 articles, and other types of studies excluded a further 335. Following all of the listed inclusion criteria, there were 13 published observational studies that included longitudinal follow-up of patients who underwent stand-alone ablative surgery for AF.

In total, the 13 included articles allowed for a total study population of 699 patients (**Table 1**). The mean age of study participants ranged from 54.2 to 65 years, with one study providing a median age of 56 years. Reported duration of follow-up data ranged from 3 to 60 months. Six studies described freedom from AF as the primary end point, and 7 designated return to NSR as the primary end point (see **Table 1**). All included studies measured recurrence of AF or return to NSR through 24-hour Holter monitoring, electrocardiogram (ECG), AF monitor device, or a combination of the 3 (see **Table 1**).

Surgical technique varied among the studies: 8 used pulmonary vein isolation (PVI), 2 used PVI with the Dallas Lesion Set,[8] and 3 performed a version of the Cox Maze procedure (**Table 2**). Reports of previous CA-based therapy varied greatly among studies. Of the studies that included this information, the percentage of patients who had received previous CA for AF ranged from 4.2% to 100%. The reported means of left atrial size ranged from 41.2 to 52.0 mm.

In-Depth Evidence Review of Stand-Alone Surgical Ablation for AF

After detailed review using the methodology described, 13 articles were included in this systematic review. An overview of each article, highlighting the main points, is given here. Descriptive characteristics of the included studies are presented in **Tables 1** and **2**.

In a study by Bagge and colleagues,[9] patients with symptomatic AF were referred for thoracoscopic off-pump epicardial PVI and ganglionated plexi ablation using radiofrequency (RF) energy. All 43 patients included in the study had an EF greater than 50%, a mean age of 57.1 years, and

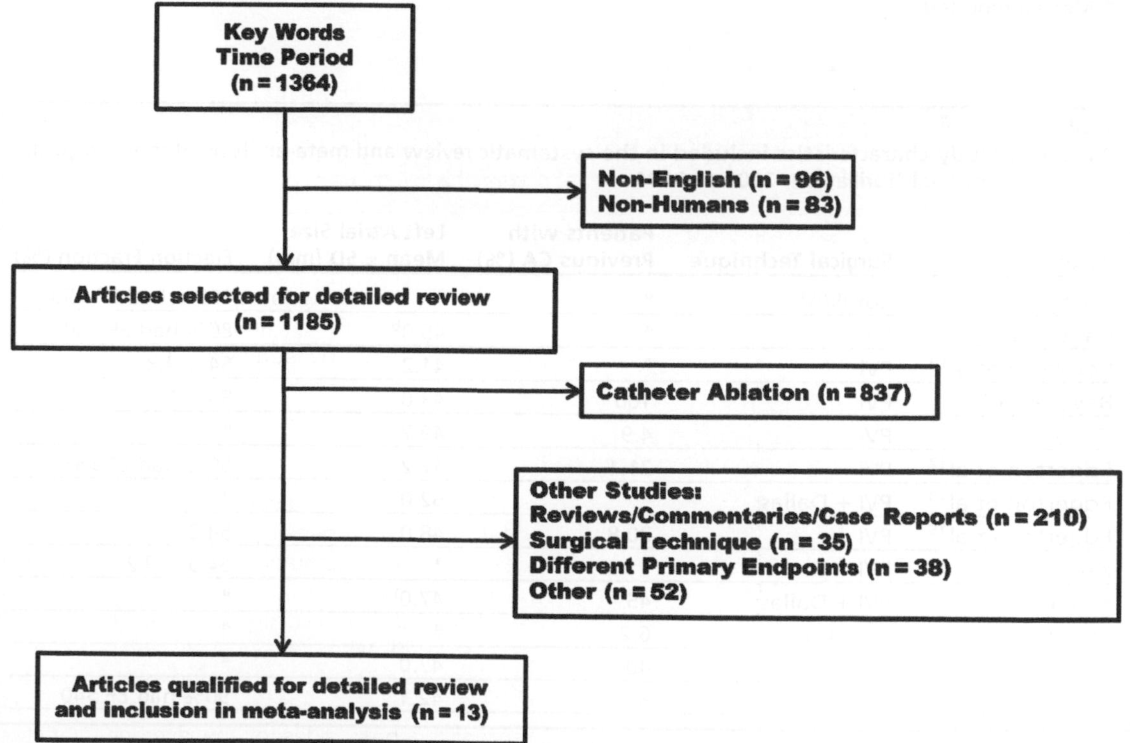

Fig. 1. Schematic breakdown of studies included within the systematic review and meta-analysis of stand-alone surgical ablation for atrial fibrillation (AF), 2009 to 2011.

Table 1
Descriptive characteristics of studies included in the systematic review and meta-analysis of lone surgical ablation for atrial fibrillation, 2009 to 2011

Authors[Ref.]	Total (N)	Included (n)	Age (Mean ± SD)	Follow-Up (Months, Minimum[a])	Outcome	Assessment Method
Albåge et al[17]	43	6	54.2	12	NSR	ECG + Holter
Bagge et al[9]	43	33	57.1	12	Freedom from AF	Holter
Beukema et al[10]	33	33	59.4 ± 8.9	3	NSR	ECG + AF alarm
Beyer et al[11]	100	100	65 ± 11	3	NSR	Holter
Cui et al[7]	80	49	57.6 ± 10	12	NSR	ECG + Holter + UCG
Edgerton et al[12]	114	114	59.5 ± 10	6	NSR	ECG + AF monitor
Edgerton et al[13]	30	30	58 ± 9	6	Freedom from AF	ECG + AF monitor
Edgerton et al[15]	52	52	60.3	12	NSR	ECG + Holter
Kron et al[14]	50	37	63.4 ± 9.3	12	NSR	ECG + AF monitor
Krul et al[18]	31	22	57	12	Freedom from AF	ECG + Holter
Stulak et al[19]	289	93	56[a]	60	Freedom from AF	ECG + Holter
Weimar et al[20]	100	100	56 ± 10	24	Freedom from AF	ECG + Holter
Yilmaz et al[16]	30	30	55.6 ± 8.6	3	Freedom from AF	ECG + Holter

Abbreviations: AF, atrial fibrillation; ECG, electrocardiography; NSR, normal sinus rhythm; UCG, ultrasonic cardiography.
[a] Median reported.

Table 2
Available study characteristics included in the systematic review and meta-analysis of lone surgical ablation for atrial fibrillation, 2009 to 2011

Authors[Ref.]	Surgical Technique	Patients with Previous CA (%)	Left Atrial Size, Mean ± SD (mm)	Ejection Fraction (%)
Albåge et al[17]	Cox III/IV	[a]	[a]	100% had EF >50
Bagge et al[9]	PVI	[a]	45.0[b]	86% had EF >50
Beukema et al[10]	PVI	[a]	41.2	54 ± 4.3
Beyer et al[11]	PVI	100	43.0	55 ± 8.5
Cui et al[7]	PVI	4.9	49.7	[a]
Edgerton et al[12]	PVI	21.1	47.2	50% had EF >55
Edgerton et al[13]	PVI + Dallas	[a]	52.0	[a]
Edgerton et al[15]	PVI	20.8	48.0	54.2
Kron et al[14]	PVI	[a]	[a]	54.9 ± 8.2
Krul et al[18]	PVI + Dallas	45	47.0	[a]
Stulak et al[19]	Cox III/IV	6.2	[a]	[a]
Weimar et al[20]	Cox III/IV	40	47.0	[a]
Yilmaz et al[16]	PVI	60	42.1	90% had EF >40

Abbreviations: CA, catheter ablation; EF, ejection fraction; PVI, pulmonary vein isolation.
[a] Information not provided.
[b] Median provided.

a median left atrial size of 45.0. Sixty-five percent of patients had paroxysmal AF, 14% had persistent AF, and 21% had LSP AF. A successful outcome was defined as no documented symptomatic AF episodes or left ATs after 12 months of follow-up, excluding the initial 3 months postoperatively. Of the 33 who had follow-up results at 12 months, 76% had no symptomatic AF recurrences or AF episodes on a 24-hour Holter monitor.

Beukema and colleagues[10] published results of 33 patients undergoing a minimally invasive PVI and left atrial appendage ligation procedure. These patients, with mean age of 59.4 ± 8.9 years, mean left atrial size of 41.2 mm, and mean EF of 54% ± 4.3%, were followed for a minimum of 3 months, and assessed by ECG, Holter monitor, and an AF-alarm device. Thirty-nine percent of the patients in this study had paroxysmal AF and 61% had persistent AF. Success was defined as sustained sinus rhythm, including atrial rhythm or an atrial-based paced rhythm. Success rates were 87% based on serial ECGs; 84% based on ECG and 24- to 48-hour Holter monitor; and 69% based on ECG, the Holter monitor, and AF-alarm device. At latest follow-up, 69% of the patients were free from AF after surgical ablation, and of those free of AF, 64% used antiarrhythmic drugs (AADs).

In 2009, Beyer and colleagues[11] discussed the results of their study on stand-alone AF. This study included 100 patients, all of whom previously underwent CA and were followed for a minimum of 3 months, with mean age of 65 ± 11 years, mean left atrial size of 43.0 mm, and mean EF of 55% ± 8.5%. Thirty-nine percent of the patients had paroxysmal AF, 29% had persistent AF, and 32% had LSP AF. These patients underwent bilateral PVI, autonomic denervation, and left atrial appendage resection, and success was defined as the absence of AF or Aflutter on follow-up ECGs and Holter-monitor recordings. Eighty-seven percent were in NSR after 3 months, antiarrhythmic therapy was discontinued in 63%, and anticoagulation therapy was discontinued in 65%.

Edgerton and colleagues[12] published a study of 114 patients with mean age of 59.5 ± 10 years, mean left atrial size of 47.2 mm, and mean EF of 54.2% ± 9.5%; 21.1% previously underwent CA. Fifty-three percent of the patients had paroxysmal AF, 28% had persistent AF, and 19% had LSP AF. These patients underwent bilateral minithoracotomies with video assistance, were assessed by an ECG and 2-week AF monitor, and were followed for a minimum of 6 months. Diagnosis before ablation indicates that 86.7% with paroxysmal AF were in sinus rhythm at 6 months. Similarly, 56.3% with persistent AF and 50.0% with LSP AF were also in sinus rhythm at 6 months.

Additionally in 2009, Edgerton and colleagues[13] published a different study that included 30 patients, with a mean age of 58 ± 9 years and left atrial size of 52.0 mm. The patients in this study underwent minimally invasive surgery with an extended lesion set and PVI, and were assessed by an ECG and 2-week AF monitor. Thirty-three percent had persistent AF and 67% had LSP AF. Success was defined as no episodes of AF, AT, or Aflutter longer than 15 seconds in duration during monitoring at 6 months. Those with persistent AF had a 90% success rate while those with LSP AF had a 75% success rate. Overall, 80.0% were free from AF while 58.3% were free from AF, AT, and Aflutter off AADs.

Kron and colleagues[14] conducted a study on 50 patients who underwent bipolar RF ablation of the pulmonary vein (PV) antrum, parasympathetic ganglionated plexi, and ligament of Marshall. Seventy-four percent of patients had paroxysmal AF and 26% had persistent AF. Of the 50 patients, 37 did not undergo electrophysiology studies and electroanatomic mapping, and therefore were included in the current analysis. These 37 patients, with mean age of 63.4 ± 9.3 years and mean EF of 54.9% ± 8.2%, were followed for a minimum of 12 months and assessed by an ECG and AF monitor device. Eighty-four percent returned to NSR at the 12-month follow-up.

In the study by Cui and colleagues,[7] 81 patients with mean age of 57.6 ± 10 years and mean left atrial size of 49.7 mm were followed for a minimum of 12 months. Of the 81 patients, 4.9% previously underwent CA, but only 49 patients had follow-up results at 12 months. Forty-nine percent of the patients had paroxysmal AF, 17% had persistent AF, and 15% had LSP AF. The main procedures performed on the patients include bilateral PV antrum isolation, obliteration of the left atrial appendage, division of the ligament of Marshall, and intraoperative electrophysiologic testing. Patients were assessed using ECG, a Holter monitor, and ultrasonic cardiography. At 12 months, 79.6% of the patients were in sinus rhythm (paroxysmal AF, 80.0%; persistent AF, 75.0%; LSP AF, 66.7%).

In 2010, Edgerton and colleagues[15] published a study on 52 patients with paroxysmal AF who underwent bilateral epicardial PVI with bipolar RF, partial autonomic denervation, and selective excision of the left atrial appendage. The definition of success for the procedure was no episodes of AF/left atrial flutter/AT longer than 30 seconds. These patients had a mean age of 60.3 years, mean left atrial size of 48.0 mm, and mean EF of 54.2%; 20.8% previously underwent CA. These patients were assessed by ECG and a 14-day Holter monitor, and were followed for a minimum of 12 months. Freedom from AF, AT, and Aflutter was 80.8%, and AADs were stopped in 33 of 37 patients in whom ablation was successful at 12 months.

Yilmaz and colleagues[16] conducted a study on 30 patients who underwent bilateral video-assisted thoracoscopy using bipolar RF energy with a minimum follow-up of 3 months. These patients had a mean age of 55.6 ± 8.6 years and a mean left atrial size of 42.1 mm. Sixty percent previously underwent CA, and 90% had an EF greater than 40%. Sixty-three percent of the patients had paroxysmal AF, 27% had persistent AF, and 10% had LSP AF. Success was defined as no episodes of AF lasting longer than 30 seconds after a blanking period of 3 months. Seventy-seven percent were free from AF, and, of those who had a successful procedure, 65% were free from AF without AADs.

In 2011, Albåge and colleagues[17] published a study on 43 patients who underwent a biatrial cryo-Maze procedure as a concomitant (n = 37) or stand-alone procedure (n = 6). The patients in the stand-alone group had a mean age of 54.2 years, and all had an EF greater than 50%. Fifty percent of the patients in the stand-alone group had paroxysmal AF, 17% had persistent AF, and 33% has LSP AF. Eighty-three percent were in sinus rhythm with no AF at 12 months, while overall, 81% had sinus/paced rhythm at 12 months with no AF and no AADs.

The study by Krul and colleagues[18] included 31 patients who underwent thoracoscopic surgery with PVI and ganglionated plexi ablation, with bipolar RF and dissection of ligament of Marshall, and were assessed by ECG and a Holter monitor. The mean age was 57 years, the mean left atrial size was 47.0 mm, and 45% previously underwent CA. Fifty-two percent of the patients had paroxysmal AF, 42% had persistent AF, and 6% had LSP AF. Twenty-two had follow-up results at 12 months, and 86% had no recurrences of AF, Aflutter, or AT and were not using AADs.

Of the 289 patients included in the study by Stulak and colleagues,[19] 194 underwent CA, 97 underwent an isolated cut-and-sew Cox Maze procedure, and 2 did not give consent for research authorization. Success was reported as "freedom from AF at last follow-up." The investigators did not delineate the type of AF experienced by study participants. The Cox-Maze group was followed for 60 months and had a median age of 60 years; 6.2% had an unsuccessful previous CA. Success rate in the Cox-Maze group was 84% while freedom from AF without AADs was 82%.

Cox Maze IV was performed as a stand-alone procedure using cardiopulmonary bypass with bicaval cannulation in the study by Weimar and colleagues[20]; patients underwent either a median sternotomy or a right mini-thoracotomy. The study included 100 patients with a mean age of 56 ± 10 years and a mean left atrial size of 47.0 mm; 40% previously had unsuccessful CA. Thirty-one percent of the patients had paroxysmal AF, 6% had persistent AF, and 63% had LSP AF. Patients were considered to be a success if they were both free from AF and free of AADs. Following patients for 24 months, freedom from AF was 90% and freedom from AF without AADs was 84%.

Meta-Analysis

The 13 described studies were then combined within a meta-analysis, the results of which can be seen in **Figs. 2** and **3**. Combined results of postoperative freedom from AF (see **Fig. 2**A) indicate an overall 84% (95% CI, 80.0–88.0) success rate for the 6 included studies. Combined results of postoperative return to NSR indicate an 83% (95% CI, 79.0–87.0) success rate (see **Fig. 2**B). Cochrane evaluation of these groups indicated no heterogeneity, with I^2 values less than 50% (P>.05).

Because of small sample size, the studies had to be combined to include both freedom from AF and return to NSR when stratified by type of AF. Those patients with paroxysmal AF who underwent stand-alone ablative surgery experienced an 85% (95% CI, 80.0–89.0) success rate when the study results were combined (see **Fig. 3**A). Patients with persistent AF had a 79% (95% CI, 70.0–86.0) success proportion (see **Fig. 3**B), but results are unstable according to the Cochrane evaluation (I^2 = 64.8%; P = .0092). The patients with LSP AF had a 64% (95% CI, 54.0–73.0) success rate in freedom from AF/return to NSR according to the 7 studies included in the analysis (see **Fig. 3**C). The funnel plot in **Fig. 4** indicates a potential for publication bias within the study group, as the included studies do not represent a symmetric pattern about the mean.

Results of Catheter Ablation Review Articles, Registries, and Meta-Analyses: The Evidence

To compare the surgical meta-analysis with catheter meta-analyses, the research team chose 3 meta-analyses of CA already published in the peer-reviewed literature. Each of these studies sought to collate published literature on the effectiveness and safety of at least one catheter-based therapy approach and used sound research methodology.

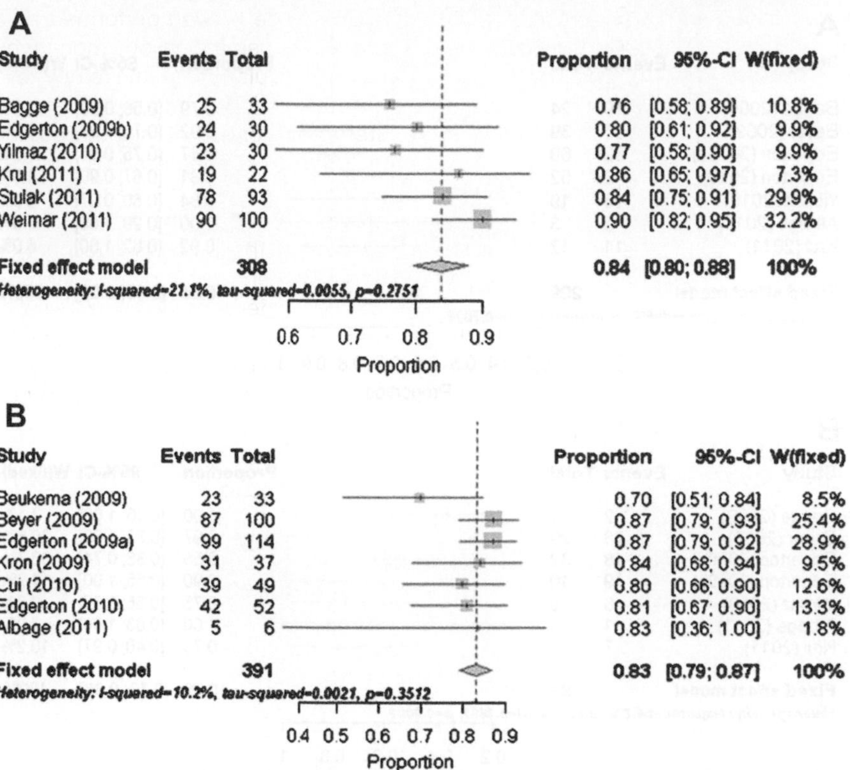

Fig. 2. Forest plots of combined studies of (*A*) freedom from AF and (*B*) return to normal sinus rhythm following stand-alone surgical ablation for AF, 2009 to 2011.

Calkins and colleagues[21] published 2 separate systematic reviews and 1 meta-analysis in one article, only a portion of which is applicable to the current discussion. To ascertain the relative safety and effectiveness of RF CA (RFA), the research group performed a review of the EMBASE and MEDLINE databases, with a follow-up review of the Cochrane Library resources. In all, this review included 9 randomized clinical trials (RCTs) and 54 observational studies (42 prospective, 12 retrospective) with a total of 8789 patients. The minimum follow-up time for inclusion was set at 7 days, and the study observed a mean age at time of ablative procedure of 55 years and duration of AF at 6.0 years. Of the study participants 35.8% had paroxysmal AF, 33.3% had persistent AF, and 30.8% had LSP AF. Success was defined as the lack of recurrence of arrhythmia throughout the follow-up period, and the combined results indicated success of following single procedure of patients either on or off AAD therapy at 72%. For patients requiring multiple procedures, the success rate was 77% (95% CI, 73–81) following RFA either on or off AADs. The mean follow-up period for these studies was 14 months, with a range of 2 to 30 months.

In 2010, Kong and colleagues[22] published a meta-analysis of 6 RCTs of success following a single catheter ablative procedure, with success defined as freedom from AF or AT, either with or without the ongoing use of AADs. All patients within this study received either PVI CA or PVI with complex fractionated atrial electrogram (CFAE) CA, and had a follow-up time of at least 3 months. A total of 538 patients were included within the analysis, 50.3% with paroxysmal AF and 49.7% with persistent AF. Combined results were stratified by length of follow-up, with 48% of the patients who underwent PVI alone and 66% who underwent PVI and CFAE free from AF/AT after one procedure with or without AAD, with a mean follow-up of 10.5 $\pm$ 1.8 months. Longer-term follow-up (14.2 $\pm$ 4.9 months) results indicated 68% success following PVI alone and 82% success following PVI plus CFAE, respectively.

Li and colleagues[23] performed and published a meta-analysis of 7 controlled clinical trials (4 with randomization, 3 without randomization) of patients following PVI plus CFAE for AF. The investigators sought to understand how CFAE following a single PVI procedure affected the maintenance of sinus rhythm. In all, 662 patients were included within the analysis, with follow-up time ranging from

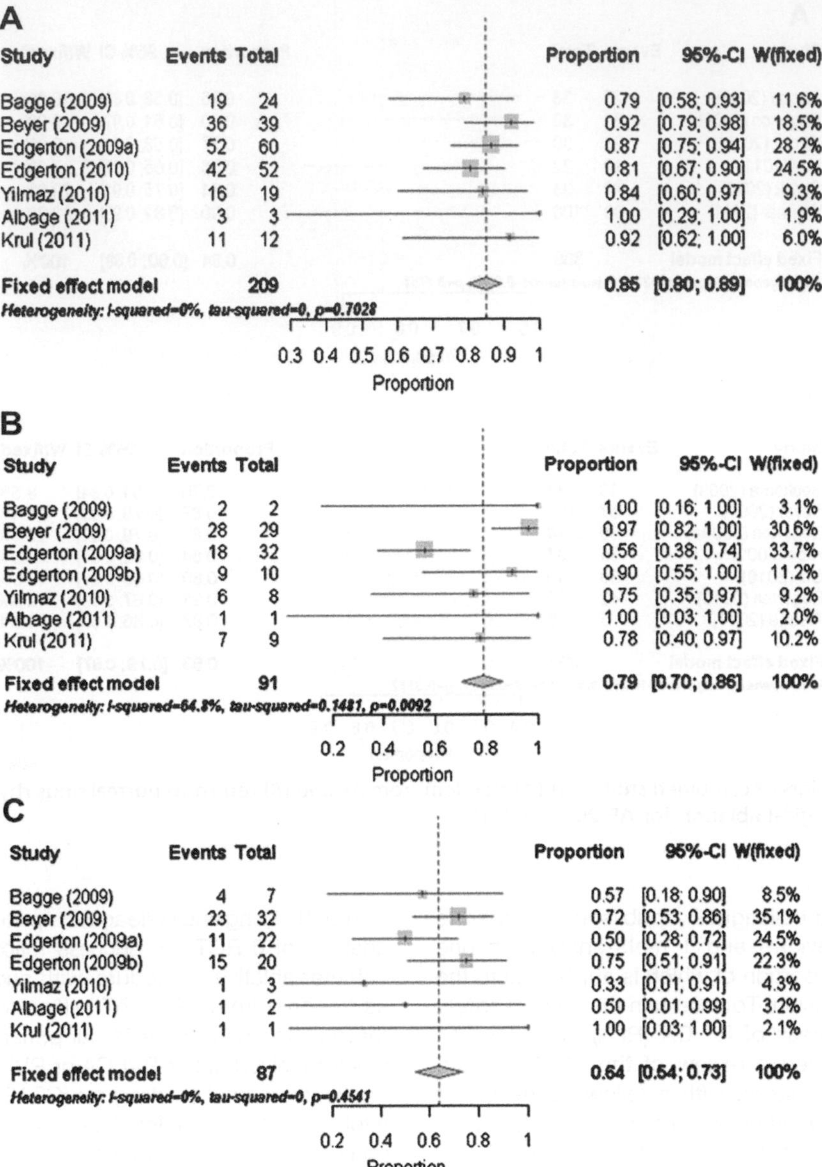

Fig. 3. Forest plots of combined studies of (*A*) paroxysmal AF, (*B*) persistent AF, and (*C*) long-standing persistent AF following stand-alone surgical ablation, 2009 to 2011.

12 to 19 months. Patients with paroxysmal AF who underwent PVI experienced 75% maintenance of sinus rhythm, and 45% of the patients with persistent or LSP AF achieved sinus rhythm maintenance, although the investigators do not delineate the proportion of patients within each AF group.

There was also a systematic review of CA for LSP AF.[24] When PVI alone was performed in these patients the success rate was 21%. When substrate ablation was added to PVI, the mean success was 47%.

Summary

The best available data from meta-analyses of catheter and surgical literature yields the following results.

Results from stand-alone surgical ablation:

- OVERALL SUCCESS
  - Postoperative freedom from AF: with/without AAD: 84%
  - Postoperative freedom of AF, AT, Aflutter: with/without AADs: 83%

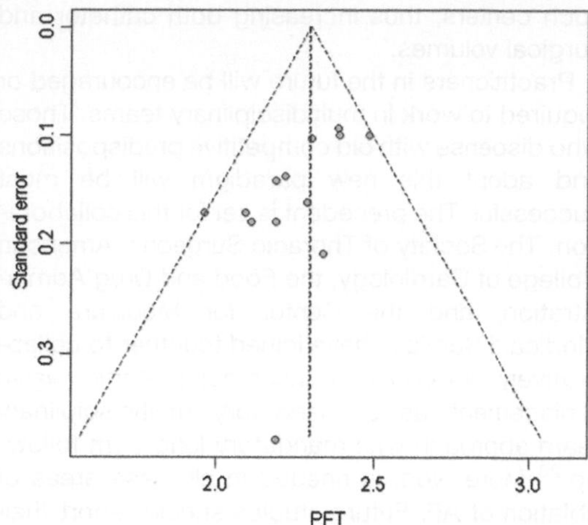

Fig. 4. Funnel plot of all studies included (n = 13) within the systematic review and meta-analysis of stand-alone surgical ablation for AF, 2009 to 2011.

- SUCCESS by AF TYPE
  - PAF: 85%
  - Persistent: 79%
  - LSP: 64%

Results from CA:

- Kong and colleagues,[22] freedom from AF/AT
  - After 1 procedure with or without AADs
    - PVI = 48%
    - PVI + CFAE = 66%
  - After all procedures, with or without AADs
    - PVI = 68%
    - PVI + CFAE = 82%
- Calkins and colleagues,[21] freedom from AF without AADs
  - Single procedure = 57%
  - Multiple procedures = 71%
- Li and colleagues[23]
  - PAF = 75%
  - Persistent/LSP = 45.25%
- Brooks, freedom from AF/AT[24]
  - LSP: 47%

It seems clear that the initial ablative approach to patients with PAF should be CA. The results of CA in this population approach those of surgery, with less morbidity. The paroxysmal patients can be treated with PVI alone, without the need for the more difficult linear ablations required for substrate modification in more advanced types of AF. In addition, improvements in catheter design and technology should further facilitate antral ablation.

For patients with persistent AF, there is insufficient evidence to argue for either catheter or surgical ablation. The ablative approach to these patients should be individualized, with the more difficult patients being referred for a minimal-access surgical approach. In the authors' hands the minimal-access approach is totally thoracoscopic, with 3 ports (two 10 mm and one 5 mm) in each side of the chest. Patient pain is minimal, and the patient is usually discharged on the third postoperative day.

Based on the data given herein, the authors believe that the appropriate initial ablative procedure for patients with LSP AF should be a totally thoracoscopic surgical Maze procedure. In the authors' hands this yields a 70% success at mean follow-up of 13 months. The surgical meta-analysis here shows a success rate of 64% in contrast to a 47% success for CA.

Limitations

Readers should note that the potential for bias in estimation is inherent in the meta-analysis design. This analytical approach allows for the collation of a large number of studies and, thereby, increased sample size and power, but results should be interpreted with caution. Publication bias and the potential for heterogeneity of included studies can lead to biased estimation of success proportions. The research team used a funnel plot (see **Fig. 4**) as a tool to understand the potential for heterogeneity of study populations, which indicate a need for caution in interpretation of results. This heterogeneity may be caused by differing definitions of AF and success. In addition, not all studies reported complete information on proportion by type of AF and defining characteristics of assessed outcomes. This lack of information does not allow for assured collation of outcomes within the meta-analysis.

DISCUSSION

In many of the surgical series, all of the patients operated on had been turned down for CA. Therefore this is not a valid comparison, as the more favorable patients, with a higher chance of success, were treated with CA. With reference to CA trials, the newly released 2012 HRS Expert Consensus Statement on Catheter and Surgical Ablation of Atrial Fibrillation states, "in considering the results of these clinical trials, it is important to recognize that the trials enrolled predominantly middle-aged white men with paroxysmal atrial fibrillation and few comorbidities." Despite taking less favorable patients, surgical ablation has a higher success rate.

Nevertheless, CA has made great strides in the treatment of patients with AF. The results in paroxysmal AF are admirable and approach those of surgical ablation. Limitations of CA technology make it difficult to reliably produce the linear transmural lesions that are usually required for success in more advanced types of AF. One of the strengths of minimal-access surgical ablation is its ability to produce linear lesions, which contributes to the higher success rate in LSP AF and justifies surgery as the ablative procedure of choice for these difficult cases.

However, the authors prefer to view CA and surgical ablation as complementary rather than competitive techniques, having found that patients who fail a surgical ablation usually fail as paroxysmal with a relatively low burden of AF. Whereas they may not have been candidates for CA preoperatively, they are now ideal candidates for a "touch-up" CA. Frequently the electrophysiologist will find a single small break in a line, which is easily completed with a catheter; thus, the patient is converted to a success.

There are other reasons that surgical (epicardial) and catheter (endocardial) ablation are complementary. Surgical devices may fail to penetrate the endocardium; catheter devices may fail to penetrate to the epicardium. Surgeons are skilled at making lines: the tools are designed for it, the smooth epicardial surface is ideal for it, and visual imaging can reveal breaks in a line. Electrophysiologists excel at "spot welding": the catheter tip is punctuated by design, it can slip off of endocardial ridges or trabeculations, resulting in breaks, and nonvisual imaging does not show continuity of burns. Surgeons may have difficulty mapping for completeness: they are constrained by pericardial reflections, they may lack formal training, and their tools may be homemade or first generation. Electrophysiologists excel at mapping for success: they have full access to the entire endocardial surface, they are formally trained in the techniques, and they have mature enabling technology. In addition, each specialty has its own unique contributions. Surgeons can fully divide the ligament of Marshall, exclude the atrial appendage, perform targeted ablation of ganglionated plexi, and isolate the superior vena cava with little risk of injury to the phrenic nerve. Electrophysiologists can easily make a cavotricuspid isthmus line, map for flutters, ablate within the coronary sinus, and map and ablate CFAEs. Recognition of the complementary nature of these techniques has led some centers to explore "hybrid" combined surgical ablation and CA, with early promising results.[25]

The most successful programs in the future will be those using an interdisciplinary collaborative team approach to the treatment of AF, resulting in higher success rates for patients. Many of these patients are well read and mobile and will seek out such centers, thus increasing both catheter and surgical volumes.

Practitioners in the future will be encouraged or required to work in multidisciplinary teams. Those who dispense with old competitive predispositions and adopt this new paradigm will be most successful. The precedent is set for this collaboration. The Society of Thoracic Surgeons, American College of Cardiology, the Food and Drug Administration, and the Center for Medicare and Medicaid Services have joined together to collaboratively introduce transcatheter aortic valve replacement as a mandatory multidisciplinary team approach with mandatory long-term follow-up.[26] More work is needed in all these areas of ablation of AF. Future studies should report their results in compliance with the HRS/EHRA/ECAS Expert Consensus Statement[27] so that results can be easily compared and conclusions more clearly made.

REFERENCES

1. Fuster V, Rydén LE, Cannom DS, et al. ACC/AHA/ESC 2006 Guidelines for the management of patients with atrial fibrillation. Circulation 2006;114:e257–354.
2. Go A, Hylek E, Phillips K, et al. Prevalence of diagnosed atrial fibrillation in adults: national implications for rhythm management and stroke prevention: the AnTicoagulation and Risk Factors in Atrial Fibrillation (ATRIA) Study. JAMA 2001;285:2370–5.
3. Cox JL, Schuessler RB, Boineau JP. The development of the Maze procedure for the treatment of atrial fibrillation. Semin Thorac Cardiovasc Surg 2000;12:2–14.
4. Edgerton ZJ, Edgerton JR. History of surgery for atrial fibrillation. Heart Rhythm 2009;6(12S):S1–4.
5. Mack MJ. Current results of minimally invasive surgical ablation for isolated atrial fibrillation. Heart Rhythm 2009;6(12S):S46–9.
6. Edgerton ZJ, Edgerton JR. Rationale for minimally invasive pulmonary vein isolation and partial autonomic denervation for surgical treatment of atrial fibrillation. Innovations 2008;3:121–4.
7. Cui YQ, Li Y, Gao F, et al. Video-assisted minimally invasive surgery for lone atrial fibrillation: a clinical report of 81 cases. J Thorac Cardiovasc Surg 2010;139:326–32.
8. Edgerton JR, Jackman WM, Mack MJ. A new epicardial lesion set for minimal access left atrial maze: the Dallas Lesion Set. Ann Thorac Surg 2009;88:1655–7.
9. Bagge L, Blomstrom P, Nilsson L, et al. Epicardial off-pump pulmonary vein isolation and vagal denervation improve long-term outcome and quality of life in patients with atrial fibrillation. J Thorac Cardiovasc Surg 2009;137:1265–71.

10. Beukema R, Beukema WP, Sie HT, et al. Monitoring of atrial fibrillation burden after surgical ablation: relevancy of end-point criteria after radiofrequency ablation treatment of patients with long atrial fibrillation. Interact Cardiovasc Thorac Surg 2009;9:956–9.
11. Beyer E, Lee R, Lam BK. Point: minimally invasive bipolar radiofrequency ablation of lone atrial fibrillation: early multicenter results. J Thorac Cardiovasc Surg 2009;137:521–6.
12. Edgerton JR, McClelland JH, Duke D, et al. Minimally invasive surgical ablation of atrial fibrillation: six-month results. J Thorac Cardiovasc Surg 2009; 138:109–14.
13. Edgerton JR, Jackman WM, Mahoney C, et al. Totally thorascopic surgical ablation of persistent AF and longstanding persistent atrial fibrillation using the "Dallas" lesion set. Heart Rhythm 2009; 6(12S):S64–70.
14. Kron J, Kasirajan V, Wood MA, et al. Management of recurrent atrial arrhythmias after minimally invasive surgical pulmonary vein isolation and ganglionic plexi ablation for atrial fibrillation. Heart Rhythm 2009;7:445–51.
15. Edgerton JR, Brinkman WT, Weaver T, et al. Pulmonary vein isolation and autonomic denervation for the management of paroxysmal atrial fibrillation by a minimally invasive surgical approach. J Thorac Cardiovasc Surg 2010;140:823–8.
16. Yilmaz A, Geuzebroek GS, Van Putte BP, et al. Completely thoracoscopic pulmonary vein isolation with ganglionic plexus ablation and left atrial appendage amputation for treatment of atrial fibrillation. Eur J Cardiothorac Surg 2010;38:356–60.
17. Albåge A, Péterffy M, Källner G. The biatrial cryomaze procedure for treatment of atrial fibrillation: a single center experience. Scand Cardiovasc J 2011;45:112–9.
18. Krul SPJ, Driessen AH, van Boven WJ, et al. Thoracoscopic video-assisted pulmonary vein antrum isolation, ganglionated plexus ablation, and periprocedural confirmation of ablation lesions: first results of a hybrid surgical-electrophysiological approach for atrial fibrillation. Circ Arrhythm Electrophysiol 2011;4:262–70.
19. Stulak JM, Dearani JA, Sundt TM, et al. Ablation of atrial fibrillation: comparison of catheter-based techniques and the Cox-Maze III operation. Ann Thorac Surg 2011;91:1882–9.
20. Weimar T, Bailey MS, Watanabe Y, et al. The Cox-maze IV procedure for lone atrial fibrillation: a single center experience in 100 consecutive patients. J Interv Card Electrophysiol 2011;31:47–54.
21. Calkins H, Reynolds MR, Spector P, et al. Treatment of atrial fibrillation with antiarrhythmic drugs or radiofrequency ablation: two systematic literature reviews and a meta-analysis. Circ Arrhythm Electrophysiol 2009;2:349–61.
22. Kong MH, Piccini JP, Bahnson TD. Efficacy of adjunctive ablation of complex fractionated atrial electrograms and pulmonary vein isolation for the treatment of atrial fibrillation: a meta-analysis of randomized controlled trials. Europace 2011;13: 193–204.
23. Li WJ, Bai YY, Zhang HY, et al. Additional ablation of complex fractionated atrial electrograms after pulmonary vein isolation in patients with atrial fibrillation: a meta-analysis. Circ Arrhythm Electrophysiol 2011;4:143–8.
24. Brooks AG, Stiles MK, Laborderie J, et al. Outcomes of long-standing persistent atrial fibrillation ablation: a systematic review. Heart Rhythm 2010;7:835–46.
25. Mahapatra S, Lapar DJ, Kamath S, et al. Initial experience of sequential surgical epicardial-catheter endocardial ablation for persistent and long-standing persistent atrial fibrillation with long-term follow-up. Ann Thorac Surg 2011;91:1890–8.
26. Mack MH, Holmes DR Jr. Rational dispersion for the introduction of transcatheter valve therapy. JAMA 2011;306:2149–50.
27. Calkins H, Brugada J, Packer DL, et al. HRS/EHRA/ECAS Expert Consensus Statement on catheter and surgical ablation of atrial fibrillation: recommendations for personnel, policy, procedures and follow-up. A report of the Heart Rhythm Society (HRS) Task Force on catheter and surgical ablation of atrial fibrillation. Heart Rhythm 2007;4:816–61.

The Emerging Role of Epicardial Ablation

Luigi Di Biase, MD, PhD, FHRS[a,b,c,*]
Pasquale Santangeli, MD[a,c], Rong Bai, MD, FHRS[a],
Roderick Tung, MD[d], J. David Burkhardt, MD, FHRS[a],
Kalyanam Shivkumar, MD, PhD, FHRS[d],
Andrea Natale, MD, FHRS[a,b,e,f,g,h,*]

KEYWORDS

- Catheter ablation • Epicardial mapping and ablation • Epicardial access • Ventricular arrhythmias
- Supraventricular arrhythmias

KEY POINTS

- Sosa and colleagues first described a percutaneous approach (via the subxiphoid area) to access the pericardial space in 1996.
- Epicardial mapping and ablation is increasingly used for the treatment of supraventricular and ventricular arrhythmias and represents an adjunctive approach for challenging arrhythmias to improve procedural success rate.
- Epicardial ablation should be considered not only after the failure of an endocardial ablation but often as a first-line approach.
- Complications may occur during percutaneous access and epicardial ablation, and these might be reduced or avoided by improved operator skills and experience.
- New tools to access the epicardial space are being evaluated.

INTRODUCTION

Endocardial mapping and ablation is the standard approach for the treatment of a variety of arrhythmias.[1–3] However, epicardial mapping and ablation are becoming more important for both the treatment of supraventricular arrhythmias, such as accessory pathways, atrial tachycardia, inappropriate sinus tachycardia, and, more importantly, for the treatment of ventricular tachycardia (VT).

Sosa and colleagues[4,5] first described a percutaneous approach (via the subxiphoid area) to access the pericardial space in 1996. Since then, epicardial access has been used in all experienced electrophysiology laboratories as an adjunctive approach for challenging arrhythmias, which has improved ablation success rates, especially after the failure of the conventional endocardial mapping and ablation approach.[6–28]

Mapping and ablation within the pericardial space require advanced skills and relevant knowledge of the anatomic structures and sinuses present in the pericardial space. Although limited to highly experienced operators, an important advantage of percutaneous pericardial access is that invasive surgical approaches can be avoided. The major limitation

[a] Texas Cardiac Arrhythmia Institute at St. David's Medical Center, Austin, TX, USA; [b] Department of Biomedical Engineering, University of Texas, 3000 North I-35, Suite 720, Austin, TX 78705, USA; [c] Department of Cardiology, University of Foggia, Foggia, Italy; [d] UCLA Cardiac Arrhythmia Center, Los Angeles, CA, USA; [e] EP Services, California Pacific Medical Center, San Francisco, CA, USA; [f] Division of Cardiology, Stanford University, Palo Alto, CA, USA; [g] Case Western Reserve University, Cleveland, OH, USA; [h] Interventional Electrophysiology, Scripps Clinic, San Diego, CA, USA
* Correspondings author.
E-mail addresses: dr.natale@gmail.com; dibbia@gmail.com

Card Electrophysiol Clin 4 (2012) 425–437
http://dx.doi.org/10.1016/j.ccep.2012.05.004
1877-9182/12/$ – see front matter

during mapping in the pericardial space is the lack of anchoring structures that can be used to direct the catheters to the intended target areas. The presence of sinuses, recesses, and reflections are important to loop the catheters and direct them to the intended location. The advent of deflectable sheaths and robotic magnetic navigation has improved the ability to navigate in the pericardial space.[29] This article discusses the importance of epicardial ablation for the commonly treated arrhythmias.

ANATOMY OF THE PERICARDIAL SPACE: A BRIEF SUMMARY

The heart and its main vessels are contained in a sack called the *pericardium*. The pericardial cavity is a virtual space between the internal serosal layer and an external fibrous layer. The cavity separates the heart from the surrounding mediastinal structures, thus allowing the heart to have free movements in the virtual cavity. In the absence of adhesions, the pericardial space is a potential space, with only 15 to 50 mL of serosal fluid. The serosal layer is also divided into 2 substructures: the *parietal* layer attached to the external fibrous layer, and the visceral layer, better known as epicardial space. The pericardial space consists of a cavity, reflections, sinuses, and recesses. During epicardial mapping and ablation, reflections are useful because they represent important landmarks for the placement and anchoring of the mapping/ablation catheter.

The main sinuses that are instrumented during electrophysiology procedures are the transverse and the oblique sinuses. The transverse sinus is attached inferiorly to the pericardial reflection and anteriorly to the left atrium, and connects with the left and the right pulmonary veins. In this sinus, the aortic recess and the right pulmonary artery are contained. When mapping in this area, the left atrium, the pulmonary veins, and the coronary cusps (noncoronary and right) can be accessed. The oblique sinus is attached anteriorly to the atria and inferiorly to the vena cava.

By navigating in the oblique sinus, epicardial mapping and ablation of the ventricles can be achieved.

In patients with previous cardiac surgery, as well as pericarditis, significant adhesions may form, rendering this space inaccessible. It is our opinion that epicardial instrumentation should not be attempted in these cases in which adhesions are suspected. However, the epicardial space can be reaccessed in the event of a recurrence following prior epicardial access for mapping and ablation.[30,31]

Methods of Obtaining Epicardial Access

Sosa and colleagues[4] first reported the subxiphoid percutaneous puncture to access the virtual space between the heart and the pericardium. Since then, 2 approaches have been described:

- Anterior: directing the needle superiorly with a shallow trajectory to enter the pericardial space anteriorly over the right ventricle (RV) to allow easy maneuverability over the left ventricle (LV)
- Posterior: directing the needle with a steeper trajectory toward the left shoulder, thus entering the epicardial space over the basal, inferior part of the ventricles

After the needle (Tuohy needle designed for epidural lumbar puncture) crosses the skin, the abdominal fascia, and the diaphragm, cardiac pulsations may be transmitted via the needle to the operator when the tip comes into contact with the pericardium. Tenting of the pericardium can be seen in fluoroscopy while injecting small amount of contrast.

Puncture of the pericardium is often felt as a popping sensation and, if puncture of the RV is avoided, no or minimal blood is aspirated. Before advancing the sheath, it is important to advance a guidewire in left anterior oblique (LAO) projection so that it loops several times around the cardiac silhouette and all the chambers of the heart (**Fig. 1**). The right anterior oblique/anteroposterior projections can be misleading because a perforation of the RV can lead the wire in the pulmonary artery or in the right atrium and this can simulate an intrapericardial location of the wire.[30,31]

After the pericardial access is obtained, a long sheath can be advanced to allow delivery of the mapping/ablation catheter. At our institution, we perform the epicardial access under general anesthesia, because this allow us better respiratory control and less diaphragmatic excursion, although, in some cases, the critical clinical condition of the patients does not allow general anesthesia. The use of conscious sedation has also been reported as a safe alternative.

COMPLICATIONS

Several major complications may occur during percutaneous access and epicardial ablation. These include[30]:

1. Cardiac tamponade and perforation, mainly caused by the inadvertent puncture of the RV
2. Intra-abdominal bleeding secondary to diaphragmatic vessel puncture/rupture

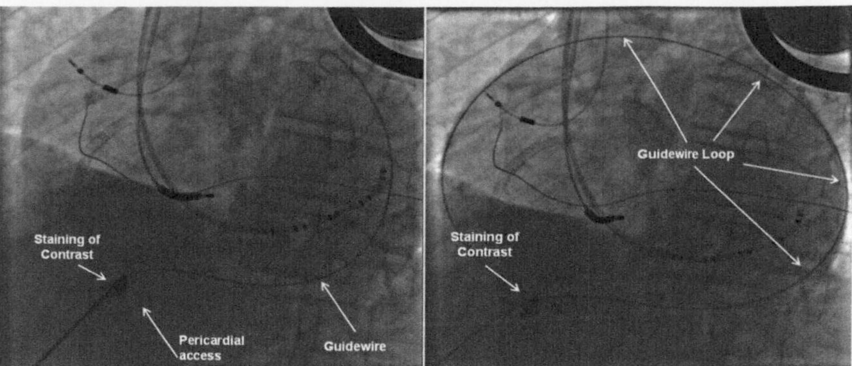

Fig. 1. Percutaneous pericardial access for epicardial mapping and ablation. Left panel: insertion of the guidewire into the pericardial space after pericardial access (*arrow*). Right panel: advancement of the guidewire within the pericardial space. Note that the guidewire loops around the outer fluoroscopic border of the heart, thereby confirming its location in the proper space.

3. Diaphragmatic paralysis caused by an injury to the phrenic nerve
4. Gastroparesis caused by damage to the vagus nerve at the level of the esophageal plexus
5. Coronary artery occlusion caused by injury to the coronary artery induced by radiofrequency energy
6. Coronary artery/vein laceration
7. Liver hematoma secondary to puncture
8. Increased defibrillation threshold mainly caused by residual air in the pericardial space
9. Pericarditis
10. Hemothorax

How to Avoid Complications

Operator experience and understanding of fluoroscopic and surrounding anatomy are critical to minimize complications. As mentioned earlier, while attempting a subxiphoid pericardial access there is risk of damaging different adjacent structures. After accessing the pericardial space, usually 30 to 50 mL of serous or serosanguinous fluid are removed. If more blood is aspirated or the bleeding is not self-contained, a cardiac perforation should be suspected. If the RV is entered with the needle tip only, it is usually inconsequential as long as the needle is promptly withdrawn. To avoid this, it is advisable to advance the needle in the LAO view and to be cautious not to go beyond the spine. In addition, the tactile feedback and the presence of premature ventricular complexes irritating the heart once touched by the needle tip are important clues to prevent this complication.

Mahapatra and colleagues[32–34] reported on a novel needle able to measure the changes in pericardial pressure once the needle enters the pericardial space and abandons the thoracic cavity. Macris and Igo[35] and Seferovic and colleagues[36] proposed a new device (PerDUCER device, Comedicus Inc., Columbia Heights, MN) to enter the pericardial space and to reduce complications associated with the pericardial access. Laham and colleagues[37] proposed a device able to deliver continuous positive pressure by using saline to push away the RV and facilitate the puncture. In the case of a double pericardial access, Nault and colleagues[38] described the injection of fluid to induce hydropericardium, thus separating the surrounding structures such as the coronary artery and the RV. Other ways to improve fluoroscopy orientation include the positioning of mapping catheters (eg, aortic root RV, coronary sinus) and the use of intracardiac echocardiography.[30]

Epicardial Ablation of Supraventricular Tachycardia

Accessory pathways

Accessory pathways (APs) may, in rare cases, have an epicardial location. Morady and colleagues[6] reported that the major reason for the failure of endocardial ablation of accessory pathways was an epicardial location of the APs (8% of the cases in their series). Several uncommon locations such as posteroseptal and left posterior pathways, as well as right atrial appendage to right ventricular pathways and left atrial appendage to left ventricular pathways, have been described as challenging pathways requiring epicardial ablation to achieve success.[7–9,11–13] It is not true that an endocardial ablation is not feasible or safe in these cases but, in the presence of an epicardial APs, the endocardial ablation has a high risk of failure.[6] In these cases, epicardial mapping and ablation should be considered or discussed with the patients as an important adjunctive strategy. The epicardial approach may include ablation within the coronary sinus and its tributaries and/or the instrumentation of the pericardial space.

In some cases, epicardial ablation may fail for the presence of a thick fat pad or because of the inability to deliver energy due to the vicinity of structures such as the coronary vessel or the phrenic nerve.

Inappropriate sinus tachycardia

Ablation of inappropriate sinus tachycardia is challenging for the risk of damaging the sinus node, because of the subepicardial location of the sinus node, and due to its vicinity to the phrenic nerve. For these reasons, different groups have proposed an endoepicardial ablation to achieve sinus node modification and to avoid phrenic nerve palsy. In this respect, an angioplasty balloon or the use of saline and air have been used as possible ways to increase the procedural success and minimize the risk for phrenic nerve damage.[14–18]

Atrial tachycardia

Only a few case reports or series have reported unsuccessful endocardial ablation of atrial tachycardia or flutter with successful epicardial ablation. Epicardial atrial tachycardia may be encountered after unsuccessful ablation of atrial fibrillation (AF) caused by an epicardial location of the triggers or caused by uncommon locations such as the right and the left atrial appendages.[13,19]

Atrial fibrillation

Despite satisfactory results for paroxysmal AF, repeat procedures are often required to achieve success in patients with nonparoxysmal AF undergoing catheter ablation. Among the possible explanations for procedural failure, the absence of lesion transmurality with conduction recovery may be the most important. This condition may occur in certain areas of the left atrium, such as the base of the left atrial appendage and thicker ridges, or in close proximity to the esophagus and or the phrenic nerve. In this scenario, an epicardial or combined endoepicardial ablation procedure may be useful.[20]

Given the rationale for epicardial ablation of AF, a few reports have recently been described. Pak and colleagues[21] showed the feasibility of adjunctive epicardial ablation to achieve success in persistent AF cases. All patients had failed previous endocardial ablation and underwent adjunctive ablation sites such as the roof, perimitral annulus, and ligament of Marshall. Such areas may require long radiofrequency times and are more amenable to treatment with epicardial ablation. Kiser and colleagues[22] reported on 28 patients with persistent or long standing persistent AF undergoing a combined surgical epicardial radiofrequency ablation with endocardial ablation with a high success rate at the short-term follow-up. Despite the enthusiasm for the short-term results, the long-term follow-up showed no improved success compared with manual ablation with a high complication rate. Mahapatra and colleagues[23] reported on an initial experience of 15 patients with persistent and long-standing persistent AF undergoing surgical epicardial and endocardial ablation following a failed endocardial ablation. At 20.7 $\pm$ 4.5 months' follow-up, 87% of the patients were free from atrial tachyarrhythmia and this was higher in a group of 30 patients undergoing repeat endocardial ablation, whose success was 53% (P = .04).

When to consider an epicardial approach for VT ablation

Several considerations need be taken into account when planning a VT ablation. An epicardial origin should always be suspected and there are characteristics on the 12-lead electrocardiogram (ECG) that can suggest an epicardial origin of the VT.[24] However, the 12-lead ECG can be misleading because of the presence of delayed activation around scar regions that may confound the ECG morphology (**Table 1**).

Several groups and investigators have tried to identify ECG features predictors of an epicardial origin. An epicardial origin of a given VT is suspected if the ECG morphology of the VT has 1 or more of the following characteristics:

- Terminal S wave in V2 and Q wave in lead 1 strongly suggest VT of subepicardial origin
- Pseudo-δ wave (slurred upstroke of QRS)
- Intrinsicoid deflection time of 85 milliseconds
- RS complex duration of greater than 120 milliseconds and/or QRS width of greater than 200 milliseconds

Berruezo and colleagues[39] analyzed the ECG recordings of VTs that were successfully ablated from the left ventricular pericardium and found that a pseudo-δ wave $\geq$34 milliseconds had a sensitivity of 83% and a specificity of 95%, an intrinsicoid deflection time $\geq$85 milliseconds had a sensitivity of 87% and a specificity of 90%, and an RS complex duration $\geq$121 milliseconds had a sensitivity of 76% and a specificity of 85% in identifying an epicardial origin of the VTs.

In addition, left ventricular outflow tract (LVOT) arrhythmias (LVOT-VT) can originate from the LV epicardium and be ablated from the coronary cusps (Epi-LVOT-VT). Among the various ECG findings,

Table 1
ECG criteria to predict the epicardial origin of VTs. The morphologic and metric criteria described are useful for recognizing the epicardial origin of the VT

ECG Criteria	Main Limitations
Berruezo criteria: Pseudo-δ wave ≥34 ms Intrinsicoid deflection V2 ≥85 ms Shortest RS complex ≥121 ms	LBBB like VT excluded
Q wave in leads that reflect local activation	Not useful if prior myocardial infarction or baseline Q waves
Precordial maximum deflection index	Described for LVOT-VT (paraseptal)

Abbreviations: LBBB, left bundle branch block; LVOT, left ventricular outflow tract; VT, ventricular tachycardia.

the R-wave duration index and R/S amplitude index in lead V1 or V2 are useful for identifying Epi-LVOT-VT. In this scenario, a delayed precordial maximum deflection index greater than or equal to 0.55 identified epicardial LVOT-VT far from the aortic sinus of Valsalva with a sensitivity of 100% and a specificity of 98.7% relative to all other sites of origin. The Q-wave ratio of lead aVL to aVR and S-wave amplitude in lead V1 are useful to differentiate between an Epi-LVOT-VT originating from the LV epicardium far from the left sinus of Valsalva (LSV) and that from the LSV (see **Table 1**). Studies led by the Marchlinski's group[40,41] show that, when a stimulus arises from the epicardial surface of the RV, the QRS is more likely to show initial negative forces (Q waves) in inferior leads, lead 1, and/or lead V2, depending on the region of origin. More specifically, the anterior epicardial sites present with Q wave or QS complex in lead 1 and V2, and the inferior RV epicardial sites show an initial Q wave in inferior leads.

Mapping and ablation in the pericardial space

Epicardial mapping is usually performed using both fluoroscopy and three-dimensional electroanatomic mapping. Areas of scar with low-amplitude abnormal electrograms (delayed and/or fractionated potentials) should also be differentiated by epicardial fat, which can simulate an area of scar.[42,43] Epicardial fat is also an obstacle for pacing (entrainment and pace mapping) as well as for ablation. For these reasons, high pacing outputs are often required.

For epicardial ablation, an open-irrigated catheter with radiofrequency energy seems the best energy source to create effective lesions. We usually use up to 50 W for at least 30 seconds with a flow rate of 30 mL/min.[44]

We have proposed cryoablation as a possible valid alternative ablation energy source in the pericardial space to minimize potential damage to the coronary artery and to the phrenic nerve. Different techniques using balloon, air, and saline have been proposed to allow epicardial or endocardial ablation by separating the phrenic nerve from the targeted ablation area. Intracardiac echo and angiography are used to avoid coronary artery damages with the ablation.[16–18]

Epicardial ablation of idiopathic VT

Idiopathic VT defines arrhythmias present in subjects with apparently structurally normal hearts. Many idiopathic VTs originate from the RV outflow tract (RVOT) in close proximity to the pulmonary valve, but others may arise from the pulmonary artery, the LVOT, the aortomitral continuity, the coronary cusps, and epicardially from the anterior interventricular vein, the great cardiac vein, and other locations overlapping the previously described endocardial site. Some of the areas described earlier constitute a triangle of close structures (anterior interventricular vein, RVOT, coronary cusps, aortomitral continuity), and, in many cases, ablation from more than 1 structure is required to achieve success, including epicardial ablation via the coronary sinus or by instrumenting the pericardial space.[45–54] Analysis of the surface ECG for characteristics that suggest epicardial sites of origin can be useful.[39–41]

Epicardial ablation of VT in idiopathic cardiomyopathy

Endocardial ablation in patients with nonischemic idiopathic cardiomyopathy has shown a poorer outcome compared with VT ablation in ischemic cardiomyopathy.[25–28,55,56] One of the possible explanations is the presence of an epicardial substrate and circuits that cannot be successfully ablated endocardially. The major challenge in these patients is the presence of low bipolar voltage in the perimitral annulus and lateral free wall, which have an epicardial predilection. Soejima and colleagues[27] first described an improved outcome following endoepicardial ablation in this subset of patients. Cano and colleagues[42] showed, in a series of patients with nonischemic idiopathic cardiomyopathy and undergoing epicardial mapping and ablation (because of the failure of the endocardial ablation or because of an ECG suggesting an epicardial origin of the VT) that these patients have a large epicardial scar (generally larger than the endocardial scar) with low voltage and fragmented bipolar electrograms suggesting scar in up to 82% of the patients (**Figs. 2–4**).[25,26,43,54–56]

Although low voltage and amplitude are secondary to the epicardial fat and or coronary vessels, the cutoff value[42] of 0.94 mV has been described as normal epicardial voltage electrograms and all values less than this as scar or fat/coronary vessels. When analyzing abnormal electrograms less than 0.94 mV, scar areas were associated with characteristics of abnormal electrograms such as delayed and split potentials. The latter seemed to be more specific in identifying epicardial areas that are suitable targets for ablation. The implementation of epicardial ablation has improved the mid-term and long-term follow-up in these patients, although the mortality and need for heart transplant remain high in patients with idiopathic cardiomyopathy.[42]

Epicardial ablation of arrhythmogenic right ventricular dysplasia

Arrhythmogenic right ventricular dysplasia (ARVD) is an autosomal dominant genetic disease

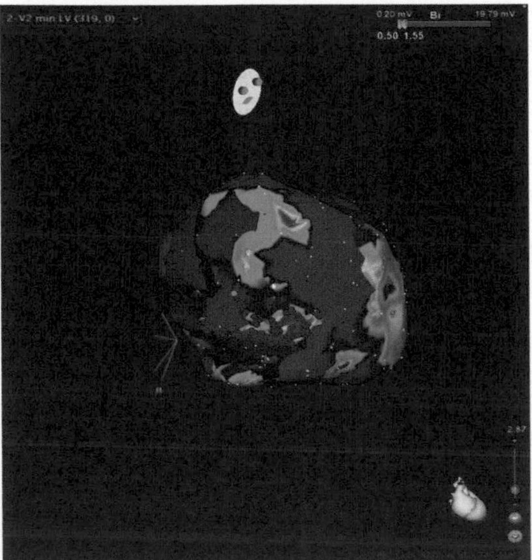

Fig. 2. Endoepicardial mapping and ablation (endocardial only) of a patient with nonischemic cardiomyopathy. Note the typical perivalvular distribution of scar. Epicardial ablation was not performed given the lack of abnormal fragmented potentials.

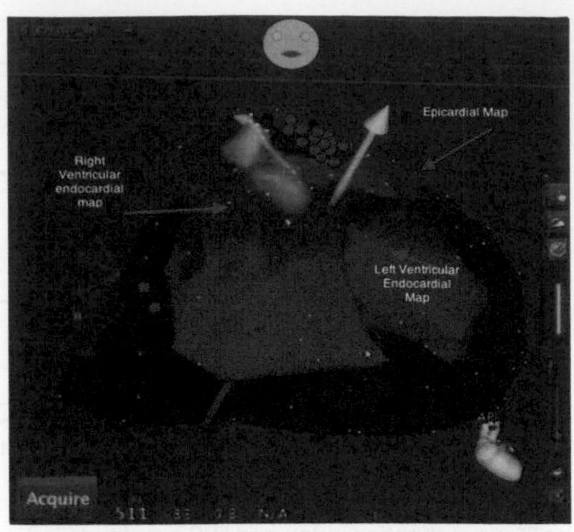

Fig. 3. Endoepicardial biventricular mapping and ablation of a patient with nonischemic idiopathic cardiomyopathy with remote magnetic navigation. The red dots indicate successful epicardial ablation sites.

characterized by progressive replacement of the right ventricular myocardium (rarely LV) with fatty and fibrous tissue. The fatty replacement is more prominent in the subepicardium and progresses to the subendocardium.[57–59] The disease is often characterized by the presence of nonsustained and sustained ventricular arrhythmias (VAs) with left bundle branch block (LBBB) morphology. Reentry around the fibrofatty areas, enhanced automaticity occurring during exercise, and trigged activity from inflammatory myocytes are the main mechanisms of VTs in patients with ARVD. Radiofrequency ablation of VA has become an effective therapeutic option in patients with ARVD with recurrent VA; however, using only an endocardial approach, the ablation success rate has shown good results at the short-term follow-up (up to 75% success rate at 3 months' follow-up) but unsatisfactory results at the long-term follow-up (25%–50% success rate).[60–65] For these reasons, epicardial ablation has been considered in patients with ARVD and associated with a better outcome at follow-up. These findings have been confirmed by surgical VT ablation in patients with ARVD.[66–70]

Several studies have tested the role of epicardial ablation after the failure of endocardial ablation. Garcia and colleagues,[71] Bakir and colleagues,[72] and, recently, Berruezo and colleagues[73] and our group[74] in a series of patients with longer follow-up proposed an endoepicardial ablation as first-line therapy in patients with ARVD. It has been noted that the epicardial scar as identified by three-dimensional voltage mapping is often larger than the endocardial scar,[42,71] suggesting that many areas of the epicardial substrate would not be targeted by an endocardial ablation alone. It is also

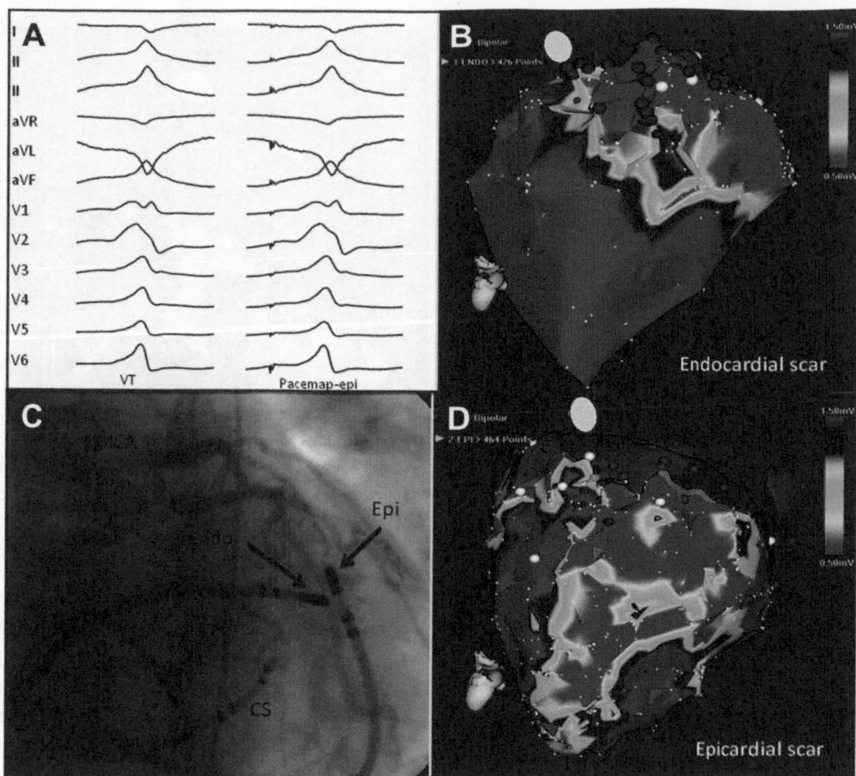

Fig. 4. Endoepicardial mapping and ablation of VT in a patient with nonischemic dilated cardiomyopathy. After endocardial ablation, the clinical VT was still inducible and epicardial mapping was performed. (*A*) 12-lead ECG of the clinical VT with 12/12 pace-map match during epicardial mapping. Endocardial (*B*) and epicardial (*D*) three-dimensional voltage mapping showing a large endoepicardial scar in the basal left ventricular lateral wall. Red dots indicate ablation lesions. VT became noninducible only after epicardial ablation. (*C*) LAO fluoroscopic view showing 2 ablation catheters, 1 inserted through a transseptal access in the LV and another inserted through an epicardial access. Both catheters target the same area (endoepicardial scar in the basal left ventricular lateral wall) to achieve a more effective lesion. Intraprocedural coronary angiography was performed to avoid delivery of ablation lesions in proximity of the coronary arteries. Endo, endocardial access; Epi, epicardial access.

our belief that abolition of any delayed, split, and fragmented abnormal electrograms is of utmost importance to improving long-term success (**Fig. 5**).

Epicardial ablation of Chagas disease

Chagas disease is an infectious disease endemic in Latin America, caused by a parasite named *Trypanosoma cruzi*. It may affect around 90 million people in Latin America and is responsible for almost 45,000 deaths per year.[75] Cardiac involvement is common in the chronic phase of the disease.[76,77] Ventricular arrhythmias as a consequence of Chagas disease represent a major cause of sudden cardiac death in Latin America. Reentry and, in some cases enhanced automaticity, are the major arrhythmic mechanisms. Sarabanda and colleagues[78] reported wall motion abnormalities as VTs predictors in patients with Chagas disease. Because the disease is characterized by the development of subepicardial fibrosis, epicardial VAs with right bundle branch block represent the prevalent morphology of arrhythmia, which explains why most of these patients require an endoepicardial ablation to improve the success rate.[79,80] Epicardial access in these patients is frequently challenging because the patients develop strong adhesions. In such cases, a surgical pericardial window should be considered.[79]

The prevalent scar location is posterolateral, in close proximity to the mitral valve. Angiography is often required in these cases to avoid coronary artery damage.

Epicardial VT Ablation for Ischemic Cardiomyopathy

Ischemic cardiomyopathy is the most common cardiac disease in the United States and Europe, leading to VT and sudden cardiac arrest. In patients at high risk for cardiac sudden death,

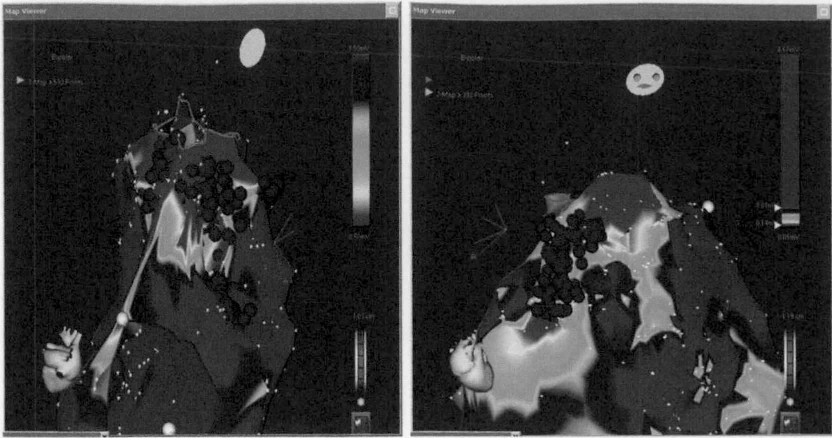

Fig. 5. Endocardial (*left side*) and epicardial (*right side*) voltage mapping in a patients with arrhythmogenic right ventricular cardiomyopathy. Red dots indicate radiofrequency applications around the scar regions displaying fragmented potentials.

the implantation of an implantable cardioverter-defibrillator (ICD) is warranted.[3] Despite the presence of the ICD, VTs remains a challenging issue in these patients. Antiarrhythmic Drugs (AADs) can be used but are often ineffective and associated with side effects.[81]

Catheter ablation of VAs in these patients represents a viable alternative to AADs, although the outcome at the long-term follow-up has not been optimal despite the introduction of open-irrigated catheters.[82–87] New technologies and tools are being investigated to improve the efficacy of ablation procedures.[88,89] Calkins and colleagues[90] in 2000 showed a success rate of 54% at 1-year follow-up in 176 patients and, similarly, Della Bella and colleagues[91] showed a success rate of 51% during a median follow-up of 36 months. Tanner and colleagues,[92] in the Euro VT study, and Rothman and colleagues[93] reported a success rate of 63% and 66% at 19 and 24 months' follow-up respectively. Carbucicchio and colleagues[82] recently reported a success rate of 66% at 22 months' follow-up. These results were slightly better than those reported in the large, multicenter Thermocool trial.[44]

The reasons for failed ablation are unclear. A possible explanation could be the inability of the current technology to create effective or transmural lesions. Although the introduction of open-irrigated catheters has increased the success rate at follow-up, it is possible that the complexity of the left ventricular scar and the thickness of the LV protect the intramyocardial and epicardial layers. Several new technologies, such as ablation catheter with a retractable needle to create deeper lesions, are being investigated.

Another possible explanation for VT recurrence might be related to the ablation technique used. The conventional approach includes pace mapping, activation mapping, and entrainment mapping to define the mechanism of the arrhythmias and to identify the target site for ablation. Following substrate mapping, clinical VT induction is attempted. Once the clinical VT is induced and when the VT is tolerated, activation/entrainment mapping is performed. The target for ablation of tolerated VTs is identified by mid-diastolic electrograms and confirmed by entrainment with concealed fusion. Short linear lesions are placed across the VT isthmus to terminate the VT.[44]

In patients with untolerated VT, a high-density three-dimensional substrate map of the chamber of interest is obtained. Once the substrate map is built, multiple pace mapping during sinus rhythm or ventricular pacing (in the case of pacemaker-dependent rhythm), predominantly along the infarct border-zone (bipolar voltages between 0.5 and 1.5 mV), is performed to select the ablation site. The site with a paced 12-lead QRS morphology matching greater than 10/12 ECG leads of the inducible clinical VT is considered the exit site and targeted for ablation with short linear lesions. Cardiopulmonary support can be used in patients who do not tolerate the VT to allow for mapping during VT.

In patients with persistent inducibility after endocardial ablation and/or after failure of endocardial ablation, epicardial ablation should be considered. The need for epicardial ablation in the setting of ischemic VT ablation is considered to be around 10% to 15%.[82] We recently proposed a more extensive ablation approach that covers the scar area both endocardially and epicardially, assuming

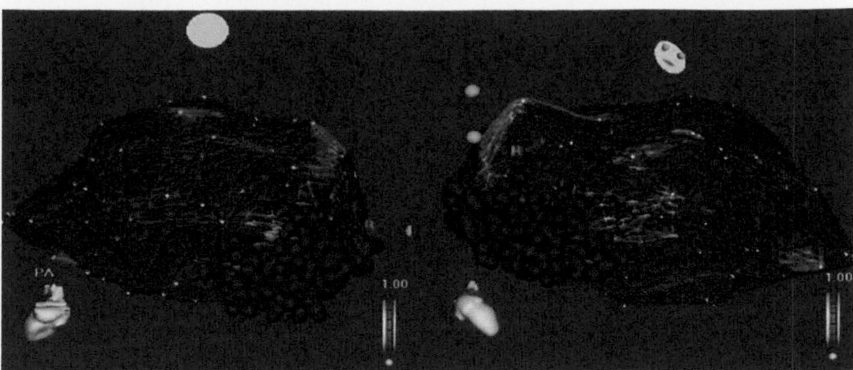

Fig. 6. Endoepicardial mapping and ablation (homogenization of scar) in a patient with scar-related postinfarct VT storm. Note the distribution of ablation dots covering the entire inferobasal scar area with fragmented/late electrograms.

that the clinical VT circuit is only 1 of the potential circuits that can be maintained within the scar areas. Therefore, in addition to voltage criteria,[94] abnormal electrograms including delayed and fragmented recordings are targeted during ablation both endocardially and epicardially. This extensive ablative technique seemed to be superior to the conventional one and to improve the success rate at follow-up (**Fig. 6**).[95]

New Tools to Access the Epicardial Space

One of the major limitations of epicardial ablation is the ability to access the pericardial space. The ideal tool would be one that reduce the operator dependency and minimizes access complications. One of the major limitations of pericardial access is the visualization of the pericardium: under fluoroscopic guidance, it is difficult to know when the needle enters the pericardial space. A pressure-sensor needle able to differentiate the pressure in the parietal pericardium (respiratory rate) from the pressure of the visceral pericardium (heart rate), would solve this issue. Mahapatra and colleagues[32] reported on an early prototype of an epicardial needle that is able via a pressure transducer to transmit the changes of pressure and frequency during pericardial access, providing additional information on the needle tip localization and thus reducing possible complications.

Horowitz and colleagues[96] tested intrapericardial echocardiography in patients undergoing pericardial access and showed the safety and the feasibility of reducing fluoroscopy use during pericardial procedures.

Nazarian and colleagues[97] reported on the use of fiberoptic endoscopy for direct visualization within the pericardial space. To achieve better visualization of the targeted sites, air is insufflated through the endoscope. If visualization is poor despite the air insufflations, an inflatable balloon is inserted and expanded with saline. This technology allows visual identification of the pericardial structures, potentially reducing fluoroscopy and procedural time.

Sumiyama and colleagues[98] tried to visualize the epicardium during gastrointestinal endoscopy. This methodology is better known as submucosal endoscopy with mucosal flap safety valve. This technology should be considered when percutaneous access is not feasible or contraindicated. In addition, Perikor technology is being investigated. Perikor technology allows better visualization of and access to the pericardial space. In addition, it allows thermal protection of anatomic structures during catheter ablations and is able to deliver therapies such as gene therapy, stem cell therapy, and biologic therapy. Larger studies are needed to assess the safety and the feasibility of these new technologies.

REFERENCES

1. Fuster V, Ryden LE, Cannom DS, et al. ACC/AHA/ESC 2006 guidelines for the management of patients with atrial fibrillation - a report of the American College of Cardiology/American Heart Association Task Force on Practice Guidelines and the European Society of Cardiology Committee for Practice Guidelines (Writing Committee to Revise the 2001 Guidelines for the Management of Patients With Atrial Fibrillation). J Am Coll Cardiol 2006;48: e149–246.
2. Blomström-Lundqvist C, Scheinman MM, Aliot EM, et al, European Society of Cardiology Committee, NASPE-Heart Rhythm Society. ACC/AHA/ESC guidelines for the management of patients with supraventricular arrhythmias–executive summary. a report of the American College of Cardiology/American Heart

Association Task Force on Practice Guidelines and the European Society of Cardiology Committee for Practice Guidelines (Writing Committee to Develop Guidelines for the Management of Patients with Supraventricular Arrhythmias) developed in collaboration with NASPE-Heart Rhythm Society. J Am Coll Cardiol 2003;15(42):1493–531.
3. Zipes DP, Camm AJ, Borggrefe M, et al, American College of Cardiology, American Heart Association Task Force, European Society of Cardiology Committee for Practice Guidelines. ACC/AHA/ESC 2006 guidelines for management of patients with ventricular arrhythmias and the prevention of sudden cardiac death: a report of the American College of Cardiology/American Heart Association Task Force and the European Society of Cardiology Committee for Practice Guidelines (Writing Committee to Develop Guidelines for Management of Patients With Ventricular Arrhythmias and the Prevention of Sudden Cardiac Death). J Am Coll Cardiol 2006;48:e247–346.
4. Sosa E, Scanavacca M, d'Avila A, et al. A new technique to perform epicardial mapping in the electrophysiology laboratory. J Cardiovasc Electrophysiol 1996;7:531–6.
5. Sosa E, Scanavacca M, D'Avila A, et al. Endocardial and epicardial ablation guided by nonsurgical transthoracic epicardial mapping to treat recurrent ventricular tachycardia. J Cardiovasc Electrophysiol 1998;9:229–39.
6. Morady F, Strickberger A, Man KC, et al. Reasons for prolonged or failed attempts at radiofrequency catheter ablation of accessory pathways. J Am Coll Cardiol 1996;27:683–9.
7. Lam C, Schweikert R, Kanagaratnam L, et al. Radiofrequency ablation of a right atrial appendage-ventricular accessory pathway by transcutaneous epicardial instrumentation. J Cardiovasc Electrophysiol 2000;11:1170–3.
8. Sapp J, Soejima K, Couper GS, et al. Electrophysiology and anatomic characterization of an epicardial accessory pathway. J Cardiovasc Electrophysiol 2001;12:1411–4.
9. Saad EB, Marrouche NF, Cole CR, et al. Simultaneous epicardial and endocardial mapping of a left-sided posteroseptal accessory pathway associated with a large coronary sinus diverticulum: successful ablation by transection of the diverticulum's neck. Pacing Clin Electrophysiol 2002;25: 1524–6.
10. Schweikert RA, Saliba WI, Tomassoni G, et al. Percutaneous pericardial instrumentation for endo-epicardial mapping of previously failed ablations. Circulation 2003;108:1329–35.
11. Valderrábano M, Cesario DA, Ji S, et al. Percutaneous epicardial mapping during ablation of difficult accessory pathways as an alternative to cardiac surgery. Heart Rhythm 2004;1:311–6.
12. de Paola AA, Leite LR, Mesas CE. Nonsurgical transthoracic epicardial ablation for the treatment of a resistant posteroseptal accessory pathway. Pacing Clin Electrophysiol 2004;27:259–61.
13. Phillips KP, Natale A, Sterba R, et al. Percutaneous pericardial instrumentation for catheter ablation of focal atrial tachycardias arising from the left atrial appendage. J Cardiovasc Electrophysiol 2008;19: 430–3.
14. Koplan BA, Parkash R, Couper G, et al. Combined epicardial-endocardial approach to ablation of inappropriate sinus tachycardia. J Cardiovasc Electrophysiol 2004;15:237–40.
15. Rubenstein JC, Kim MH, Jacobson JT. A novel method for sinus node modification and phrenic nerve protection in resistant cases. J Cardiovasc Electrophysiol 2009;20:689–91.
16. Buch E, Vaseghi M, Cesario DA, et al. A novel method for preventing phrenic nerve injury during catheter ablation. Heart Rhythm 2007;4:95–8.
17. Matsuo S, Jaïs P, Knecht S, et al. Images in cardiovascular medicine. Novel technique to prevent left phrenic nerve injury during epicardial catheter ablation. Circulation 2008;117:e471.
18. Di Biase L, Burkhardt JD, Pelargonio G, et al. Prevention of phrenic nerve injury during epicardial ablation: comparison of methods for separating the phrenic nerve from the epicardial surface. Heart Rhythm 2009;6:957–61.
19. Yamada T, McElderry HT, Allison JS, et al. Focal atrial tachycardia originating from the epicardial left atrial appendage. Heart Rhythm 2008;5:766–7.
20. Buch E, Shivkumar K. Epicardial catheter ablation of atrial fibrillation. Minerva Med 2009;100:151–7 Review.
21. Pak HN, Hwang C, Lim HE, et al. Hybrid epicardial and endocardial ablation of persistent or permanent atrial fibrillation: a new approach for difficult cases. J Cardiovasc Electrophysiol 2007;18:917–23.
22. Kiser AC, Landers M, Horton R, et al. The convergent procedure: a multidisciplinary atrial fibrillation treatment. Heart Surg Forum 2010;13:E317–21.
23. Mahapatra S, LaPar DJ, Kamath S, et al. Initial experience of sequential surgical epicardial-catheter endocardial ablation for persistent and long-standing persistent atrial fibrillation with long-term follow-up. Ann Thorac Surg 2011;91:1890–8.
24. Daniels DV, Lu YY, Morton JB, et al. Idiopathic epicardial left ventricular tachycardia originating remote from the sinus of Valsalva: electrophysiological characteristics, catheter ablation, and identification from the 12-lead electrocardiogram. Circulation 2006;113:1659–66.
25. Hsia HH, Marchlinski FE. Characterization of the electroanatomic substrate for monomorphic ventricular tachycardia in patients with nonischemic cardiomyopathy. Pacing Clin Electrophysiol 2002;25:1114–27.

26. Hsia HH, Callans DJ, Marchlinski FE. Characterization of endocardial electrophysiological substrate in patients with nonischemic cardiomyopathy and monomorphic ventricular tachycardia. Circulation 2003;108:704–10.
27. Soejima K, Stevenson WG, Sapp JL, et al. Endocardial and epicardial radiofrequency ablation of ventricular tachycardia associated with dilated cardiomyopathy: the importance of low-voltage scars. J Am Coll Cardiol 2004;43:1834–42.
28. Cesario DA, Vaseghi M, Boyle NG, et al. Value of high-density endocardial and epicardial mapping for catheter ablation of hemodynamically unstable ventricular tachycardia. Heart Rhythm 2006;3:1–10.
29. Di Biase L, Santangeli P, Astudillo V, et al. Endo-epicardial ablation of ventricular arrhythmias in the left ventricle with the Remote Magnetic Navigation System and the 3.5-mm open irrigated magnetic catheter: results from a large single-center case-control series. Heart Rhythm 2010;7:1029–35.
30. Shivkumar K, Boyle NG, Thakur RK, et al. Epicardial intervention in electrophysiology. Card Electrophysiol Clin 2011;1:1–150.
31. D'Avila A, Scanavacca M, Sosa E, et al. Pericardial anatomy for the interventional electrophysiologist. J Cardiovasc Electrophysiol 2003;14:422–30.
32. Mahapatra S, Tucker-Schwartz J, Wiggins D, et al. Pressure frequency characteristics of the pericardial space and thorax during subxiphoid access for epicardial ventricular tachycardia ablation. Heart Rhythm 2010;7:604–9.
33. Tucker-Schwartz JM, Gillies GT, Scanavacca M, et al. Pressure-frequency sensing subxiphoid access system for use in percutaneous cardiac electrophysiology: prototype design and pilot study results. IEEE Trans Biomed Eng 2009;56:1160–8.
34. Tucker-Schwartz JM, Gillies GT, Mahapatra S. Improved pressure-frequency sensing subxiphoid pericardial access system: performance characteristics during in vivo testing. IEEE Trans Biomed Eng 2011;58:845–52.
35. Macris MP, Igo SR. Minimally invasive access of the normal pericardium: initial clinical experience with a novel device. Clin Cardiol 1999;22(1 Suppl 1):I36–9.
36. Seferovic PM, Ristic AD, Maksimovic R, et al. Initial clinical experience with PerDUCER device: promising new tool in the diagnosis and treatment of pericardial disease. Clin Cardiol 1999;22(1 Suppl 1):I30–5.
37. Laham RJ, Simons M, Hung D. Subxyphoid access of the normal pericardium: a novel drug delivery technique. Catheter Cardiovasc Interv 1999;47(1):109–11.
38. Nault I, Nguyen BL, Wright M, et al. Double pericardial access facilitated by iatrogenic pneumopericardium. J Cardiovasc Electrophysiol 2009;20:1068–9.
39. Berruezo A, Mont L, Nava S, et al. Electrocardiographic recognition of the epicardial origin of ventricular tachycardias. Circulation 2004;109:1842–7.
40. Vallès E, Bazan V, Marchlinski FE. ECG criteria to identify epicardial ventricular tachycardia in nonischemic cardiomyopathy. Circ Arrhythm Electrophysiol 2010;3:63–71.
41. Bazan V, Bala R, Garcia FC, et al. Twelve-lead ECG features to identify ventricular tachycardia arising from the epicardial right ventricle. Heart Rhythm 2006;3:1132–9.
42. Cano O, Hutchinson M, Lin D, et al. Electroanatomic substrate and ablation outcome for suspected epicardial ventricular tachycardia in left ventricular nonischemic cardiomyopathy. J Am Coll Cardiol 2009;54:799–808.
43. Tung R, Nakahara S, Ramirez R, et al. Distinguishing epicardial fat from scar: analysis of electrograms using high-density electroanatomic mapping in a novel porcine infarct model. Heart Rhythm 2010;7:389–95.
44. Stevenson WG, Wilber DJ, Natale A, et al. Irrigated radiofrequency catheter ablation guided by electroanatomic mapping for recurrent ventricular tachycardia after myocardial infarction: the Multicenter Thermocool Ventricular Tachycardia Ablation Trial. Multicenter Thermocool VT Ablation Trial Investigators. Circulation 2008;118:2773–82.
45. Sekiguchi Y, Aonuma K, Takahashi A, et al. Electrocardiographic and electrophysiologic characteristics of ventricular tachycardia originating within the pulmonary artery. J Am Coll Cardiol 2005;45:887–95.
46. Tada H, Tadokoro K, Miyaji K, et al. Idiopathic ventricular arrhythmias arising from the pulmonary artery: prevalence, characteristics, and topography of the arrhythmia origin. Heart Rhythm 2008;5:419–26.
47. Tada H, Tadokoro K, Ito S, et al. Idiopathic ventricular arrhythmias originating from the tricuspid annulus: prevalence, electrocardiographic characteristics, and results of radiofrequency catheter ablation. Heart Rhythm 2007;4:7–16.
48. Kanagaratnam L, Tomassoni G, Schweikert R, et al. Ventricular tachycardias arising from the aortic sinus of Valsalva: an under-recognized variant of left outflow tract ventricular tachycardia. J Am Coll Cardiol 2001;37:1408–14.
49. Iwai S, Cantillon DJ, Kim RJ, et al. Right and left ventricular outflow tract tachycardias: evidence for a common electrophysiologic mechanism. J Cardiovasc Electrophysiol 2006;17:1052–8.
50. Kim RJ, Iwai S, Markowitz SM, et al. Clinical and electrophysiological spectrum of idiopathic ventricular outflow tract arrhythmias. J Am Coll Cardiol 2007;49:2035–43.
51. Stellbrink C, Diem B, Schauerte P, et al. Transcoronary venous radiofrequency catheter ablation of ventricular tachycardia. J Cardiovasc Electrophysiol 1997;8:916–21.
52. Meininger GR, Berger RD. Idiopathic ventricular tachycardia originating in the great cardiac vein. Heart Rhythm 2006;3:464–6.

53. Obel OA, d'Avila A, Neuzil P, et al. Ablation of left ventricular epicardial outflow tract tachycardia from the distal great cardiac vein. J Am Coll Cardiol 2006;48:1813–7.
54. Wright M, Hocini M, Ho SY, et al. Epicardial ablation of left ventricular outflow tract tachycardia via the coronary sinus. Heart Rhythm 2009;6:290–1.
55. Nakahara S, Tung R, Ramirez RJ, et al. Characterization of the arrhythmogenic substrate in ischemic and nonischemic cardiomyopathy implications for catheter ablation of hemodynamically unstable ventricular tachycardia. J Am Coll Cardiol 2010;55:2355–65.
56. Maury P, Escourrou G, Guilbeau C, et al. Histopathologic effects of endocardial and epicardial percutaneous radiofrequency catheter ablation in dilated nonischemic cardiomyopathy. Pacing Clin Electrophysiol 2008;31:1218–22.
57. El Masry HZ, Yadav AV. Arrhythmogenic right ventricular dysplasia/cardiomyopathy. Expert Rev Cardiovasc Ther 2008;6:249–60.
58. Thiene G, Basso C, Calabrese F, et al. Pathology and pathogenesis of arrhythmogenic right ventricular cardiomyopathy. Herz 2000;25:210–5.
59. Basso C, Thiene G, Corrado D, et al. Arrhythmogenic right ventricular cardiomyopathy. Dysplasia, dystrophy, or myocarditis? Circulation 1996;94:983–91.
60. Dalal D, Jain R, Tandri H, et al. Long-term efficacy of catheter ablation of ventricular tachycardia in patients with arrhythmogenic right ventricular dysplasia/cardiomyopathy. J Am Coll Cardiol 2007;50:432–40.
61. Aliot EM, Stevenson WG, Almendral-Garrote JM, et al, European Heart Rhythm Association (EHRA), Registered Branch of the European Society of Cardiology (ESC), Heart Rhythm Society (HRS), American College of Cardiology (ACC), American Heart Association (AHA). EHRA/HRS Expert Consensus on Catheter Ablation of Ventricular Arrhythmias: developed in a partnership with the European Heart Rhythm Association (EHRA), a registered branch of the European Society of Cardiology (ESC), and the Heart Rhythm Society (HRS); in collaboration with the American College of Cardiology (ACC) and the American Heart Association (AHA). Heart Rhythm 2009;6:886–933.
62. Arbelo E, Josephson ME. Ablation of ventricular arrhythmias in arrhythmogenic right ventricular dysplasia. J Cardiovasc Electrophysiol 2010;21:473–86.
63. Verma A, Kilicaslan F, Schweikert RA, et al. Short- and long-term success of substrate-based mapping and ablation of ventricular tachycardia in arrhythmogenic right ventricular dysplasia. Circulation 2005;111:3209–16.
64. Satomi K, Kurita T, Suyama K, et al. Catheter ablation of stable and unstable ventricular tachycardias in patients with arrhythmogenic right ventricular dysplasia. J Cardiovasc Electrophysiol 2006;17:469–76.
65. Wijnmaalen AP, Schalij MJ, Bootsma M, et al. Patients with scar-related right ventricular tachycardia: determinants of long-term outcome. J Cardiovasc Electrophysiol 2009;20:1119–27.
66. Francis J, Fontaine G. Role of catheter ablation in arrhythmogenic right ventricular dysplasia. Indian Pacing Electrophysiol J 2005;5:81–5.
67. Yao Y, Zhang S, He DS, et al. Radiofrequency ablation of the ventricular tachycardia with arrhythmogenic right ventricular cardiomyopathy using non-contact mapping. Pacing Clin Electrophysiol 2007;30:526–33.
68. Miljoen H, State S, de Chillou C, et al. Electroanatomic mapping characteristics of ventricular tachycardia in patients with arrhythmogenic right ventricular cardiomyopathy/dysplasia. Europace 2005;7:516–24.
69. Fontaine G. The ablative techniques from surgery to catheter ablation in the treatment of cardiac arrhythmias: a 20 year experience. Acta Cardiol 1995;50:467–8.
70. Marcus FI, Fontaine GH, Guiraudon G, et al. Right ventricular dysplasia: a report of 24 adult cases. Circulation 1982;65:384–98.
71. Garcia FC, Bazan V, Zado ES, et al. Epicardial substrate and outcome with epicardial ablation of ventricular tachycardia in arrhythmogenic right ventricular cardiomyopathy/dysplasia. Circulation 2009;120:366–75.
72. Bakir I, Brugada P, Sarkozy A, et al. A novel treatment strategy for therapy refractory ventricular arrhythmias in the setting of arrhythmogenic right ventricular dysplasia. Europace 2007;9:267–9.
73. Berruezo A, Fernández-Armenta J, Mont L, et al. Combined endocardial and epicardial catheter ablation in arrhythmogenic right ventricular dysplasia incorporating scar dechanneling technique. Circ Arrhythm Electrophysiol 2012;5(1):111–21.
74. Bai R, Di Biase L, Shivkumar K, et al. Ablation of ventricular arrhythmias in arrhythmogenic right ventricular dysplasia/cardiomyopathy: arrhythmia-free survival after endo-epicardial substrate based mapping and ablation. Circ Arrhythm Electrophysiol 2011;4:478–85.
75. Rassi A Jr, Rassi A, Rassi S. Predictors of mortality in chronic Chagas disease: a systematic review of observational studies. Circulation 2007;115:1101–8.
76. Bestetti R, Theodoropoulos T. A systematic review of studies on heart transplantation for patients with end-stage Chagas's heart disease. J Card Fail 2009;15:249–55.
77. Rassi A Jr. Implantable cardioverter defibrillators in patients with Chagas heart disease: misperceptions,

may questions and the urgent need for a randomized clinical trial. J Cardiovasc Electrophysiol 2007;18: 1241–3.

78. Sarabanda AV, Sosa E, Simoes MV, et al. Ventricular tachycardia in Chagas's disease: a comparison of clinical, angiographic, electrophysiologic and myocardial perfusion disturbances between patients presenting with either sustained or nonsustained forms. Int J Cardiol 2005;102(1):9–19.
79. Sosa E, Scanavacca M, D'Avila A. Surgery and catheter ablation for the treatment of ventricular tachycardia in Chagas' disease. In: Tentori MC, Segura EL, Hayes DL, editors. Arrhythmia management in Chagas' disease. Armonk (NY): Futura Publishing; 2000. p. 117–28.
80. Sosa E, Scanavacca M, D'Avila A, et al. Radiofrequency catheter ablation of ventricular tachycardia guided by nonsurgical epicardial mapping in chronic chagasic heart disease. Pacing Clin Electrophysiol 1999;22(1 Pt 1):128–30.
81. Kowey PR, Levine JH, Herre JM, et al. Randomized, double-blind comparison of intravenous amiodarone and bretylium in the treatment of patients with recurrent, hemodynamically destabilizing ventricular tachycardia or fibrillation. Circulation 1995;92: 3255–63.
82. Carbucicchio C, Santamaria M, Trevisi N, et al. Catheter ablation for the treatment of electrical storm in patients with implantable cardioverter defibrillators. Circulation 2008;117:462–9.
83. Kozeluhova M, Peichl P, Cihak R, et al. Catheter ablation of electrical storm in patients with structural heart disease. Europace 2011;13:109–13.
84. Verma A, Kilicaslan F, Marrouche NF, et al. Prevalence, predictors and mortality significance of the causative arrhythmia in patients with electrical storm. J Cardiovasc Electrophysiol 2004;15:1265–70.
85. Bänsch D, Böcker D, Brunn J, et al. Clusters of ventricular tachycardias signify impaired survival in patients with idiopathic dilated cardiomyopathy and implantable cardioverter defibrillators. J Am Coll Cardiol 2000;36:566–73.
86. Marrouche ND, Verma A, Wazni O, et al. Mode of initiation and ablation of ventricular fibrillation storms in patients with ischemic cardiomyopathy. J Am Coll Cardiol 2004;43:1715–20.
87. Bänsch D, Oyang F, Antz M, et al. Successful catheter ablation of electrical storm after myocardial infarction. Circulation 2003;108:3011–6.
88. Sapp JL, Cooper JM, Zei P, et al. Large radiofrequency ablation lesions can be created with a retractable infusion-needle catheter. J Cardiovasc Electrophysiol 2006;17:657–61.
89. Sapp JL, Cooper JM, Soejima K, et al. Deep myocardial ablation lesions can be created with a retractable needle-tipped catheter. Pacing Clin Electrophysiol 2004;27:594–9.
90. Calkins H, Epstein A, Packer D, et al. Catheter ablation of ventricular tachycardia in patients with structural heart disease using cooled radiofrequency energy: results of a prospective multicenter study. Cooled RF Multi Center Investigators Group. J Am Coll Cardiol 2000;35:1905–14.
91. Della Bella P, De Ponti R, Uriarte JA, et al. Catheter ablation and antiarrhythmic drugs for haemodynamically tolerated post-infarction ventricular tachycardia; long-term outcome in relation to acute electrophysiological findings. Eur Heart J 2002;23: 414–24.
92. Tanner H, Hindricks G, Volkmer M, et al. Catheter ablation of recurrent scar-related ventricular tachycardia using electroanatomical mapping and irrigated ablation technology: results of the prospective multicenter Euro-VT-study. J Cardiovasc Electrophysiol 2010;21:47–53.
93. Rothman SA, Hsia HH, Cossú SF, et al. Radiofrequency catheter ablation of postinfarction ventricular tachycardia: long-term success and the significance of inducible nonclinical arrhythmias. Circulation 1997;96:3499–508.
94. Cassidy DM, Vassallo JA, Miller JM, et al. Endocardial catheter mapping in patients in sinus rhythm: relationship to underlying heart disease and ventricular arrhythmias. Circulation 1986;73:645–52.
95. Di Biase L, Burkhardt JD, Sanchez JE, et al. Endo-epicardial homogeneization of the scar versus limited endocardial substrate ablation for the treatment of electrical storms in patients with ischemic cardyomiopathy. Circulation 2010;122:A17371.
96. Horowitz BN, Vaseghi M, Mahajan A, et al. Percutaneous intrapericardial echocardiography during catheter ablation: a feasibility study. Heart Rhythm 2006;3:1275–82.
97. Nazarian S, Kantsevoy SV, Zviman MM, et al. Feasibility of endoscopic guidance for nonsurgical transthoracic atrial and ventricular epicardial ablation. Heart Rhythm 2008;5:1115–9.
98. Sumiyama K, Gostout CJ, Rajan E, et al. Pilot study of transesophageal endoscopic epicardial coagulation by submucosal endoscopy with the mucosal flap safety valve technique (with videos). Gastrointest Endosc 2008;67:497–501.

Premature Ventricular Contraction Ablation
How Aggressive Should We Be?

Rakesh Latchamsetty, MD, Frank Bogun, MD*

KEYWORDS

• Premature ventricular contraction • Catheter ablation • Cardiomyopathy

KEY POINTS

- Frequent premature ventricular contractions (PVCs) may be a result or cause of a cardiac or systemic disease process.
- Initial management of frequent or symptomatic PVCs focuses on identification and modification of reversible triggers.
- Medical or catheter-based therapy for PVC reduction is indicated when there is an expected improvement in symptoms, cardiac function, or ventricular tachyarrhythmias.
- Elimination of frequent PVCs often restores cardiac function in patients with PVC-induced cardiomyopathy.

INTRODUCTION

Premature ventricular contractions (PVCs) can present with a wide spectrum of symptoms in patients with and without structural heart disease. In patients with structural heart disease, they may cause or aggravate the disease process, or be a consequence of the disease process itself. Determining optimal management of the PVCs can be a challenge, especially in asymptomatic patients. PVC frequency, site of origin, presence and prevalence of pleomorphic PVCs, presence of underlying cardiac disease, left ventricular function and dimensions, and presence of comorbidities all have an impact on the optimal therapeutic strategy.

Ablation of PVCs has gained more interest recently and has been used as a first-line therapeutic option when chances of procedural success with clinical improvement are high. Advances in ablation catheter design together with the introduction of three-dimensional electroanatomical mapping systems have greatly enhanced the ability to accurately map and eliminate ventricular arrhythmias. These technological innovations paired with a better understanding of PVCs and their pathologic potential have contributed to the current prominent role of ablation in the management of frequent PVCs.

This article explores the prevalence of PVCs and their association with underlying heart disease; examines proposed indications for therapy, particularly for catheter ablation; and evaluates the existing data regarding outcomes of ablation in these patients. Ultimately, the aim is to highlight the subset of patients most likely to benefit from catheter ablation targeting PVCs.

HISTORY AND EPIDEMIOLOGY

History

Extrasystoles and irregularities in the cardiac pulse have been recognized for many centuries and theories as to their significance have been well debated. As early as the fifth century BCE, a Chinese physician by the name of Pien Ts'io recognized that frequent pulse irregularities can be associated with a shorter life span.[1] Claudius

Division of Cardiovascular Medicine, University of Michigan, Ann Arbor, MI, USA
* Corresponding author. Cardiovascular Center, SPC 5856, 1500 East Medical Center Drive, Ann Arbor, MI 48109.
E-mail address: fbogun@med.umich.edu

Card Electrophysiol Clin 4 (2012) 439–445
http://dx.doi.org/10.1016/j.ccep.2012.05.009
1877-9182/12/$ – see front matter

Galen, a Greek physician in the second century CE, spent much effort scrutinizing the circulatory system and classifying rhythm abnormalities.[1] He proposed that an intermittent pulse was a sign of underlying disease that predicted poor clinical outcome.[2] The teachings of Galen prevailed for centuries until, ultimately, technological advances fostered more rigorous monitoring of electrocardiographic abnormalities and clinical follow-up.

Prevalence

Determining the prevalence of PVCs is naturally dependent on the duration of monitoring and the patient population studied. In 1962, Hiss and Lamb[3] published one of the larger observational series reporting on ECG findings of 122,043 healthy individuals obtained by routine screening in the United States Air Force. Using only 48 seconds of monitoring, 7.8 people per thousand were found to have PVCs. Among these, most had 1 to 4 PVCs with no correlation between age and PVC frequency. Multifocal PVCs were extremely rare and were only seen in three patients.

In 2002, an analysis by Simpson and colleagues,[4] as part of the Atherosclerosis Risk in Communities study, evaluated 15,070 participants between the ages of 45 and 64 with 2 minute ECGs. PVCs were seen in more than 6% of patients, with complex PVC patterns seen in fewer than 1%. Increased prevalence of PVCs was seen with older age, heart disease, male gender, African American race, and hypertension. In 1969, Hinkle and colleagues[5] studied 301 asymptomatic men with a median age of 55 years using 6 hours of continuous monitoring during routine daily activity and found a prevalence of 62% for at least a single PVC. Most subjects had rare PVCs and only 9% had at least a 1% PVC burden. PVCs occurred more frequently in men with, or at high risk for, coronary heart disease.

In general, PVCs are common throughout the population and prevalence increases with increased monitoring times, advanced age, and in the presence of structural heart disease. Whether these PVCs manifest clinically will depend on multiple factors, one of which is PVC burden or frequency.

PVC Frequency

Different definitions classifying frequent PVCs have been used in the literature and are often based on the clinical scenario or the outcome being measured. For example, a PVC burden of more than 10 per hour has been found to correlate with adverse outcome in postinfarction patients and has been used in this population for risk stratification.[6]

In the Framingham study, complex or frequent PVCs were defined as more than 30 PVCs per hour and were seen in 7% of patients without coronary heart disease as well as 18% of patients with coronary heart disease. In men without coronary disease, the prevalence of a significant ventricular arrhythmia burden was associated with an increase in mortality, whereas in women without coronary disease and in all patients with coronary disease there was no such correlation.[7] A higher burden of more than 60 PVCs per hour was less frequent and occurred in 1% to 4% of the general population.[8]

The incremental implications of an increasing PVC burden as well as the prevalence of very frequent PVCs (>20% of all QRS complexes) is not well defined. However, case reports and several case series have implicated very frequent PVCs as a potential cause of cardiomyopathy[9–13] that can be reversed with ablation or at times pharmacotherapy. In addition to frequency, other characteristics of PVCs may also affect their potential to alter cardiac performance, including location and timing.

In general, once the presence of frequent PVCs is verified, five critical questions must be answered in determining whether medical or ablative therapy should be entertained:

- Are there any modifiable triggers?
- Does the patient have symptoms that correlate temporally with the PVCs?
- Does the patient have structural heart disease, and is the left ventricular function compromised?
- Is the patient at high risk for developing structural heart disease?
- Is treatment likely to provide a clinical improvement?

The remainder of this article discusses the implications of symptoms, underlying heart disease, and characteristics of PVCs on clinical management.

PRESENTATION AND EVALUATION

Patients with symptomatic PVCs with or without structural heart disease can present with a variety of complaints, including palpitations, lightheadedness, dizziness, presyncope, chest pain, dyspnea, fatigue, and exercise intolerance. In addition to quantifying the PVC burden in these patients, it is important to establish a temporal correlation between the symptoms and the arrhythmia, usually through patient-activated ambulatory monitoring or exercise testing, both class I indications in such patients.[14]

All patients with frequent ventricular arrhythmias should also receive an evaluation for underlying structural heart disease and undergo an ischemic work-up. For certain disease processes, PVC characteristics can even constitute part of the diagnosis. For example, a PVC burden of more than 500 PVCs per 24 hours is a minor criterion in the diagnosis of arrhythmogenic right ventricular dysplasia[15]; the same is true for cardiac sarcoidosis.[16]

When an underlying structural abnormality is discovered, initial management should focus on treating the most likely cause; that is, revascularization and/or medical management for ischemia or potential surgery for severe valvular disease. Following this, if PVCs are felt to contribute or even be the primary cause of impaired left ventricular function, or if they continue to cause significant symptoms, therapy should be tailored to target the PVCs.

It is important to note that patients present with quite variable degrees of symptoms from PVCs; while some patients sense each PVC, others remain asymptomatic despite a high PVC burden. Although symptoms are important in guiding therapy, patients with frequent asymptomatic PVCs may be more likely to develop cardiomyopathy because they seek medical attention later.[17] It is therefore important to perform an adequate cardiac evaluation of all patients with frequent PVCs regardless of symptoms.

MANAGEMENT

If a clear clinical trigger is identified, life style or medical changes can help to diminish the PVC burden. Some potential reversible triggers include hypoxia, hypercapnia, ischemia, drug therapy, caffeine, electrolyte abnormalities, alcohol, recreational drugs, hormonal changes, or emotional stress. If no such reversible triggers are uncovered, lifestyle modification and/or medical management with beta-blockers or calcium channel blockers may result in an acceptable symptomatic response. Further management with antiarrhythmic medications may also be considered.

Although the details of pharmacologic management are not the focus of this article, it is worth noting that medical management should center on improving symptoms and, in some settings (such as prior infarction), certain antiarrhythmic drugs can even result in increased mortality.[18] Medical management may be preferable in patients with significant comorbidities or contraindications to catheter ablation procedures or in patients with frequent pleomorphic PVCs in whom there is no predominant PVC morphology. If the PVCs in the setting of left ventricular dysfunction can be pharmacologically suppressed, there is some evidence of an associated improvement in left ventricular function.[19] In the Survival Trial of Antiarrhythmic Therapy in Congestive Heart Failure study, 674 patients with left ventricular dysfunction, heart failure, and more than or equal to 10 PVCs per hour were randomized to amiodarone versus placebo. Amiodarone decreased ventricular arrhythmias and improved ventricular function, but failed to prolong survival.[20]

When medical management is insufficient or undesirable and there is a predominant PVC morphology, catheter ablation can be a very attractive option with the potential to eliminate the PVCs. The two most common mapping techniques used during ablation are activation mapping and pace mapping. During activation mapping, the earliest electrical activation is sought with the mapping catheter (**Fig. 1**). During pace mapping, pacing is performed with the mapping catheter in an attempt to identify a site where the 12-lead ECG of the pace map matches the 12-lead ECG of the spontaneous PVC (**Fig. 2**). Activation mapping is the preferred technique owing to its higher accuracy.[21] Pace mapping is used predominantly in the presence of infrequent PVCs.

Results of catheter ablation depend on many factors, including the location of the arrhythmogenic focus within the myocardium (endocardial, epicardial, or intramural) and within the heart (eg, outflow

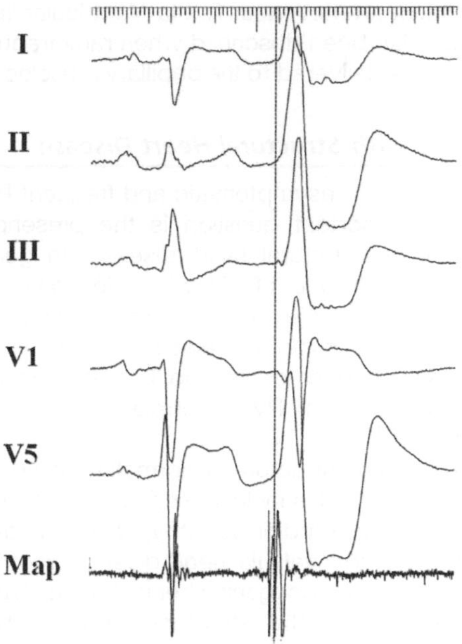

Fig. 1. Surface and intracardiac recordings (Map) from the site of origin of a PVC that originated in the left aortic cusp. The dashed line indicates the beginning of the QRS complex during the PVC. The activation time measured from the bipolar recordings of the mapping catheter (Map) precedes the QRS onset by 25 milliseconds.

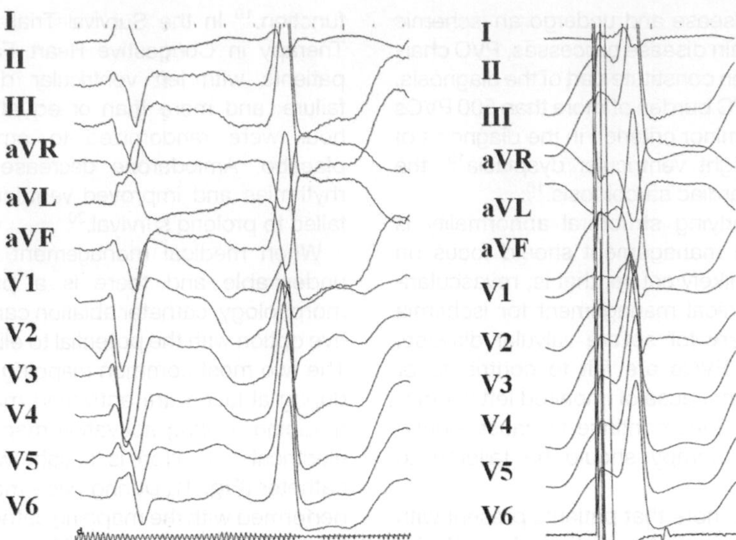

Fig. 2. Spontaneous PVC (*left panel*) and the matching paced-QRS complex at the site of origin of a PVC originating from an aortic cusp.

tract, papillary muscles, aortic cusps), as well as the number of PVC foci and their relative prevalence. The success rate in selected series is greater than 80%[11,17] and may be higher when limited to the right ventricular outflow tract.[10] Major complications are rare but can include cardiac perforation, heart block, stroke or transient ischemic attack, groin hematoma, or arteriovenous fistula. Ventricular fibrillation has also been described when radiofrequency energy was delivered to the papillary muscles.[22]

Patients with Structural Heart Disease

In patients with asymptomatic and frequent PVCs, the next important question is the presence or absence of structural heart disease. In general, patients with frequent PVCs with evidence of other cardiac abnormalities have a worse prognosis than those without structural disease. Particularly in patients with prior acute and healed myocardial infarction, frequent PVCs correlate with a higher mortality.[6,23]

The common structural abnormalities associated with frequent PVCs include ischemic cardiomyopathy, infiltrative cardiomyopathy, idiopathic dilated cardiomyopathy, valvular heart disease, ventricular hypertrophy, and congenital heart disease. Optimal management of the structural abnormality (ie, revascularization for ischemia or beta blockers for cardiomyopathy) is indicated, and this can often improve the PVC burden in itself.

However, frequent PVCs may contribute to a preexisting cardiomyopathy by further aggravating left ventricular dilatation or decreasing ejection fraction. It can be challenging to establish the impact of the PVCs in such a setting, but certain clues may aid in the assessment. For example, in a series of postinfarction patients with and without frequent PVCs, MRI data identified patients in whom the ejection fraction was out of proportion to the amount of scar tissue, indicating that the PVCs were predominantly responsible for the abnormal left ventricular function.[24] In patients with preexisting nonischemic cardiomyopathy, elimination of frequent PVCs may still result in some improvement of left ventricular function.[25]

Another scenario in which targeting PVCs may prove beneficial is in patients with cardiomyopathy and cardiac resynchronization therapy in whom frequent PVCs prevent true biventricular pacing.[26] Biventricular pacing less than 93% has been linked with diminished benefit[27] and there have been reports suggesting that elimination of PVCs and restitution of biventricular pacing can result in improvement of left ventricular function and heart failure symptoms in these patients.[28]

PVCs originating from the Purkinje fiber system can also trigger ventricular fibrillation. If this triggering PVC can be identified, ablation can eliminate recurrences of ventricular fibrillation. This scenario has been described in patients with structural heart disease, particularly postinfarction,[29] but also in patients with idiopathic ventricular fibrillation.[30]

Patients Without Structural Heart Disease

The significance of PVCs in association with ischemic and other structural heart disease has been evident for some time. However, the significance of PVCs and the role for their elimination in patients with minimal or no structural heart disease has only recently been recognized. The concept that PVCs in such a setting are benign was based largely on a report of 73 healthy asymptomatic patients in whom no increased mortality was observed over a mean follow-up period of 6.5 years.[8] However, other important clinical parameters, such as cardiac function during follow-up, were not provided. Studies have since suggested the importance of PVC burden and other characteristics that can identify patients at high risk for future deterioration of cardiac function.

A PVC burden of greater than 24% has been found to best separate patients with and without left ventricular dysfunction.[13] Such patients are found to have cardiomyopathy with a sensitivity and specificity of about 80%. However, 25% of patients with PVC-induced cardiomyopathy had a lower PVC burden and about 20% of patients with a burden greater than 24% had normal left ventricular function, indicating that the PVC burden is not the only factor determining PVC-induced cardiomyopathy. It is important to note that even a burden as low as 4% to 10% has been reported to cause a PVC-induced cardiomyopathy.[12,13]

In addition to frequency, duration of PVCs is likely to contribute to development of cardiomyopathy. In patients with frequent symptomatic PVCs, those with cardiomyopathy were found to have a longer duration of symptoms. Furthermore, patients with frequent PVCs and cardiomyopathy were also more likely to be asymptomatic because these patients probably remained undiagnosed for longer periods of time.[17]

The site of origin of PVCs is also likely to be a factor in determining the propensity for developing cardiomyopathy, although more data will be needed to clarify this. Initial reports limited to patients with frequent PVCs originating from the right ventricular outflow tract suggested that ventricular dyssynchrony secondary to delayed left ventricular activation are responsible and, therefore, left bundle branch block PVCs are more likely to cause cardiomyopathy than PVCs from other sites.[10] This has not been confirmed in larger studies that included consecutive patients with PVCs originating from other sites.[11] The presence of frequent interpolated PVCs seems to be an aggravating factor and these patients seem to have a higher risk of developing cardiomyopathy (**Fig. 3**).[31]

The decision to pursue PVC ablation in patients without structural heart disease in the absence of left ventricular dysfunction or dilatation relies on identifying risk factors for progression to PVC-induced cardiomyopathy. Patients with a particularly high PVC burden (>24%) and interpolated PVCs may be at a higher risk of developing cardiomyopathy and would likely benefit from PVC suppression. This has to be weighed against a strategy of watchful waiting during which left ventricular function and dimensions are assessed in regular intervals. This may be a reasonable option, especially if other potential aggravating factors are absent and the patient is not an ideal candidate for an ablation procedure.

The mechanism by which PVCs cause cardiomyopathy is not fully understood.[32] The suspicion that left ventricular dysfunction is caused by dyssynchrony due to left bundle branch block PVCs[10] was not confirmed in larger studies.[11] A better understanding of the mechanism will help to further improve risk assessment for the development of

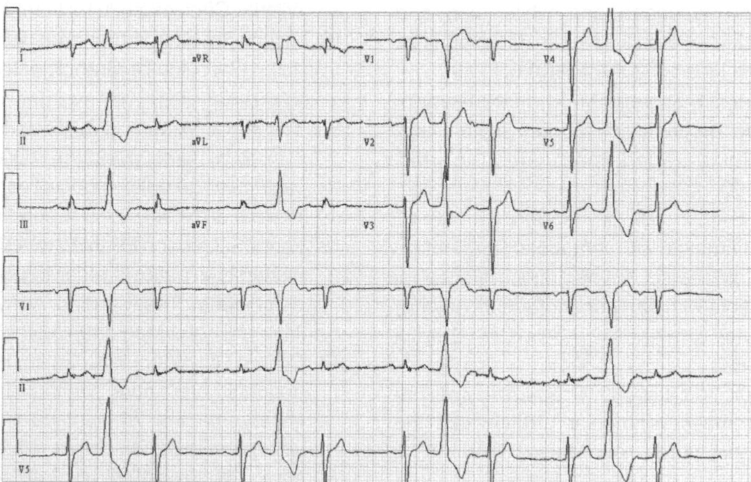

Fig. 3. The 12-lead ECG from a patient with PVC-cardiomyopathy. The patient has frequent PVCs that are interpolated. The PP interval during sinus rhythm remains unchanged despite the presence of PVCs.

PVC-mediated cardiomyopathy and, thereby, facilitate the process for selecting which patients to treat more aggressively with ablation procedures.

SUMMARY

In patients with frequent PVCs, catheter ablation should be considered for

- Patients with idiopathic PVCs and left ventricular dilatation and/or left ventricular dysfunction regardless of their symptoms
- Patients with known structural heart disease and congestive heart failure with worsening left ventricular function or heart failure due to frequent PVCs
- Patients with ventricular fibrillation in whom a PVC trigger can be identified
- Symptomatic patients who fail medical therapy or in whom medical therapy is not desired
- Suppression of PVCs (vs medical therapy) in patients with a high PVC burden (>24%)
- Patients in whom response to cardiac resynchronization therapy is limited owing to frequent PVCs.

REFERENCES

1. Luederitz B. History of the disorder of cardiac rhythm. 3rd edition. Armonk (NY): Futura Publishing Company; 2002.
2. Ruskin JN. Ventricular extrasystoles in healthy subjects. N Engl J Med 1985;312(4):238–9.
3. Hiss RG, Lamb LE. Electrocardiographic findings in 122,043 individuals. Circulation 1962;25:947–61.
4. Simpson RJ, Cascio W, Schreiner P, et al. Prevalence of premature ventricular contractions in a population of African American and white men and women: the Atherosclerosis Risk in Communities (ARIC) study. Am Heart J 2002;143(3):6.
5. Hinkle LE, Carver ST, Stevens M. The frequency of asymptomatic disturbances of cardiac rhythm and conduction in middle-aged men. Am J Cardiol 1969;24(5):629–50.
6. Hallstrom AP, Bigger JT Jr, Roden D, et al. Prognostic significance of ventricular premature depolarizations measured 1 year after myocardial infarction in patients with early postinfarction asymptomatic ventricular arrhythmia. J Am Coll Cardiol 1992;20(2):259–64.
7. Bikkina M, Larson MG, Levy D. Prognostic implications of asymptomatic ventricular arrhythmias: the Framingham Heart Study. Ann Intern Med 1992; 117(12):990–6.
8. Kennedy H, Witlock J, Sprague M, et al. Long-term follow-up of asymptomatic healthy subjects with frequent and complex ventricular ectopy. N Engl J Med 1985;312:193–8.
9. Chugh SS, Shen WK, Luria DM, et al. First evidence of premature ventricular complex-induced cardiomyopathy: a potentially reversible cause of heart failure. J Cardiovasc Electrophysiol 2000;11(3):328–9.
10. Yarlagadda RK, Iwai S, Stein KM, et al. Reversal of cardiomyopathy in patients with repetitive monomorphic ventricular ectopy originating from the right ventricular outflow tract. Circulation 2005;112(8):1092–7.
11. Bogun F, Crawford T, Reich S, et al. Radiofrequency ablation of frequent, idiopathic premature ventricular complexes: comparison with a control group without intervention. Heart Rhythm 2007;4(7):863–7.
12. Shanmugam N, Chua TP, Ward D. 'Frequent' ventricular bigeminy—a reversible cause of dilated cardiomyopathy. How frequent is 'frequent'? Eur J Heart Fail 2006;8(8):869–73.
13. Baman TS, Lange DC, Ilg KJ, et al. Relationship between burden of premature ventricular complexes and left ventricular function. Heart Rhythm 2010; 7(7):865–9.
14. Zipes DP, Camm AJ, Borggrefe M, et al. ACC/AHA/ESC 2006 Guidelines for Management of Patients With Ventricular Arrhythmias and the Prevention of Sudden Cardiac Death: a report of the American College of Cardiology/American Heart Association Task Force and the European Society of Cardiology Committee for Practice Guidelines (writing committee to develop Guidelines for Management of Patients With Ventricular Arrhythmias and the Prevention of Sudden Cardiac Death): developed in collaboration with the European Heart Rhythm Association and the Heart Rhythm Society. Circulation 2006;114(10):e385–484.
15. Marcus FI, McKenna WJ, Sherrill D, et al. Diagnosis of arrhythmogenic right ventricular cardiomyopathy/dysplasia: proposed modification of the task force criteria. Circulation 2010;121(13):1533–41.
16. Diagnostic standard and guidelines for sarcoidosis. Jpn J Sarcoidosis Granulomatous Disorders 2007; 27:89–102.
17. Yokokawa M, Kim HM, Good E, et al. Relation of symptoms and symptom duration to premature ventricular complex-induced cardiomyopathy. Heart Rhythm 2012;9(1):92–5 [Epub 2011 Aug 17].
18. Echt DS, Liebson PR, Mitchell LB, et al. Mortality and morbidity in patients receiving encainide, flecainide, or placebo. The Cardiac Arrhythmia Suppression Trial. N Engl J Med 1991;324(12):781–8.
19. Duffee DF, Shen WK, Smith HC. Suppression of frequent premature ventricular contractions and improvement of left ventricular function in patients with presumed idiopathic dilated cardiomyopathy. Mayo Clin Proc 1998;73(5):430–3.
20. Singh SN, Fletcher RD, Fisher SG, et al. Amiodarone in patients with congestive heart failure and

asymptomatic ventricular arrhythmia. Survival Trial of Antiarrhythmic Therapy in Congestive Heart Failure. N Engl J Med 1995;333(2):77–82.
21. Bogun F, Taj M, Ting M, et al. Spatial resolution of pace mapping of idiopathic ventricular tachycardia/ectopy originating in the right ventricular outflow tract. Heart Rhythm 2008;5(3):339–44.
22. Yamada T, McElderry HT, Allred JD, et al. Ventricular fibrillation induced by a radiofrequency energy delivery for idiopathic premature ventricular contractions arising from the left ventricular anterior papillary muscle. Europace 2009;11(8):1115–7.
23. Wilson AC, Kostis JB. The prognostic significance of very low frequency ventricular ectopic activity in survivors of acute myocardial infarction. BHAT Study Group. Chest 1992;102(3):732–6.
24. Sarrazin JF, Labounty T, Kuehne M, et al. Impact of radiofrequency ablation of frequent post-infarction premature ventricular complexes on left ventricular ejection fraction. Heart Rhythm 2009;6(11):1543–9.
25. Mountantonakis SE, Frankel DS, Gerstenfeld EP, et al. Reversal of outflow tract ventricular premature depolarization-induced cardiomyopathy with ablation: Effect of residual arrhythmia burden and preexisting cardiomyopathy on outcome. Heart Rhythm 2011;8(10):1608–14.
26. Mullens W, Grimm RA, Verga T, et al. Insights from a cardiac resynchronization optimization clinic as part of a heart failure disease management program. J Am Coll Cardiol 2009;53(9):765–73.
27. Koplan BA, Kaplan AJ, Weiner S, et al. Heart failure decompensation and all-cause mortality in relation to percent biventricular pacing in patients with heart failure: is a goal of 100% biventricular pacing necessary? J Am Coll Cardiol 2009;53(4):355–60.
28. Herczku C, Kun C, Edes I, et al. Radiofrequency catheter ablation of premature ventricular complexes improved left ventricular function in a non-responder to cardiac resynchronization therapy. Europace 2007;9(5):285–8.
29. Bansch D, Oyang F, Antz M, et al. Successful catheter ablation of electrical storm after myocardial infarction. Circulation 2003;108(24):3011–6.
30. Haissaguerre M, Shah DC, Jais P, et al. Role of Purkinje conducting system in triggering of idiopathic ventricular fibrillation. Lancet 2002;359(9307):677–8.
31. Olgun H, Yokokawa M, Baman T, et al. The role of interpolation in PVC-induced cardiomyopathy. Heart Rhythm 2011;8(7):1046–9.
32. Huizar JF, Kaszala K, Potfay J, et al. Left ventricular systolic dysfunction induced by ventricular ectopy: a novel model for premature ventricular contraction-induced cardiomyopathy. Circ Arrhythm Electrophysiol 2011;4(4):543–9.

Renal Denervation

A New Approach to an Old Problem

J. Brachmann, MD, PhD*, S. Schnupp, MD, B. Blüm, MD

KEYWORDS

• Renal sympathetic denervation • Symplicity trial • Resistant hypertension

KEY POINTS

- The aim of treatment for resistant hypertension is prevention of hypertensive end-organ damage and reduction of cardiovascular morbidity and mortality.
- A vast amount of evidence suggests beneficial effects of renal sympathectomy on life expectancy in patients with severe or malignant hypertension and in the prevention of cardiovascular complications in patients with milder forms of hypertension.
- Contraindications to renal denervation include patients with renal artery diameter of less than 4 mm and/or length shorter than 20 mm; severe stenosis of renal artery; fibromuscular dysplasia; and chronic renal disease with glomerular filtration rate less than 45 mL/min/1.73 m^2 as measured by the Modification of Diet in Renal Disease formula. Patients with secondary hypertension should not undergo renal denervation.

Over the last few decades, understanding and treatment of hypertension have increased rapidly. Arterial hypertension is one the most frequent chronic diseases in industrialized nations. Arterial hypertension is also one of the major risk factors for cardiovascular diseases and the second most common factor leading to end-stage renal disease, which also continues to increase in frequency. Levels of hypertension control with medical therapy have been noted to vary. In one study, only 29% of patients in the United States and 10% of patients in Europe had their blood pressure controlled.[1] Resistant arterial hypertension is defined as high blood pressure that cannot be adequately controlled according to the current guidelines (ie, pressure of <140/90 mm Hg in general; <130–139/80–85 mm Hg in patients with diabetes mellitus; <130/80 mm Hg in patients with chronic renal disease) despite concurrent use of 3 or more antihypertensive drugs of different classes, including a diuretic, at their maximum or highest tolerated doses.[2] Resistant hypertension is not synonymous with uncontrolled hypertension. Uncontrolled hypertension includes patients with pseudoresistance or inadequate treatment.[2]

Resistant hypertension may be present in 5% to 15% of patients with high blood pressure.[2] It is important to exclude pseudoresistance and secondary hypertension as underlying causes before reaching the diagnosis of resistant hypertension. Pseudoresistance may result from insufficient compliance with treatment, incorrect choice of medications, or situationally induced high blood pressure.

EPIDEMIOLOGY

The prevalence of arterial hypertension is rising worldwide. In Germany, for example, in the age group 30 to 59 years the prevalence ranges between 10% and 35%, and there is a noticeable increase to 65% in patients older than 60 years.[3]

Conflict of interest statement: The authors do not have any conflicts of interest.

2. Med. Klinik, Klinik für Kardiologie, Angiologie und Pulmonologie, Klinikum Coburg, Ketschendorfer Straße 33, 96450 Coburg

* Corresponding author.

E-mail address: Johannes.brachmann@klinikum-coburg.de

Card Electrophysiol Clin 4 (2012) 447–454

http://dx.doi.org/10.1016/j.ccep.2012.06.009

1877-9182/12/$ – see front matter

Unfortunately, the real prevalence of resistant hypertension is unknown.[2] Clinical trials suggest that perhaps 20% to 30% of study participants have resistant hypertension.[2] Resistant hypertension is influenced by multiple etiologic factors including age, weight, diabetes mellitus, and renal disease. It is likely that the incidence of resistant hypertension will increase because of the aging population and concomitant increase in the incidence of these covariates. In an analysis of the National Health and Nutrition Examination Survey (NHANES), only 53% of treated patients were controlled to blood pressure of less than 140/90 mm Hg.[4] In the Seventh Report of the Joint National Committee on Prevention, Detection, Evaluation, and Treatment of High Blood Pressure (JNC 7) for patients with diabetes mellitus or chronic kidney disease (CKD), the proportion of uncontrolled patients was even higher.

ETIOLOGY

The etiology of resistant hypertension comprises a variety of causative factors. There are many hypertensive patients with poorly controlled blood pressure. Several factors are linked to therapy resistance: elderly patients, high baseline systolic blood pressure, obesity, high salt consumption, and chronic renal disease. Diabetes mellitus, female gender, and left ventricular hypertrophy also have an effect on therapy resistance.[2] An additional aspect may be incorrect use of antihypertensive medication.[5] Berlowitz and colleagues[6] noted that control of blood pressure varied because of differences in treatment. This study showed that blood pressure declined by 6.3 mm Hg with the most intensive treatment but increased by 4.8 mm Hg with the least intensive treatment. Another study evaluated the use of medication, and showed that 18% to 27% of hypertensive patients with uncontrolled blood pressure received at least 3 different medications.[7] Not only compliance but also concomitant use of other medications can influence the effect of antihypertensive medications, especially the combination with nonsteroidal anti-inflammatory drugs (NSAIDs). NSAIDs can increase renal sodium retention, resulting in hypervolemia and therefore causing an increase in blood pressure.[7] The consumption of too much salt or alcohol has a negative influence on hypertension control as well.

Definition

Resistant hypertension is a diagnosis of exclusion, after ruling out noncompliance, inadequate treatment, and secondary causes of hypertension.[2]

Secondary Causes of Hypertension

There exist common and uncommon secondary causes of hypertension. The common causes are more prevalent in older patients because of other comorbidities and higher prevalence of other diseases, including CKD and sleep apnea among others. Pheochromocytoma, Cushing syndrome, hyperparathyroidism, aortic coarctation, and intracranial tumor are uncommon causes of secondary hypertension.[2] Two studies have shown that obstructive sleep apnea syndrome is linked to resistant arterial hypertension.[8,9] The underlying pathophysiology for this association may be elevated sympathetic activity, primary hyperaldosteronism, and obesity.[8] Hypertension treatment guidelines recommend consideration of sleep apnea screening in patients with resistant hypertension. Chronic renal failure is also often associated with resistant hypertension. CKD evokes, and is also a complication of, hypertension. In a recent cross-sectional analysis of patients with CKD it was shown that fewer than 15% had their blood pressure controlled to less than 130/80 mm Hg despite the use of, on average, 3 different antihypertensive drugs.[10] In the ALLHAT trial, CKD (defined by a serum creatinine of >1.5 mg/dL) was a strong predictor of failure to accomplish normal blood pressure.[11] The mechanism of treatment resistance in patients with CKD is sodium and water retention, and intravascular volume expansion.

Resistant arterial hypertension may be associated with primary hyperaldosteronism. Douma and colleagues[12] showed that about 10% to 20% of patients with resistant hypertension have primary hyperaldosteronism. The prevalence appears high, yet is lower than previously reported.

The incidence of hemodynamically significant renal artery stenosis (obstruction >70% luminal diameter) was seen in more than 20% of hypertensive patients.[13] Prevalence may increase with age.[14] The cause of renal artery stenosis is atherosclerosis in more than 90% of patients.[2] Fibromuscular dysplasia is an uncommon cause of renal artery stenosis, which may be seen in women younger than 50 years.

IDENTIFICATION OF RESISTANT ARTERIAL HYPERTENSION

Essential hypertension is rarely truly resistant. If treatment of hypertension despite using 3 antihypertensive medications with maximal doses, including a diuretic, does not reach goal blood pressure, causes other than resistance must be looked for first. Secondary cause of hypertension, pseudoresistance, and pseudohypertension must be ruled out. Self-measurement or 24 hours' measurement of blood pressure can distinguish between situational hypertension (eg, "white coat hypertension") and true hypertension. Noncompliance is a frequent cause of therapy resistance and must be ruled out. Essential are the improvement of lifestyle factors (weight reduction, salt reduction, exercise, smoking cessation), suboptimal antihypertensive therapy, and side effects of other medications. After exclusion of all these factors, patients with resistant hypertension should undergo laboratory testing (including serum creatinine, electrolytes, and glucose) and urinary testing (including salt excretion and protein determination). Secondary causes such as primary hyperaldosteronism and pheochromocytoma in patients with episodic hypertension must also be excluded. Ultrasonography of the renal arteries is recommended in young patients with suspected fibromuscular dysplasia and patients with an elevated risk of atherogenesis to exclude atherosclerotic renal artery stenosis.

TREATMENT

Resistant hypertension is a common clinical problem and increases the risk of target-organ damage. The intention of treatment is prevention of hypertensive end-organ damage, and reduction of cardiovascular morbidity and mortality. In addition to the proven and tested treatments, renal denervation is a new and promising approach to an old problem.

Pharmacologic Treatment

Treatment of hypertension includes the use of up to 3 or more antihypertensive drugs of different classes, including a diuretic, at their maximum or highest tolerated doses. Comorbidities and possible end-organ damage influence the choice of medications and their combination. Combination antihypertensive drugs improve compliance and constitute a reasonable therapeutic strategy.[15] However, only a few randomized controlled trials of antihypertensive therapy are available. The initial treatment should begin with angiotensin-converting enzyme inhibitors/angiotensin receptor blockers, diuretics (especially aldosterone antagonists), calcium-channel blockers, and/or β-receptor blockers. If the goal blood pressure cannot be reached with this approach, a renin inhibitor (aliskiren) may be added as well as direct vasodilators (minoxidil, dihydralazine), central α2-receptor agonists (moxonidine, clonidine), α1-receptor antagonists (urapidil), α-receptor blockers, and/or endothelin antagonists (darusentan, atrasentan).

Percutaneous Renal Denervation

History

The kidneys play a very important role in the regulation of blood pressure, and sympathetic nervous innervation of the renal arteries offers another therapeutic target in patients with therapy-resistant hypertension. Kidneys invoke the sympathetic nervous system: efferent sympathetic innervation augments Na^+ reabsorption, followed by increased renin secretion and reduction of renal blood flow. The efferent nerve fibers are found in the adventitia of the renal arteries. The afferent sympathetic fibers are located in the dorsal root of the spinal cord. In addition, the kidneys induce an enhancement of central sympathetic nervous activity.[16] Thus the afferent and efferent sympathetic nerve fibers tie the kidneys and the central nervous system together, and play an important role in control of blood pressure.

Method

With the identification of the renal sympathetic nerves as a major contributor to the complex pathophysiology of hypertension, the method of renal sympathetic denervation (RSD) is a new therapeutic option for the treatment of resistant arterial hypertension in selected drug-resistant patients. RSD is a minimally invasive procedure to modulate the activity of the sympathetic nervous system.[17,18] Ablation of afferent and efferent sympathetic nervous innervation of both renal arteries disrupts the neural connections. First, it is necessary to obtain femoral artery access (6F) followed by angiography of the renal arteries and vascular anatomic measurements. The ablation can only be done when the renal artery diameter is more than 4 mm and the length more than 20 mm. Via a 55-cm long guiding catheter (IMA or 3D catheter), a special ablation catheter (Symplicity Catheter System; Ardian/Medtronic Inc, Palo Alto, CA, USA) with an electrode tip is introduced and located in the distal segment of the renal artery. Patients should be fully heparinized once vascular access is obtained, and the activated clotting time (ACT) should be monitored during the procedure. Attention must be paid that the ablation catheter is placed 5 mm proximal to the first bifurcation of the renal artery (**Fig. 1**), which should be done under imaging guidance. The vessel wall is locally heated to 50° to 70°C by means of radiofrequency (RF) energy (maximum 8 W) for 120 seconds. It is important to cool the catheter tip during ablation to maximize lesion size and depth. The heating of the vessel wall causes ablation of the sympathetic nerve fibers in

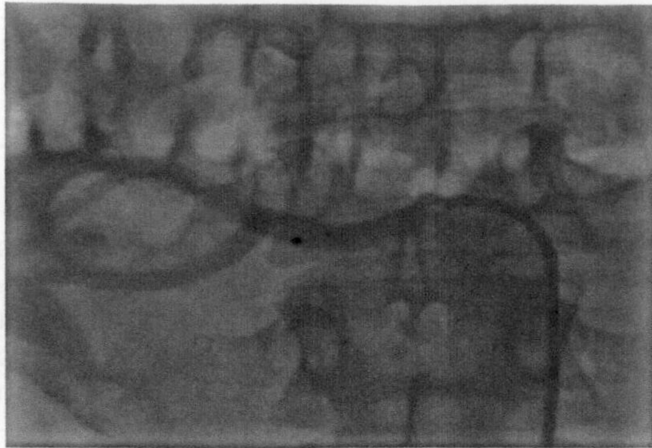

Fig. 1. Ablation catheter placed 5 mm proximal the first bifurcation of the renal artery.

the adventitia. The ACT should be maintained around 250 seconds during the procedure. In small steps (minimum 5 mm), the catheter is pulled back toward the renal artery ostium. The aim is to ablate 4 to 6 points in a helical distribution along the renal artery. The last ablation point should be on the superior proximal segment. Typically the whole procedure lasts about 40 to 60 minutes.

Contraindications

Patients with renal artery diameter of less than 4 mm and/or length shorter than 20 mm should not undergo a renal denervation. Other contraindications are severe renal artery stenosis and fibromuscular dysplasia. In the presence of anatomic abnormalities, such as accessory renal arteries, the ablation may be undertaken cautiously. Another common contraindication to renal denervation is a chronic renal disease with a glomerular filtration rate (GFR) of less than 45 mL/min/1.73 m^2 as measured by the Modification of Diet in Renal Disease (MDRD) formula. Patients with secondary hypertension should not undergo renal denervation.

Complications

Renal denervation is a new procedure with limited worldwide experience, and the full spectrum of complications has yet to be described. Thus far, the procedure appears to be relatively safe. The procedure should be performed in a center with expertise both in the management of hypertension and in complex cardiac and vascular interventions. The incidence of local complications of femoral artery cannulation, such as pseudoaneurysms, arteriovenous fistula, and local and retroperitoneal bleeding are similar to those for other cardiovascular interventions. Most of those problems are treated conservatively.[19] The occurrence of catheter-induced dissection of renal artery is rare. The solution is to stent the dissection. Other uncommon complications after ablation are early edema (**Fig. 2**), hematoma and, later on, severe renal artery stenosis.

Complications during renal denervation are hypotension, asystole, and back pain. Infrequent minor complications after ablation may include back pain, urinary tract infection, paresthesia, and postoperative hypotension. Early experience suggests that major and minor complications are infrequent and that the procedure of renal denervation is safe.

Recent studies

Interventional treatment of resistant arterial hypertension was successfully evaluated in the multicenter proof-of-principle study Symplicity HTN-1 and the randomized controlled trial Symplicity HTN-2. In the Symplicity HTN-1 study,[17] 50 patients (systolic blood pressure $\geq$160 mm Hg on $\geq$3 antihypertensive drugs, including a diuretic) were enrolled at 5 Australian and European centers; 5 patients were excluded for anatomic reasons, mainly because of dual renal artery systems (**Box 1**). The trial was designed to determine the safety and effectiveness of catheter-based renal artery denervation with the Symplicity Catheter System in reducing blood pressure in patients with drug-resistant hypertension. Patients received percutaneous radiofrequency catheter-based treatment between June 2007, and November 2008, with follow-up to 1 year.[17] Primary end points were office blood pressure and long-term safety data up to 12 months after the procedure. Postprocedural renal function and norepinephrine spillover rate were defined as secondary end points.

Radiofrequency ablation was performed at 4 points in the superior, posterior, inferior, and anterior position of about 2 minutes' duration with energy of 8 W.[17,18] After treatment, angiography of the renal vessel was performed to exclude a stenosis or dissection of the vessel. Thereafter the same procedure was done on the contralateral renal vessel. In treated patients, baseline mean

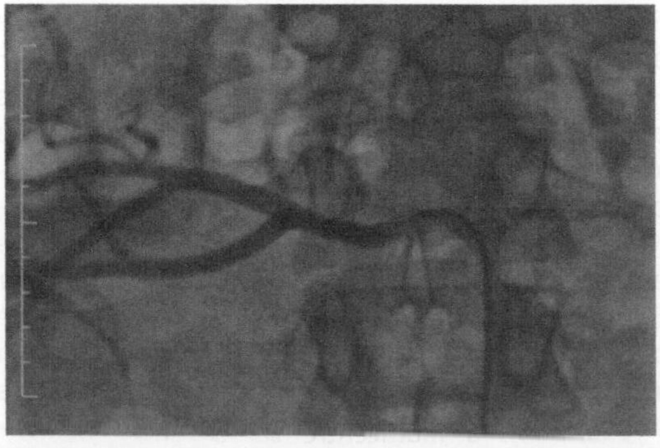

Fig. 2. Early edema after ablation at the ostium of the left renal artery.

Box 1
Inclusion and exclusion criteria of Symplicity HTN-1 study

Key Inclusion Criteria

- Office systolic blood pressure at least 160 mm Hg despite 3+ antihypertensive medications (including diuretic), or confirmed intolerance to medications
- Estimated GFR (MDRD formula) of at least 45 mL/min/1.73 m^2

Key Exclusion Criteria

- Known secondary cause of hypertension
- Type 1 diabetes mellitus
- Currently taking clonidine, moxonidine, or rilmenidine
- Renovascular abnormalities: significant renal artery stenosis, prior renal stenting or angioplasty, dual renal arteries

office blood pressure was 177/101 mm Hg and estimated GFR (eGFR) was 81 mL/min/1.73 m^2.[17,20] Renal denervation resulted in significant reductions in systolic and diastolic blood pressure, first observed at 1 month, by 14 mm Hg and 10 mm Hg, respectively, and persisting to 1 year (−27/−17 mm Hg, P = .001) (**Fig. 3**).[17,20] Decrease in blood pressure was accompanied by a marked reduction in renal norepinephrine spillover by 47%, 6 months after the procedure (n = 10), indicating effective ablation of efferent renal sympathetic fibers (secondary end point).[20]

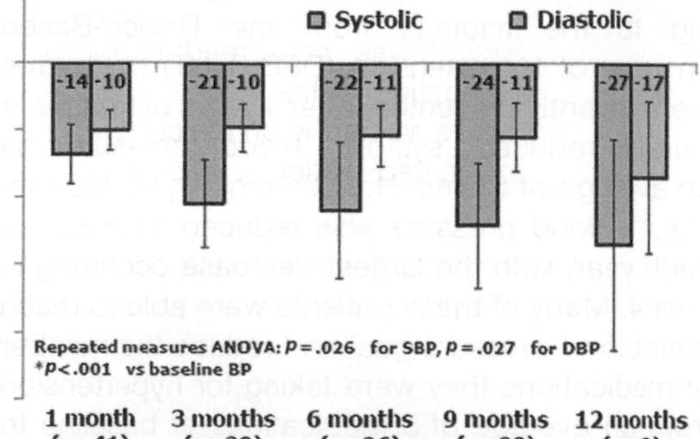

Fig. 3. The decrease in systolic and diastolic blood pressure up to 12 months after renal denervation. ANOVA, analysis of variance; BP, blood pressure; DBP, diastolic blood pressure; SBP, systolic blood pressure. (*From* Krum H, Schlaich M, Whitbourn R, et al. Catheter-based renal sympathetic denervation for resistant hypertension: a multicentre safety and proof-of-principle cohort study. Lancet 2009;373:1275–81; with permission.)

One intraprocedural renal artery dissection occurred before radiofrequency energy delivery, without further sequelae. There were no other renovascular complications. Of note, eGFR was reported to be stable from baseline (79 ± 21 mL/min/1.73 m^2) to 6 months' follow-up (83 ± 25 mL/min/1.73 m^2), with 6 of 25 patients having an increase of more than 20% in eGFR and only 1 patient with a decrease in eGFR.[20] Sympathetic nerves have been demonstrated to regrow over time. Therefore, the long-term safety and durability of blood-pressure reduction after renal denervation were anticipated with great interest. The findings from the extended follow-up further support the efficacy of renal nerve ablation, with post-procedure office blood pressure being reduced by 32/14 mm Hg up to 24 months, without affecting other pelvic, abdominal, or lower extremity innervation, making functional reinnervation unlikely.[20–23]

The Symplicity HTN-2 trial[24] was the first randomized controlled trial to evaluate catheter-based renal denervation for the treatment of hypertension. In this recently published multicenter, prospective study 106 patients, who had a baseline systolic blood pressure of 160 mm Hg or more (≥150 mm Hg for patients with type 2 diabetes), despite taking 3 or more antihypertensive drugs, were randomly allocated in a 1-to-1 ratio to undergo renal denervation with previous treatment or to maintain previous treatment alone (control group) at 24 participating centers, using the same inclusion and exclusion criteria as those of the proof-of-concept study.[24] The primary-effectiveness end point was changed to seated office-based measurement of systolic blood pressure at 6 months. Patients who met initial screening criteria were subsequently excluded from the trial if their blood pressure fell below eligibility criteria at a second clinic visit after a 2-week screening phase. During this phase, patients were required to document medication compliance and twice-daily home monitoring of blood pressure. Patients were also excluded if they were found to have unfavorable renal artery anatomy on imaging; other exclusion criteria included an eGFR of less than 45 mL/min/1.73 m^2 and type 1 diabetes.[24] After this period, patients were randomized 1:1 to maintain previous treatment alone (control group) or to undergo renal denervation. Patients and treating physicians were instructed not to change antihypertensive medication during 6 months of follow-up, except when medically required. Forty-nine (94%) of 52 patients who underwent renal denervation and 51 (94%) of 54 controls were assessed for the primary end point at 6 months.[24] After 6 months the office-based blood pressure in the treatment group had decreased significantly by 32/12 mm Hg (P<.0001) compared with the control group, and this was confirmed by home-based blood-pressure measurements and ambulatory blood-pressure recordings.[20,24] The blood pressure at home also decreased by 20/12 mm Hg (P<.0001, n = 32), compared with an unchanged result in the control group. This reduction in blood pressure alone can be anticipated to have significant impact on long-term cardiovascular risk in these patients.[25] In 84% of the patients, renal denervation resulted in reduction in systolic blood pressure of greater than10 mm Hg, subsequently defined as a response.[24] In 20% of patients the reduction in blood pressure permitted a decrease in the number or dosage of antihypertensive medications. There were no serious procedure-related or device-related complications and occurrence of adverse events between groups; one patient who had renal denervation developed possible progression of an underlying atherosclerotic lesion, but required no treatment. There was no significant difference in frequency of the combined cardiovascular end point between the treatment group and the control group (3 vs 2 cases).

Because of the low nonresponse rate (currently estimated to be 12%), no factors predicting lack of response have been identified.[24] By contrast, higher baseline systolic blood pressure and use of central sympatholytic agent were identified as independent predictors of response. The results demonstrate a dramatic reduction in blood pressure in patients with severe drug-resistant hypertension. A reduction in office blood pressure of 32/12 mm Hg, if sustained, would be expected to dramatically reduce cardiovascular morbidity and mortality in this high-risk group. Thus, Symplicity HTN-2 has become a landmark study in the rapidly developing field of invasive device–based therapy for hypertension.

Effect on glucose metabolism and insulin sensitivity

The benefit of renal denervation may not be restricted to lowering of blood pressure alone, because chronic activation of the sympathetic nervous system has been associated with the components of the metabolic syndrome, such as hyperinsulinemia, type 2 diabetes, and obesity.[26] More than 50% of patients with essential hypertension are hyperinsulinemic. It is well known that insulin resistance is related to sympathetic drive by a positive feedback mechanism.[27] There is a bidirectional relationship between sympathetic overactivity inducing insulin resistance and hyperinsulinemia producing sympathetic activation, thus initiating a vicious cycle. A recently published pilot study[28] and a case series[29–31] investigated the effect of renal denervation on glucose metabolism and insulin resistance in patients with resistant hypertension. Besides significant reduction in blood pressure observed in the treatment group (−32/−12 mm Hg) after 3 months, fasting glucose level (from 118 ± 3.4 mg/dL to 108 ± 3.8 mg/dL; P = .039) and insulin level (from 20.8 ± 3.0 μIU/mL to 9.3 ± 2.5 μIU/mL; P = .006) also improved significantly after 3 months.[28] In addition, mean 2-hour glucose levels during an oral glucose tolerance test were reduced by 27 mg/dL (P = .012), whereas there were no significant changes in blood pressure or any of the aforementioned metabolic markers in the control group.[28]

Baroreflex Stimulation of the Carotid Sinus

Stimulation of the baroreceptor afferents leads, via a negative feedback system, to stimulation of the vagus nerve, which causes a lower blood pressure and heart rate.[32,33] Baroreceptor stimulation is achieved through a pulse generator implanted subcutaneously (much like a pacemaker), which is connected to 2 leads placed around the carotid sinus bulb. One of these devices is the Rheos device (CVRx, Maple Grove, MN, USA), which stimulates the carotid baroreceptors for better control of blood pressure by taking advantage of chronic electrical activation of the afferent limb of the carotid baroreflex. The device consists of a pulse generator and bilateral perivascular carotid sinus leads that are implanted under narcotic anesthesia. The 2 early studies that include about 110 patients demonstrated significant efficacy of the device, with up to 30/18 mm Hg reduction in blood pressure, which can be maintained long term. According to the findings from the Device-Based Therapy of Hypertension (DEBuT-HT) study that were recently presented, after 4 years of treatment Rheos reduced systolic blood pressure by an average of 53 mm Hg (193 mm Hg vs 140 mm Hg).[34] Blood pressure was reduced significantly each year, with the largest decrease occurring in year 4. Many of these patients were able to reach their blood-pressure goal and reduce the number of medications they were taking for hypertension from an average of 5 medications at baseline to 3.4 medications at 4 years. Baroreflex activation therapy also improved functional capacity and reduced left ventricular mass without any evidence of carotid injury or stenosis. In the recently published randomized, placebo-controlled Rheos study[35] of 265 patients, a significant reduction in blood pressure was found in the group with baroreflex stimulation; however, the end points for acute response and technical safety were not attained.

SUMMARY

Resistant hypertension remains a challenging clinical problem, and its incidence is increasing. Catheter-based renal denervation appears to be a promising approach to improve control of blood pressure in patients with resistant hypertension. A vast amount of evidence suggests beneficial effects of renal sympathectomy on life expectancy in patients with severe or malignant hypertension and in the prevention of cardiovascular complications in patients with milder forms of hypertension. Renal denervation will significantly enrich the therapeutic future for hypertension treatment and control. If renal denervation proves to have long-lasting beneficial effects, patients' quality of life can be improved using this interventional therapy to cure hypertension and avoid life-long drug therapy with its associated expense and potential side effects.

REFERENCES

1. Wolf-Maier K, Cooper RS, Kramer H, et al. Hypertension treatment and control in five European countries, Canada, and the United States. Hypertension 2004;43:10–7.
2. Calhoun DA, Jones D, Textor S, et al. Resistant hypertension: diagnosis, evaluation, and treatment: a scientific statement from the American Heart Association Professional Education Committee of the Council for High Blood Pressure Research. Circulation 2008;117:e510–26.
3. Lowel H, Meisinger C, Heier M, et al. Epidemiology of hypertension in Germany. Selected results of population-representative cross-sectional studies. Dtsch Med Wochenschr 2006;131:2586–91 [in German].
4. Hajjar I, Kotchen TA. Trends in prevalence, awareness, treatment, and control of hypertension in the United States, 1988-2000. JAMA 2003;290:199–206.
5. Thoenes M, Tebbe U, Rosin L, et al. Blood pressure management in a cohort of hypertensive patients in Germany treated by cardiologists. Clin Res Cardiol 2011;100(6):483–91.
6. Berlowitz D, Arlene S, Hickey EC, et al. Inadequate management of blood pressure in a hypertensive population. N Engl J Med 1998;339(27):1957–63.
7. Amar J, Chamontin B, Genes N, et al. Why is hypertension so frequently uncontrolled in secondary prevention? J Hypertens 2003;21:1199–205.
8. Goncalves SC, Martinez D, Gus M, et al. Obstructive sleep apnea and resistant hypertension: a case-control study. Chest 2007;132:1858–62.
9. Pratt-Ubunama MN, Nishizaka MK, Boedefeld RL, et al. Plasma aldosterone is related to severity of obstructive sleep apnea in subjects with resistant hypertension. Chest 2007;131:453–9.
10. Saelen MG, Prøsch LK, Gudmundsdottir H, et al. Controlling systolic blood pressure is difficult in patients with diabetic kidney disease exhibiting moderate-to-severe reductions in renal function, 14. Blood Press; 2005. p. 170–6.
11. Cushman WC, Ford CE, Cutler JA, et al, for the ALLHAT Collaborative Research Group. Success and predictors of blood pressure control in diverse North American settings: the antihypertensive and lipid-lowering and treatment to prevent heart attack trial (ALLHAT). J Clin Hypertens 2002;4:393–404.
12. Douma S, Petidis K, Doumas M, et al. Prevalence of primary hyperaldosteronism in resistant hypertension: a retrospective observational study. Lancet 2008;371:1921–6.
13. Aqel RA, Zoghbi GJ, Baldwin SA, et al. Prevalence of renal artery stenosis in high-risk veterans referred to cardiac catheterization. J Hypertens 2003;21: 1157–62.
14. Crowley JJ, Santos RM, Peter RH, et al. Progression of renal artery stenosis in patients undergoing cardiac catheterization. Am Heart J 1998;136: 913–8.
15. Hill MN, Miller NH, Degeest S. Adherence and persistence with taking medication to control high blood pressure. J Am Soc Hypertens 2011;5:56–63.
16. Mahfoud F, Böhm M. Interventional renal sympathetic denervation—a new approach for patients with resistant hypertension. Dtsch Med Wochenschr 2010;135:2422–5 [in German].
17. Krum H, Schlaich M, Whitbourn R, et al. Catheter-based renal sympathetic denervation for resistant hypertension: a multicentre safety and proof-of-principle cohort study. Lancet 2009;373:1275–81.
18. Schlaich MP, Sobotka PA, Krum H, et al. Renal sympathetic-nerve ablation for uncontrolled hypertension. N Engl J Med 2009;361:932–4.
19. Lenartova M, Tak T. Iatrogenic pseudoaneurysm of femoral artery: case report and literature review. Clin Med Res 2003;1:243–7.
20. Symplicity HTN-1 Investigators. Catheter-based renal sympathetic denervation for resistant hypertension: durability of blood pressure reduction out to 24 months. Hypertension 2011;57:911–7.
21. Doumas M, Douma S. Interventional management of resistant hypertension. Lancet 2009;373:1228–30.
22. Peet MM. Results of subdiaphragmatic splanchicectomy for arterial hypertension. N Engl J Med 1947; 236:270–6.
23. Schlaich MP, Sobotka PA, Krum H, et al. Renal denervation as a therapeutic approach for hypertension: novel implications for an old concept. Hypertension 2009;54:1195–201.
24. Esler MD, Krum H, Sobotka PA, et al. Renal sympathetic denervation in patients with treatment-resistant hypertension (the Symplicity HTN-2 Trial): a randomised controlled trial. Lancet 2010;376:1903–9.

25. Lobodzinski SS. New developments in the treatment of severe drug resistant hypertension. Cardiol J 2011;18(6):707–11.
26. Grassi G, Seravalle G, Cattaneo BM, et al. Sympathetic activation in obese normotensive subjects. Hypertension 1995;25(4 Pt 1):560–3.
27. Huggett RJ, Scott EM, Gilbey SG, et al. Impact of type 2 diabetes mellitus on sympathetic neural mechanisms in hypertension. Circulation 2003;108(25):3097–101.
28. Mahfoud F, Schlaich M, Kindermann I, et al. Effect of renal sympathetic denervation on glucose metabolism in patients with resistant hypertension: a pilot study. Circulation 2011;123:1940–6.
29. Lima NK, Abbasi F, Lamendola C, et al. Prevalence of insulin resistance and related risk factors for cardiovascular disease in patients with essential hypertension. Am J Hypertens 2009;22(1):106–11.
30. Vollenweider P, Tappy L, Randin D, et al. Differential effects of hyperinsulinemia and carbohydrate metabolism on sympathetic nerve activity and muscle blood flow in humans. J Clin Invest 1993;92(1):147–54.
31. Mancia G, Bousquet P, Elghozi JL, et al. The sympathetic nervous system and the metabolic syndrome. J Hypertens 2007;25(5):909–20.
32. Krum H, Sobotka P, Mahfoud F, et al. Device-based antihypertensive therapy: therapeutic modulation of the autonomic nervous system. Circulation 2011; 123:209–15.
33. Heusser K, Tank J, Engeli S, et al. Carotid baroreceptor stimulation, sympathetic activity, baroreflex function, and blood pressure in hypertensive patients. Hypertension 2010;55:619–26.
34. Scheffers IJ, Kroon AA, Schmidli J, et al. Novel baroreflex activation therapy in resistant hypertension: results of a European multi-center feasibility study. J Am Coll Cardiol 2010;56:1254–8.
35. Bisognano JD, Bakris G, Nadim MK, et al. Baroreflex activation therapy lowers blood pressure in patients with resistant hypertension results from the double-blind, randomized, placebo-controlled Rheos pivotal trial. J Am Coll Cardiol 2011;58(7): 765–73.

Atrial Tachyarrhythmias After Cardiac Transplantation

Daniel J. Cantillon, MD

KEYWORDS

- Cardiac transplantation • Atrial tachycardia • Atrial fibrillation • Supraventricular tachycardia

KEY POINTS

- Surgical modification of the atria during transplantation has antiarrhythmic effects, including pulmonary vein isolation and vagal denervation, as well as proarrhythmic effects, including the creation of atriotomy scar.
- Cavotricuspid isthmus (CTI)-dependent right atrial flutter is the most common macroreentrant atrial arrhythmia, possibly owing to isolation of the right atrial posterior wall in some transplant recipients.
- Atrial fibrillation (AF) is markedly less common among transplant recipients, except in cases of allograft rejection. AF can occur in a few stable transplant recipients and studying these patients has provided insight into important nonpulmonary vein triggers.
- Donor hearts containing pre-existing accessory pathways or dual atrioventricular (AV) nodal physiology can also develop supraventricular tachycardia for which adenosine treatment is not recommended but catheter ablation is highly curable.

Medical and surgical advancements in cardiac transplantation have extended median survival beyond 10 years, creating steady growth in the number of cardiac transplant patients despite stability in the number of transplant surgeries.[1] Cardiac transplant recipients are well known to carry increased risk for postoperative bradyarrhythmias and have a favorable prognosis with pacemaker therapy.[2,3] Atrial tachyarrhythmias occurring in this population, however, have only been recently explored in the literature. Older data have been limited to arrhythmias resulting from pre-existing donor heart substrate, such as dual AV nodal physiology or AV accessory pathways.[4] Recent data from US transplant centers demonstrate that supraventricular tachycardia affects between 7% and 12% of heart transplant recipients and that complex modification of atrial substrate during cardiac transplant surgery results in both proarrhythmic and antiarrhythmic effects depending on the technique used and other parameters.[5,6]

MODIFICATION OF ATRIAL SUBSTRATE RESULTING FROM CARDIAC TRANSPLANT SURGERY

The bicaval surgical technique is the dominant method for contemporary cardiac transplantation. This involves a complete recipient cardiectomy at the level of the great vessels and posterior left atrium, which leaves only a small cuff of recipient left atrial tissue containing the pulmonary venous antrum.[7,8] The donor heart is implanted largely intact and connected at the level of the great vessels and the partially cleaved donor left atrium to the small recipient left atrial cuff. Advantages of this technique include a lower incidence of postoperative bradyarrhythmias, owing to a largely unperturbed donor heart and possibly overall improved survival outcomes.[9,10] In contrast, the biatrial technique connects the donor heart to a much larger cuff of recipient right and left atrial tissue by a running anastomosis. Disadvantages of this technique include larger atrial chambers,

Cardiac Electrophysiology and Pacing, Heart and Vascular Institute, Lerner College of Medicine, Cleveland Clinic, 9500 Euclid Avenue, Desk J2-2, Cleveland, OH 44195, USA
E-mail address: cantild@ccf.org

Card Electrophysiol Clin 4 (2012) 455–460
http://dx.doi.org/10.1016/j.ccep.2012.05.006
1877-9182/12/$ – see front matter

a higher incidence of pacemaker-requiring bradyarrhythmias, and some data that suggest overall worse outcomes.[7–10] Advantages include a slightly shorter donor heart ischemic time on average due to a simplified operation, which can be performed expediently.[7,8] Both techniques alter atrial substrate in different ways to create both proarrhythmic and antiarrhythmic substrate (**Table 1**).

Pulmonary Vein Isolation

Both surgical transplant techniques result in obligatory pulmonary vein isolation owing to cut-and-sew anastomosis of the pulmonary venous antrum. Data from the Cleveland Clinic demonstrate a markedly lower incidence of postoperative AF among cardiac transplant recipients when compared with low-risk coronary bypass surgery patients.[11] This observation is not surprising because atrial ectopy originating from muscular sleeves within the pulmonary veins are known to represent an important trigger for AF.[12] These findings provide an example of an antiarrhythmic modification of atrial substrate resulting from cardiac transplant surgery, albeit nonintended.

Right Atriotomy and Suture Line

Biatrial surgical transplant technique results in an enlarged transplanted right atrium due to inclusion of both donor and recipient tissue and also extensive posterior wall scar due to the obligatory running anatomosis suture line. The posterior wall of the right atrium is commonly electrically isolated in such patients and thus capable of remaining in sinus rhythm while the rest of the heart races in an atrial arrhythmia (shown in **Fig. 1**). Use of a bicaval technique solves this problem by largely preserving the architecture of the donor right atrium. It remains unclear, however, if bi-caval transplant recipients are less likely to develop atrial arrhythmias. Scar in the high right atrium can develop along the superior vena cava and right atrial suture line and has been shown to promote arrhythmias (discussed later).[5]

Left Atriotomy and Suture Line

Both surgical transplant techniques compel left atriotomy and anastamosis in the donor heart. The bicaval technique minimizes resultant chamber enlargement by connecting only a minimal cuff of recipient left atria connecting the pulmonary venous antrum to the cleaved donor heart. The biatrial technique results in a significantly enlarged left atrium with a wider circumferential scar border zone. As discussed later, left atrial scar can result in macroreentrant arrhythmias, including perimitral flutter.[5]

Cardiac Denervation

An increase in resting heart rate, loss of heart rate variability, and sensitization to the effects of adenosine and isoproterenol result from denervation of parasympathetic ganglia owing to cardiac transplant surgery.[13,14] Data obtained from Holter monitoring in cardiac transplant recipients demonstrate a marked loss of heart rate variability compared with age-matched and gender-matched control groups.[5] There are few data, however, regarding how cardiac denervation specifically influences substrate for atrial tachyarrhythmias despite an abundance of data on the important role of the autonomic nervous system, in particular vagal input, in promoting AF in the general population.[15,16] It is possible that vagal denervation may be at least partially responsible for the low incidence of AF in the transplant population. It is also possible that the loss of vagal inputs to the AV node may facilitate induction AV nodal-dependent supraventricular tachycardias when dual AV nodal physiology or an accessory pathway is present in the donor heart. Unfortunately, there are no data to validate either of these concepts.

Table 1
Overview of proarrhythmic and antiarrhythmic effects resulting from cardiac transplantation using the bicaval technique, biatrial technique, or both

Antiarrhythmic Effects	Proarrhythmic Effects
Pulmonary vein isolation (both techniques)	Right atriotomy • Superior vena cava—right atrial suture line (bicaval) • Posterior right atrial wall and suture line (biatrial)
Cardiac denervation (both techniques)	Left atriotomy (both techniques) • Perimitral flutter • Scar-related macroreentry

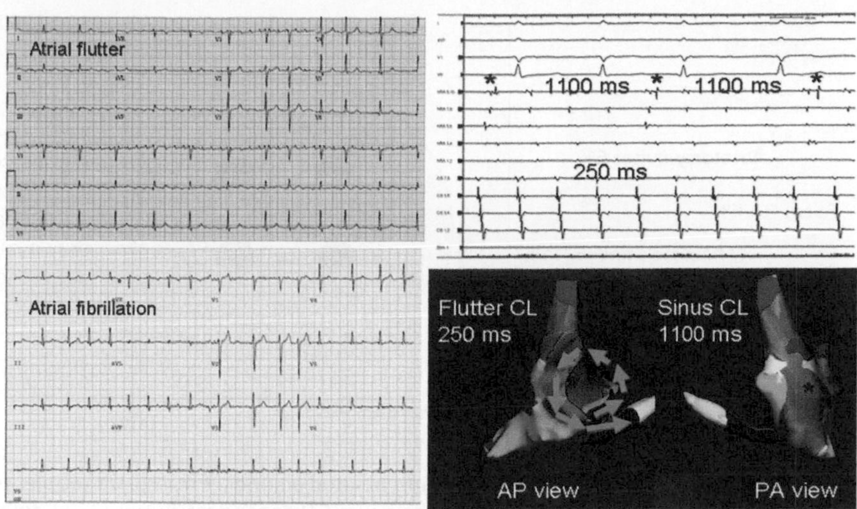

Fig. 1. Illustrative case example of atrial flutter occurring in a biatrial transplanted patient, which had clinically degenerated into AF as shown on the ECG tracings. Intracardiac tracings demonstrate electrical dissociation of the recipient right atrial cuff in sinus rhythm (cycle length 1100 milliseconds [ms]) denoted by the corresponding asterisks on the tracings from the posterior right atrium, as shown on the map. The rest of the heart is in a typical, counterclockwise right atrial flutter (cycle length 250 ms) using the CTI, as shown on the activation map with arrows tracing the wavefront path around the annulus and into the coronary sinus. Ablation of the CTI resulted freedom from both atrial flutter and fibrillation in this patient.

ATRIAL FIBRILLATION

As discussed previously, AF is uncommon in the cardiac transplant population, with the 5-year incidence ranging between 1% and 7.5% among major transplant centers.[5,6,11] Obligatory pulmonary vein isolation and vagal denervation of the transplanted heart are thought to represent important mechanisms yet there are no definitive data to confirm either principle. The clinical experience of cardiac transplant surgeons and cardiologists has led to the long-standing belief that AF occurring in the transplanted heart is pathognomonic for allograft rejection, purportedly resulting from an acute increase in atrial ectopy and heterogeneity of conduction resulting from the inflammatory myopathy. Published data on supraventricular tachycardia occurring after cardiac transplantation from the University of California, Los Angeles (UCLA), support this principle because there were no cases of AF occurring in patients without rejection beyond the early postoperative period.[5] These data thus also indirectly support the hypothesis that some aspect of cardiac transplant surgery itself must render the hearts less amenable to AF, whether obligatory pulmonary vein isolation, vagal denervation, or some other yet undiscovered influence.

Data from the Cleveland Clinic have identified a small cohort of stable post-transplant AF patients without overt evidence of allograft rejection.[6] In a small study of 13 stable transplant recipients with both an organized atrial tachycardia and AF referred for electrophysiology (EP) study, ablation of the atrial tachycardia resulted in long-term AF freedom in 9 of 13 patients (69%), raising the possibility that the atrial tachycardia served as a nonpulmonary vein trigger for AF in these patients. These arrhythmias included focal atrial tachycardias (58%), CTI flutter (32%), right atriotomy flutter (5%), or left atriotomy flutter (5%). Focal atrial tachycardias originated from the coronary sinus (36%), tricuspid annulus (18%), posterior left atrium (18%), left atrial appendage (18%), and posterior right atrium scar border zone (9%) (**Fig. 2**).[17] One of these cases, involving a focal atrial tachycardia originating from the coronary sinus repeatedly triggering AF that was immediately cured by focal ablation, was published separately as a case report.[18] Although not definitive, these data are consistent with the notion that nonpulmonary vein triggers are also important in initiating AF, as is known to be the case in the general population. Such data perhaps provide insight into the importance of considering the atrial appendage, coronary sinus, tricuspid annulus, and posterior wall as potential triggers for AF among patients presenting with recurrence after successful pulmonary vein isolation in the general population.

RIGHT ATRIAL TACHYARRHYTHMIAS

Typical CTI-dependent right atrial flutter is by far the most common macroreentrant arrhythmia in the transplant population, occurring in almost

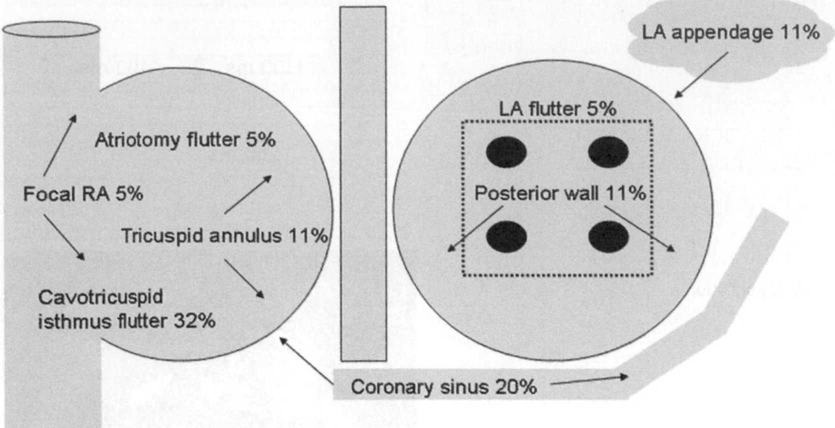

Fig. 2. Distribution of atrial tachyarrhythmias mapped and ablated among 13 transplant recipients taken for EP study at the Cleveland Clinic. The most common arrhythmia was CTI-dependent flutter (32%), followed by focal arrhythmias involving the coronary sinus (20%). Left atrial (LA) arrhythmias were less common, accounting for less than one-third of the cumulative total.

two-thirds of the patients referred for EP study in the UCLA data set[5] and almost half of the patients in the Cleveland Clinic data set.[6] It remains unclear, however, if the chosen surgical transplant technique influences the likelihood for developing CTI-dependent flutter because the proportion of patients with a biatrial and bicaval technique were similar in the UCLA series. As shown in **Fig. 1**, counterclockwise CTI-dependent flutter was facilitated by the surgically isolated posterior right atrium in this biatrial transplant recipient by serving as a large nonconducting anatomic barrier. During flutter, any conduction across the posterior wall might have allowed the leading wavefront to collide with the excitable gap, thus terminating the tachycardia.

Focal right atrial tachycardias can also occur in transplant recipients. The UCLA data set includes 6 cases of focal right atrial tachycardia successfully mapped and ablated along the suture line in the high posterior right atrium.[5] Focal atrial tachycardia originating from the tricuspid annulus (**Fig. 3**) and also the right atrial suture line were present in the Cleveland Clinic data set.[6,17]

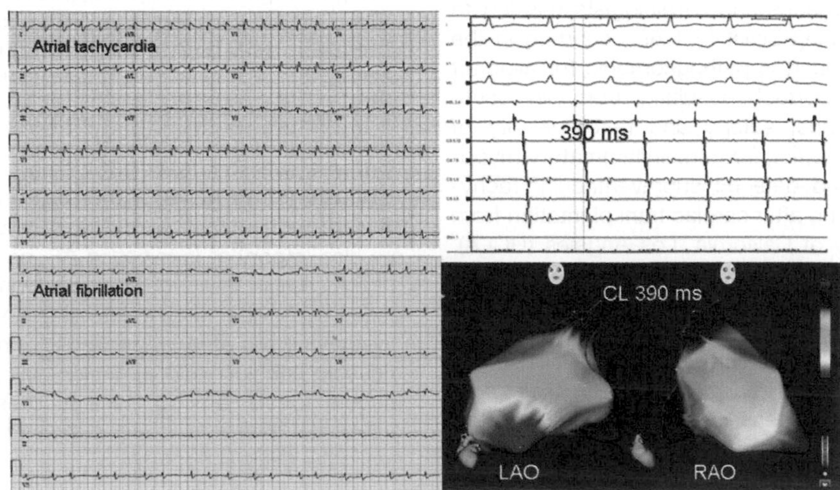

Fig. 3. Illustrative case example of a bicaval transplanted patient with focal atrial tachycardia (cycle length [CL] 390 ms) mapped and ablated at approximately the 9 o'clock position on the tricuspid annulus from the left anterior oblique (LAO) perspective, as demonstrated in the activation map. Before EP study, the arrhythmia had clinically degenerated into AF as shown by the ECG tracings. Catheter ablation resulted in freedom from both atrial tachycardia and fibrillation in follow-up.

LEFT ATRIAL TACHARRHYTHMIAS

Both bicaval and biatrial transplant techniques require anastamosis of the recipient left atrial cuff to the donor left atrium. This atriotomy scar can be proarrhythmic, as demonstrated in 1 of the 13 cases in the Cleveland Clinic series, where re-isolation of the posterior left atrium resulted in termination of an atrial tachycardia and also freedom from subsequent AF.[17] Two of the cases in the UCLA series included perimitral flutter that was demonstrated by both entrainment pacing and mapping in the left atrium.[5] These data are not surprising given the bulk of data demonstrating the proarrhythmia potential for left atrial flutters resulting from left atriotomy in the maze operation and mitral valve corrections.[19,20] The Cleveland Clinic series also demonstrated a left atrial tachycardia originating from the atrial appendage, which is a finding also present in the general population.[17]

ATRIOVENTRICULAR REENTRY AND ATRIOVENTRICULAR NODAL REENTRY

In the UCLA data set, AV nodal-dependent arrhythmias originating from pre-existing donor substrate accounted for 12% of the patients taken for EP study, including 1 case of AV nodal reentry tachycardia (AVNRT) and 2 cases of orthodromic AV reciprocating tachycardia—1 right-sided and 1 left-sided accessory pathway.[5] In the Cleveland Clinic data set, this category accounted for 15% of the patients taken for EP study, including 3 cases of AVNRT and 1 patient with an accessory pathway.[6] It remains uncertain whether vagal denervation of the AV node in the transplanted heart facilitates induction of these AV nodal-dependent arrhythmias, particularly given the common use of vagal maneuvers to terminate these arrhythmias in the general population. In contrast to the general population, an extreme sensitization to adenosine makes its use contraindicated.[14] Catheter ablation is highly effective in curing AV nodal-dependent arrhythmias, according to both UCLA and Cleveland Clinic data sets.[5,6]

SUMMARY

Cardiac transplant recipients demonstrate a unique substrate for atrial tachyarrhythmias owing to the surgical techniques involved, with differences noted between the more common bicaval technique and the classic biatrial technique. Surgical modification of the atria during transplantation has antiarrhythmic effects, including pulmonary vein isolation and vagal denervation, as well as proarrhythmic effects, including the creation of atriotomy scar. AF is markedly less common among transplant recipients, except in cases of allograft rejection. AF can occur in a few stable transplant recipients and studying these patients has provided insight into important nonpulmonary vein triggers. CTI-dependent right atrial flutter is the most common macroreentrant atrial arrhythmia, possibly owing to isolation of the right atrial posterior wall in some transplant recipients. Donor hearts containing pre-existing accessory pathways or dual AV nodal physiology can also develop supraventricular tachycardia for which adenosine treatment is not recommended but catheter ablation is highly curable.

REFERENCES

1. Taylor DO, Stehlik J, Edwards LB, et al. Registry of the internatioanl society for heart and lung transplantation: twenty-sixth official adult heart transplant report-2009. J Heart Lung Transplant 2009;28(10): 1007–22.
2. Cantillon DJ, Gorodeski EZ, Caccamo M, et al. Long-term outcomes and clinical predictors for pacing after cardiac transplantation. J Heart Lung Transplant 2009;28(8):791–8.
3. Cantillon DJ, Tarakji KT, Tu T, et al. Long-term outcomes and clinical predictors for pacemaker-requiring bradyarrhythmias after cardiac transplantation: analysis of the UNOS/OPTN cardiac transplant database. Heart Rhythm 2010;7(11):1567–71.
4. Magnano AR, Garan H. Catheter ablation of supraventricular tachycardia in the transplanted heart: a case series and literature review. Pacing Clin Electrophysiol 2003;26:1878–86.
5. Vaseghi M, Boyle NG, Kedia R, et al. Supraventricular tachycardia after orthotopic cardiac transplantation. J Am Coll Cardiol 2008;51(23):2241–9.
6. Cantillon DJ, Tarakji KG, Hu T, et al. Supraventricular tachycardia after cardiac transplantation: clinical chracteristics and outcomes for medical and ablative therapy. Heart Rhythm 2011;8(5):S355–86.
7. Miniati DN, Robbins RC. Techniques in orthotopic cardiac transplantation: a review. Cardiol Rev 2001; 9:131–6.
8. Lia KK, Bolman RM. Operative techniques in orthotopic heart transplantation. Semin Thorac Cardiovasc Surg 2004;16:370–7.
9. Meyer SR, Modry DL, Bainey K, et al. Declining need for permanent pacemaker insertion with the bicaval technique of orthotopic heart transplantation. Can J Cardiol 2005;21:159–63.
10. Schnoor M, Schafer T, Luhmann D, et al. Bicaval versus standard technique in orthotopic heart transplantation: a systematic review and meta-analysis. J Cardiovasc Thorac Surg 2009;9(2):333–42.
11. Khan M, Kalahasti V, Rajagopal V, et al. Incidence of atrial fibrillation in heart transplant patients: long-term

follow-up. J Cardiovasc Electrophysiol 2006;17(8): 827–31.

12. Haïssaguerre M, Jaïs P, Shah DC, et al. Spontaneous initiation of atrial fibrillation by ectopic beats originating in the pulmonary veins. N Engl J Med 1998;339(10):659–66.
13. Yusuf S, Theodoropoulos S, Mathias CJ, et al. Increase sensitivity of the denervated transplanted human heart to isoprenaline both before and after beta-adrenergic blockade. Circulation 1989;75: 696–704.
14. Ellenbogen KA, Thames MD, DiMarco JP, et al. Electrophysiological effects of adenosine in the transplanted human heart: evidence of super-sensitivity. Circulation 1990;81:821–8.
15. Park HW, Shen MJ, Lin SF, et al. Neural mechanisms of atrial fibrillation. Curr Opion Cardiol 2012;27(1): 24–8.
16. Ng J, Villuendas R, Cokic I, et al. Autonomic remodeling in the left atrium and pulmonary veins in heart failure: creation of a dynamic substrate for atrial fibrillation. Circ Arrhythm Electrophysiol 2011;4(3): 388–96.
17. Cantillon DJ, Fowler J, Bianco C, et al. Novel insight into non-pulmonary vein triggers for atrial fibrillation derived from electrophysiologic study and catheter ablation of atrial tachycardia after cardiac transplantation. Heart Rhythm 2011;8(5):S58–102.
18. Kanj M, Di Biase L, Wazni O, et al. Coronary sinus focus acting as a trigger for atrial fibrillation in a patient with orthotopic heart transplantation. J Cardiovasc Electrophysiol 2008;19(11):1208–11.
19. Wazni OM, Saliba W, Fahmy T, et al. Atrial arrhythmias after surgical maze: findings during catheter ablation. J Am Coll Cardiol 2006;48(7):1405–9.
20. Hussein AA, Wazni OM, Harb S, et al. Radiofrequency ablation of atrial fibrillation in patients with mechanical mitral valve prostheses: safety, feasibility, electrophysiologic findings and outcomes. J Am Coll Cardiol 2011;58(6):596–602.

Index

Note: Page numbers of article titles are in **boldface** type.

Card Electrophysiol Clin 4 (2012) 461–468
http://dx.doi.org/10.1016/S1877-9182(12)00087-1

Q

R

Printed and bound by CPI Group (UK) Ltd, Croydon, CR0 4YY
03/10/2024
01040350-0001